THE PRICE OF HEALTH

THE
PRICE
OF
HEALTH

The Modern Pharmaceutical Enterprise
and the Betrayal of a History of Care

MICHAEL KINCH
AND LORI WEIMAN

FOREWORD BY MARK CUBAN

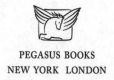

PEGASUS BOOKS
NEW YORK LONDON

THE PRICE OF HEALTH

Pegasus Books, Ltd.
148 West 37th Street, 13th Floor
New York, NY 10018

First Pegasus Books edition April 2021

Interior design by Maria Fernandez

Library of Congress Cataloging-in-Publication Data is available.

ISBN: 978-1-64313-680-6

10 9 8 7 6 5 4 3 2 1

Printed in the United States of America
Distributed by Simon & Schuster
www.pegasusbooks.com

*This book is dedicated to all the hard-working
scientists, researchers, medical professionals, pharmacists,
manufacturing engineers, and public health and policy experts
who entered their professions with the goal of improving health,
and who continue to dedicate their lives toward that mission.*

CONTENTS

FOREWORD

by Mark Cuban

Trust. It is at the heart of how all of us deal with pharmaceuticals and the companies that produce them.

We want to trust that these companies are making products that do what the label says it does. We want to trust that the companies which create the drugs we take properly educate the doctors that write our prescriptions. And we want to trust that when we get those drugs from our pharmacists they are priced fairly, even though all evidence suggests otherwise.

Examples of extreme pricing abound, including the nauseating exploits of the now jailed "Pharma Bro," Martin Shkreli, who exploited unique features of the pharmaceutical industry to hike the prices of needed medicines by outrageous amounts simply because he could. Likewise, for out-of-patent and overpriced insulin and EpiPens. Overpricing has led to far too many of us not being able to afford our medications or resorting to rationing or having to choose between eating or acquiring the drugs we need to survive. It is no surprise that as a country we are outraged at how the pharmaceutical industry has violated our trust and put profits over the health and safety of their fellow citizens.

It is not that we all haven't benefited from the many technological and scientific advancements in new drugs, vaccines, and therapies. We certainly have. We have seen diseases conquered and the quality and quantity of our lives improve and expand.

For most of recent history, these benefits were affordable and accessible, albeit sometimes with the help of government interventions, such as those that subsidize the costs of childhood vaccines or, at the other end of the spectrum, to help the elderly gain access to medicines via Medicare Part D. That is no longer the case.

The unanswered questions, or the questions that the pharmaceutical industry does it's best to keep unanswered, are: "Why, despite all the technological advances and their resultant improved efficiencies and lower costs have the prices for drugs continued to skyrocket?" "Why, if the taxpayer-funded National Institute of Health research accounts for the basis of one third of medicines discovered in recent years, are those drugs unaffordably priced?"

In order to change the pricing of the pharmaceutical industry we have to get at the heart of why pricing is so outrageous. With funding from my foundation, Michael Kinch (from Centers for Research Innovation in Biotechnology at Washington University in St. Louis) and the team at the nonprofit 46brooklyn Research have exposed many issues. These are just a few of the questions *The Price of Health* tries to finally answer.

This is a must-read book for those who want to change the course of healthcare in our country.

INTRODUCTION

T hink back ten, five, or even two years ago: What if we told you that
a new, deadly viral disease was going to take over the world and kill
500,000 people within just six months and infect nearly ten million
more around the globe? What if we told you that the virus would puzzle
leading infectious disease experts and global public health officials because
this virus would not behave like any other before it? And what if we told you
that as the infection spread, the symptoms would mutate, becoming more
varied and complicated? And what would you think if we told you that this
disease would hit the United States worse than it would other parts of the
world?[1] The disease would create panic so systemic the government would
shut down public life; businesses everywhere would be told to close and
people restricted to their homes. Such actions would topple the economy,
devastate Wall Street, and put strains on access to food and consumer goods.
After months of isolation, grappling with the loss of jobs, school, and health
insurance, tensions would flare, leading to riots and community outrage.

But wait, there's more. What if, in the grips of all of this terror and crisis,
you learned that as the dedicated scientists and researchers were rushing to
find a cure, treatment, or vaccine, their bosses were working largely in secret
with Wall Street and the government? And, despite the fact that American

taxpayers would underwrite most of the costs of development and production, the government left decisions about pricing to the companies, who could charge prices thousands of times higher than their cost to manufacture it? This approach was part of a goal to charge as much as possible and maximize profits, even as pharma executives knew it would cost the lives of the poor and less fortunate, including any without insurance—even those who had lost their insurance when their jobs were eliminated due to the virus itself! What would you do if such a scenario occurred? Would you take to the streets in protest? Would you demand to know how much it cost to develop and make the drugs, which, by the way, were largely subsidized by your own tax dollars? Would you demand that everyone have equal access to this information and that everyone knew what the price was and that they would be charged the exact same price regardless which pharmacy, hospital, or doctor they went to? Would you hold those accountable who had profited unfairly off this healthcare crisis and enact transparency laws to prevent such things from ever happening again? Would you even believe this scenario could happen in the United States, or would you have chalked it up as the storyline for a new horror movie?

This is sadly not fiction, but a recitation of the COVID-19 pandemic that, in 2020, we are all enduring together. Through a very publicized process, the general public was exposed to the scientific and medical processes typically needed to obtain regulatory approvals for drugs and vaccines, albeit occurring at an accelerated basis. While not everyone appreciated the uncertainties of the scientific endeavor or latched onto the fine details, these products provided greater clarity and insight to many as to how drugs and vaccines are developed: who funds the work; where technology originates; and who conducts the actual research and testing. We also experienced a collective glimpse into the murky world of drug pricing, a process that in this instance, as with drugs developed on a regular basis, is purposefully hidden from view. A cynic will say that's because those involved are maximizing personal wealth and not public health. But the truth is that the pricing question is more complicated than that, especially in the United States, whose citizens pay the highest prices for the same drugs used throughout the world. The process by which drugs are developed, manufactured, distributed, and priced in the United States is the very focus of this book, although we will look abroad for comparison purposes and potential ideas on how certain adjustments could benefit the American consumer without destroying the industry dedicated to advancing human healthcare. For instance, we will discuss a particularly creative experiment underway in Germany where legislation has been introduced to reward innovative new medicines that provide clear medical benefits, while controlling the prices of less innovative or nonbeneficial drugs.

While the COVID-19 pandemic has taken thousands of lives and had a dramatic worldwide impact, it may have provided us with the necessary learnings and insight and an opportunity to do something about the broken and imbalanced system that increasingly results in greater numbers of Americans not having access to lifesaving and life-enhancing cures, therapies, or vaccines due to our complicated and opaque pricing practices. Yet a theme that will resonate throughout this book is the concept that "sunshine is the best disinfectant." The idea that greater transparency as to why the prices of medicines continue to rise will help initiate the conversations and actions needed to address this growing issue. But the opacity that blocks this sunlight does not have to be this way. Some countries, such as Australia, provide comprehensive information about the prices of new medicines, and their citizens pay a fraction of what Americans do and for the exact same medicines. Were such disparities more widely known, surely pressure would mount to address the fundamental lack of fairness that Americans face and pay for daily. In this book, we look to history and track how we got to this place. Remember, the COVID-19 pandemic was not the first time the world has experienced such worries. Forgotten are tales of smallpox, Spanish flu, polio, and many other nemeses. Likewise, the Second World War was the first American conflict in which the number of deaths attributable to infectious disease was lower than those caused by combat—a direct consequence of the development of vaccines for typhoid fever and other infectious agents.[2] Contrast this outcome with the Civil War a half-century earlier, when boys from farms and cities around the nation cohabitated in tents; infectious disease spread by this close contact caused nearly five deaths for every horrific battlefield loss.

The culture of the late 1940s and 50s had the type of angst that revisited us in early 2020. Fascist powers may have been defeated on the battlefields of the European and the Pacific theaters, but a very different kind of enemy had not relented and would, without warning, strike home in a literal and debilitating sense. Polio is a disease of clean and modern societies.[3] In unsanitary conditions, poliovirus infects children within their first year and, paradoxically, is often not particularly impactful. When exposure to the infectious agent is delayed until later in life, even by just a few years, infection can be devastating, leading to lifelong paralysis and death. As such, polio inspired considerable dread among parents in the mid-20th century.[4] Rumors of a local outbreak were sufficient to cause social isolation or quarantine of entire regions, not unlike the scenes that characterized 2020.

In the early 1950s, a young scientist by the name of Jonas Salk developed a vaccine candidate to prevent polio. He managed to do so by killing viruses with chemicals.[5] Funded heavily by the American government and the precursor to today's March of Dimes, Salk's work on the vaccine candidate was anxiously monitored by an expectant public. The announcement of promising results from an early clinical trial, conveyed in a live radio bulletin broadcast on all major stations and heard by millions in the United States alone, was sufficient to trigger church bells to be rung across the nation and, indeed, around the world.[6] The eventual approval of this vaccine was so anticipated that photographs of long lines of children, waiting to be vaccinated, routinely accompanied the headlines of major newspapers.[7]

Given all this attention, it is perhaps not surprising that Salk broke the world's record for the fastest development of a vaccine (a record pace that likely will be eclipsed by the more contemporary development of a vaccine against SARS-CoV2). The tireless clinical effort needed to identify an effective polio vaccine clocked in at just over four years of arduous work. Yet the same vaccine that served as the central hope for fearful parents would in an instant morph into a source of paralytic fear. In rushing the rollout of Salk's vaccine, one particular manufacturing facility in California somehow blundered the production of the vaccine, failing to properly inactivate the virus.[8] The results were disastrous. The bad batch of this much-anticipated vaccine was administered to at least 200,000 children and caused at least 40,000 to suffer symptoms of polio. Two hundred children would suffer lifelong paralysis and eleven would die. Salk's many professional enemies pounced, forcing the replacement of Salk's killed vaccine with a vaccine consisting of a weakened virus, which had been developed by his rival, Albert Sabin.

For contemporary society, the story of the Sabin and Salk vaccines not only serve as a model and warning about the risks in rushing to a

COVID-19 vaccine, but it is remarkable for who paid for these vaccines. The research and development of both vaccines were largely underwritten by philanthropists and the American government.[9] The vaccines cost pennies to make and even these costs were absorbed largely by federal resources. Indeed, a little-known fact is that the US federal government still pays for the majority of childhood or pandemic vaccines (including the billions of dollars funneled from the government to pharmaceutical industry coffers for a SARS-CoV2 vaccine).[10]

The idea of government-sponsored childhood vaccination contrasts sharply with the cost of vaccines that are administered to teens and adults. For example, the vaccine Gardasil was launched in 2006 to immunize teens and prevent them from being infected by human papillomavirus infection, a major cause of several types of cancer. Despite the incredible benefits arising from the elimination of cervical, anal, and many oral cancers, the rollout of the vaccine was met with protest when it was announced that it would retail with a hefty price tag of more than $400.[11] Just over a decade later, the price of the HPV vaccine now commands nearly twice that amount.[12] Other vaccines for adults are comparably expensive: a vial of the shingles vaccine will set you back a few hundred dollars and a boost of the measles, mumps, and rubella (MMR) vaccine for adults costs roughly the same.[13][14] Depending upon insurance provider, consumers can expect to pay some or all of these comparatively high prices to obtain these vaccines, keeping in mind that insurance companies typically pass on increased drug pricing to their plan participants in the form of rising premiums.

Fast-forwarding to the recent crisis, the COVID-19 outbreak raised very real and important questions about how much a vaccine or a drug to treat or prevent the virus should cost and whether pricing might limit access. Indeed, in regard to the drugs that were being tested for use against COVID-19, such as remdesivir, the federal government announced that its developer alone (Gilead Sciences) should determine the price to be charged to consumers,[15] even though the research on this drug was heavily underwritten using taxpayer dollars. Even more outrageously, Gilead attempted to exploit a law meant to incentivize the development of drugs to treat rare diseases, but public scorn shamed them into rescinding an exploit that would have made the companies millions more.[16]

Such questions about cost and access are not unique to COVID-19, but apply to vaccines and medicines writ large. The price of medicines in the United States has been climbing rapidly, particularly in the past few decades, compelling frequent news stories to abound of families unable to afford lifesaving medications.[17] While politicians grumble that these medicines could derail an already-fragile public health infrastructure,[18] the fundamental question that must be asked is, "How do we slow, stop, or reverse the rising costs of medicines?" A silver lining to the COVID-19 pandemic is that it may provide an opportunity to begin addressing this underlying problem. How, you may ask? By the very enormity and transparency of the carnage caused by the infection itself. The danger associated with COVID-19 was driven largely by the fact that it could inflict damage to all peoples and societies, regardless of their geography, ethnicity, or net worth. No one was immune in both a literal and figurative sense. It thus seemed possible, perhaps for the first time in years, that these universal fears might compel measured discussions about drug pricing and availability. Thus, we might finally be nearing the point where we can discuss such concerns openly and honestly.

It is regrettable that these conversations were necessarily sparked by the sheer terror and carnage, both human and economic, as COVID-19 quickly enveloped the world. Nonetheless, such conversations did and would continue. Yet, there is comparatively little unbiased reporting of how we arrived at the present situation, where medicines have become unaffordable, especially in the United States. Amid the accumulating deaths and health complications of the COVID pandemic in the summer of 2020, even President Trump and the GOP (which had a long-standing history opposing regulation of the pharmaceutical enterprise) introduced executive orders to reduce drug pricing in an attempt to make this a key issue in the 2020 election.

The coronavirus crisis provided further evidence of an antiscience bias that had been growing for years. Alternatives to conventional science in general, and the pharmaceutical industry in particular, abound, ranging from herbal supplements to the concept, advanced by the President himself, of injecting bleach and disinfectants, or somehow directing internal ultraviolet light into the body to combat the virus, all baseless and dangerous suggestions that were tragically attempted by some in the public. Trump's suggestions gained momentum that lingered in public discourse for weeks when the story was picked up by the media. Some people condemned the comments, while others went to great lengths to defend them. Such extreme measures in part reflect widespread suspicions about conventional medicines and the individuals and organizations that develop them, a symptom of a growing pandemic of a different sort. Indeed, if one inquired about the most problematic infectious disease crisis in January 2020, they would be met with a response of measles or mumps, outcomes of the burgeoning antivaccine movement that was a subject of *Between Hope and Fear,* a book that one of us (Michael Kinch) published in 2018.[19]

In social media and even many mainstream news stories, biomedical and insurance companies are often portrayed as evil conspirators, intent upon wreaking havoc to line the pockets of the residents of their lush executive boardrooms. Such tales are an embellishment upon truly high profile villains, such as Martin Shkreli and Elizabeth Holmes. Another example, of course, is the disaster resulting from the overaggressive marketing of addictive opioids. As COVID was beginning its destructive rise, the CEO of one of the major malefactors, John Kapoor of Insys, was sentenced in early 2020 to a sixty-six-month prison term.[20] However, a malevolent characterization of the healthcare sector as populated with rapacious vermin is an inaccurate oversimplification.

We will show that the truth is much more complex and interesting. A theme that runs throughout this book is that the dysfunctional system that continually pushes up the price of medicines is the unintended consequence of an arrangement that evolved, paradoxically, to ensure that medicines are safe, effective, widely available, and affordable. Appreciating this fact requires an objective assessment of the history that led to our present situation. Such understanding is crucial at this particular point in time, not merely because of the COVID-19 disaster, but because it seems inevitable that questions about drug pricing and accessibility will remain a crucial issue facing the winners of the 2020 American elections. Healthcare costs have been rising disproportionately in the United States and the deficits and budgetary constraints that will inevitably follow the unprecedented outlay of federal monies to stabilize the economy in 2020 will create a key reckoning. All people, including and perhaps especially politicians, are more scared, motivated, pliable, and frankly discombobulated than they have been at any time since the end of the Second World War. Healthcare, and how to pay for it, will remain at the top of the agenda for years to come.

This combination of fear along with calls for action are likely to propel much-needed conversations about drug pricing and affordability. Just as the Spanish influenza of a century ago ended the First World War, the COVID-19 pandemic of the 20th century holds the potential to be the coup de grâce to end a malaise long-suffered by the American consumer: the ever-escalating prices of medicines.

CHAPTER ONE

The Law of Unintended Consequences

The price of medicines has been increasing at a disturbing rate, triggering alarmed responses by American consumers. Stories abound of people skipping vital medicines, not because they do not work or cause unwanted side effects, but simply because the high prices of vital medicines would preclude other expenses, such as food or shelter. In response some consumers routinely embark upon a relatively new form of travel known as "medical tourism." An example came to the fore early in the 2020 presidential election campaign, when then-candidate Bernie Sanders accompanied a busload of diabetic American passengers on a day trip to Canada, a destination chosen because the price of insulin for our northern neighbors is far less expensive than in the United States.[1]

The concept of medical tourism was not new to the Vermont senator, as he had similarly joined a busload of breast cancer survivors on a 1999 shopping trip across the northern border to access affordable oncology drugs. And Sanders was not the only one venturing on such journeys. According

1

to the Kaiser Family Foundation, more than nineteen million Americans (8 percent of the population) similarly import medicines using full-fledged medical tourism, mail-order prescriptions, and internet orders.[2]

Most Americans do not view Canada as a particularly foreign country. We largely share the same lifestyle and culture. The difference in drug prices cannot be accounted for by the difference of the two nations' currency value. The American and Canadian currencies remain relatively locked together, distinguished primarily by changes in the price of oil. Yet, Americans pay far more for drugs than Canadians.

These higher prices are taking a dire toll on the health of the United States. Fully one in five American consumers admits to having skipped vital medications simply because they cost too much.[3] This statistic is nearly twice the rate reported by Canadians. Looking further afield, the rate of American avoidance of medicines due to cost is ten times higher than that experienced in the United Kingdom.[4]

The Greedy, Needy American

A commonly held misperception is that American spending on medicines reflects the fact that Americans simply take more medicines. This presumption is an extension of the international stereotype of the overindulged and overweight American, impatient for quick solutions and willing to pop a pill for anything.[5]

Americans are rather unique in one way (with the exception of New Zealand) in that we are constantly bombarded with a flurry of drug advertisements. It seems impossible to recall a time before the countless television commercials portraying smiling, happy people presumably made that way by the miraculous remedies being pitched.

Given the media saturation of advertisement, along with the fast-talking announcers legally required to convey the potential risks of the product, it may come as a surprise to learn that Americans do not consume any more medicines than our international peers.[6] This fact might even serve as an indictment of the advertising industry because one would presume an efficient use of this media, given the billions of dollars spent, would at least increase the number of doses sold. Instead, we contend that advertisement costs have primarily served as contributing factors to the ever-escalating prices of medicines.

Stated simply, the higher spending per capita of the American consumer on medicine reflects nothing other than the higher costs that we pay for each pill, injection, or infusion we receive.

Interestingly, the elevated rates of American consumer spending are a relatively recent phenomenon. As recently as the mid-1990s, the average costs paid by Americans for medicines were in a middling position as compared with other developed-world nations.[7] This all began to change with the approach of the new millennium, when the pace of price increases far surpassed those paid by our international colleagues. These differences have continued to accelerate ever since, creating an unwanted form of American exceptionalism.

The Rise of the Pharmaceutical Enterprise

The causes for the excessive prices Americans pay for medicine are the subject of this book. The problem of high drug prices is in part a consequence of increasing complexity of both the scientific and business strategies used to develop, distribute, and market new medicines. Moreover, we will observe that the prices also reflect a unique perversion of general capitalistic tendencies.

The "pharmaceutical enterprise" has been metastasizing in both the number of industries involved as well as the number of individual companies in each industry. The overall enterprise has increasingly fractured in terms of the activities performed (discovery of new medicines is often distinct from their early or later-stage clinical development, manufacturing, distribution, and payment for the resulting products). The new industries that have joined the broader enterprise have often focused specifically on key aspects of the drug development and delivery process with the initial intent to reduce costs. Yet, over time each industry has undergone their own remodeling, as evidenced by waves of consolidation. The result has been an increase in expenses and a decrease in the efficiency of overall drug development and distribution, thereby contributing to rising costs. Unsurprisingly, each new company and industry that has been created seeks to optimize its own profitability. Thus, an already complex system, needed to apply cutting-edge science to derive and deliver new medicines, has spawned waves of entirely new industries and organizations, each of which seeks to maximize its revenues. All of this costs money, which we collectively refer to as "the price of health."

Let us be clear, we are not advocating against a free market. Indeed, an emphasis upon a free market has historically distinguished the United States from many of its international peers, allowing the nation to prosper and become the world's leading economic, military, and, yes, biopharmaceutical power. Yet these same positive characteristics have been twisted to create the morass of drug pricing that the United States faces today.

We will see that American dominance is not limited merely to geopolitical or economic hegemony, but extends to scientific and entrepreneurial prowess as well. Since the conclusion of the Second World War, a disproportionate number of new medical breakthroughs have resulted from research and development activities conducted at American universities and corporations alike. As we will see, the knowledge gained has been capitalized by both old and new industries, domestic and international companies. The outcomes of this tireless work have included the introduction of waves of extraordinary new medicines to prevent or treat a variety of maladies that had plagued humankind from time immemorial.

Long gone are the days that parents dreaded the coming of summertime and the inevitable accompaniment of polio or winter and the inevitable risks for influenza and pneumonia. And prior to COVID-19, many other infectious diseases had been dismissed as relics only important for the writers of history books. Moreover, as emphasized in *The End of the Beginning* (which Michael published in 2019), promising recent advancements suggest that cancer likewise could be considered a manageable illness within our lifetime. Many challenges remain, but even in the face of COVID-19, it has never been a better time to be sick, old, or both. Yet, it increasingly helps to be wealthy if one wants to gain access to these new miracle drugs.

The same mainstays of the American experience that helped propel the biopharmaceutical industry to greatness unintentionally contributed to unsustainable increases in the price of health. These rising costs now pose threats to both the American consumer and the entire healthcare infrastructure. We are rapidly approaching a point where both the cost to develop drugs as well as the ability of consumers to afford it may prevent new medicines from being effectively developed or distributed. Such an outcome would be disastrous at any time, but is particularly relevant given that the nation's (and indeed the entire planet's) population continues to get older and fatter, arguably the two greatest risk factors for chronic disease. Moreover, the COVID-19 pandemic is a reminder that infectious diseases are still with us and can and will periodically revisit us and with devastating consequences.

In planning this book, the authors centered upon the fundamental question of why the prices of medicines have bloated so disproportionately over the past few years. We both have a long history in a biotechnology industry. We love and respect this industry, where our work has allowed us to contribute to the development and introduction of new products that have fundamentally improved the quality and quantity of life. Yet, both of us were increasingly troubled and frankly confused by the fact that the prices of these innovations have been escalating so rapidly, particularly in the United States. Though neither of us have a background in economics, we presumed the widespread importance of the subject would offer many resources that would reveal the causes responsible for rising prices. If needed, we believed it would be comparatively simple to draw upon a limitless collection of academic studies of the field.

Despite the fact there is no lack of popular opinion on the subject, relatively few objective resources could help explain the phenomenon of drug pricing, much less how this system evolved. Worse still, the manifold enterprises, indeed entire industries, that are responsible for the discovery, development, distribution, and payment for drugs have remained frustratingly opaque. This lack of transparency was the indirect result of an evolution in how new medicines are discovered, developed, and distributed.

We were surprised to find that each step of the process, from early concepts through marketing and distribution, has fractured into a complexity of layered systems, many of which are comparatively new and all of which are designed to maximize profit margins. Moreover, we learned that most of these layers were originally created in an attempt to increase efficiency and restrain prices. Although the word is frequently misused, we can sincerely invoke the term "irony" to reflect the fact that our contemporary and highly troubled system for delivering medicines involves a complex series of private sector and governmental initiatives meant to increase the efficiencies of delivering safe and effective medicines to the American public.

Layer upon layer of new initiatives ultimately created a dense meshwork that has confounded reform and limited accountability. This complexity has rendered an outcome in which each element of a convoluted system (i.e., investors, regulators, biotechnology upstarts, established pharmaceutical companies, pharmacies, insurers) can individually and, with a straight face, profess their powerlessness in bringing down costs. The results of this complexity strangely facilitated an absence of accountability and, as we will see, has allowed many embattled corporate executives to point their fingers at others (with a presumed wink and a nod). Yet, each member of this circular firing squad is loaded with blanks (hence the winks) as they know that the complexity is so intense that it will confound even the largest investor, regulator, and consumer of medicines: the American government and by proxy, the American public writ large. We will see that the federal bureaucracy functions in many roles. It is the primary organization responsible for the discovery, regulation, and payment of medicines, and yet is mostly hamstrung by constraints of its own making.

Modern-Day Simon Bar Sinisters?

As Americans and as humans, we naturally seek a simple answer to this crisis and to punish the evil-doers. Indeed, there has been no lack of suitable candidates. The headlines of the past few years have been filled with high-profile villains straight out of central casting. Malevolent actors abound, such as Martin Shkreli, the ever-smirking and self-ascribed "pharma bro" (who raised the price of one drug by fifty-six times), Elizabeth Holmes (the con-artist founder of Theranos, a smoke-and-mirrors medical diagnostics company that bilked its investors out of billions), and Heather Bresch (CEO of Mylan and daughter of a prominent senator, who used her connections to create the perception of an expanded market need for the EpiPen and then escalated the costs of a hundred-year-old drug to absurd levels). Although each of these characters is quite colorful, they have been thoroughly covered by investigative journalists and federal prosecutors. Although we might reflect at times upon exploits, it is not our purpose to retell these lurid tales or to overemphasize the behaviors, bad or good, of any particular individuals, organizations, or even industries.

Quite the opposite. In each case, actions taken to improve the efficiency were invariably despoiled. In particular, we will witness the steady accumulation of new industries, mouths that need to be fed and composed of companies seeking to maximize profits. The added complexity contributed to a consistent subterfuge enabled by the progressively increasing opacity. Indeed, the actions and transparency of the legal drug trade might easily be confused with its illicit counterparts.

To put this into perspective, it is useful to contrast two different types of medicines, a recurring theme throughout this book. When we purchase an over-the-counter drug at a neighborhood grocery store or pharmacy, there are usually three major organizations involved in the transaction: the consumer, the retailer (i.e., the store from which you buy the medicine), and the manufacturer (the pharmaceutical company that made and marketed the medicine).

For a medicine requiring a doctor's prescription, these same entities are often joined by many others. First, the drug was likely discovered by one or more academic organizations and/or biotechnology companies. These entities usually participate in the early stages of the product's development, each of which seeks to be rewarded in some fashion, typically with generous royalties for their groundbreaking activities. These biotech companies are invariably backed by venture capital funds, which invest millions of dollars often over a long time frame with the intent of maximizing the returns of their investment. Second, a large pharmaceutical company will most likely have acquired the product at some point to complete its development and regulatory approval before manufacturing it at large scale for distribution. Most of the pharmaceutical companies are publicly traded, which means they are owned by investors who demand a regular healthy return on their invested dollars. Add to this complex group of characters your insurance company, your doctor, the pharmacy where you pick up your drug, and an organization known as a pharmacy benefits manager. With this laundry list of players involved in getting you your drug, is it any wonder why things are so complicated? The most disturbing fact of this entire process is that the medicine you end up with is not determined by you, your doctor, or even your insurer, but by backroom, complex deals cut between these various entities all under the pretense of keeping prices down. We will evaluate each of these layers and find they all seek to maximize profitability.

In aggregate, these many layers of added complexity contribute to the rising costs of a prescription. Worse still, the manifold layers can and do allow each to blame the other layer for rising prices.

How Did We Get Here?

How and why did such a system evolve?

Escalating prices have become so familiar to modern consumers that many of us simply accept them as a sad fact of life. Yet, the same trends that are merely irritating to a lucky and wealthy few have proven devastating to those with fewer resources. We are all aware that the impact of rising drug costs has destroyed many family budgets and could soon overwhelm our nation's collective public health and economic well-being.

Beyond the individual tragedies suffered as a result of improper treatment, escalating rates of omitting certain medicines can convey dire consequences well beyond the borders of our nation. For example, it is quite well established that even seemingly minor interruptions in the treatment of certain infectious diseases, such as the pathogen responsible for AIDS, provide an opportunity for the virus to adapt in a manner that renders it resistant to further treatment. Similar outcomes can arise in cancer patients. These two particular exemplars are relevant to our story, as HIV/AIDS and cancer are among the most prominent examples of disease management suffering from the consequences of high treatment costs.

Although the overall structure of the system is exceedingly complex and impervious, the individual components of this complex enterprise can be easily understood. Surprisingly, it seems many of these components were created in an effort to help the American consumer; to protect the safety and efficacy of medicines, as well as to rein in costs. Yet the law of unintended consequences has always predominated.

It is crucial to reiterate that the story you are about to embark upon is one composed mostly of well-intended and noble individuals, organizations, and industries, each contributing to the formation of structures meant to improve the quality and quantity of life. (It is the belief of the authors that the Martin Shkrelis of the world are red herrings, as abhorrent as they are.) All too often, however, systems created to do good have become distorted or been manipulated in ways that have often been contradictory to the original motivations of their creators.

Among the unintended consequences we will encounter is evidence that even the most principled measures, such as the creation of incentives to address rare diseases, have instead been twisted and exploited in a manner that has dramatically escalated the prices charged for medicines, new and old. Likewise, an intent to inform consumers of the opportunities for less expensive competitor products gave rise to ceaseless pharmaceutical advertising, creating a situation where many companies now spend more money on television advertisements than for research and development. Even incentives meant to increase generic medicines as competition for branded drugs have had a boomerang effect. Approaches to increase competition among generic drug manufacturers to drive down the costs of medicines instead enabled multithousand percent increases in the price of these medicines and worse still, they spawned shortages in vital pediatric oncology medicines. Another unintended consequence arose with the creation of an entirely new industry, pharmacy benefit managers (PBMs), in an attempt to control rising drug prices. Yet PBMs are today often regarded to be the largest single contributor to rising drug prices today (especially by their pharmaceutical industry counterparts).

We will see that individual components of the health enterprise interact and have metastasized in ways that were both unexpected and, in retrospect, inevitable. The resulting system became so convoluted that original intentions have given way to perverted and opaque systems that have themselves been manipulated to provide plausible deniability for the rising price of drugs. We now face a troubling future where the many parts of the healthcare enterprise control life-or-death decisions, both for individual American consumers and the overall American economy, where healthcare spending captures nearly one in five dollars of the nation's gross domestic product.[8] At the same time, the system itself is teetering and could soon tumble, either as a result of hasty political moves by canny legislators or, more likely, by benign neglect. Either way, the coming disruption could be cataclysmic, by disrupting access to new and existing medicines and by curtailing our ability to introduce new medicines.

With this in mind, we will begin our story by conveying how the increasing complexity of the American system for drug discovery and distribution evolved, a process that in many ways parallels the rise and evolution of the United States as a nation.

CHAPTER TWO

A History of Medicine Men (and Women)

The rationale for this book is a presumption that understanding how and why systems evolved to their contemporary forms can inform their future improvement. In this chapter, we seek to understand why the distribution of medicines through modern-day pharmacies (whether conventional brick and mortar, super chain, or online mail order) evolved to their current state as this knowledge will later help explain how this system contributes to rising costs.

The story of medicines is far older than written history. Recommendations to "eat this, not that" were passed along in oral form from generation to generation and it was essential to convey clear advice, lest a selection of the wrong plant or its improper preparation transform a remedy into a lethal toxin. In this spirit, it seems obvious that some of the oldest papyri, dating back nearly four millennia and preserved by dry desert air, are ancient Egyptian instruction manuals for the preparation of medicinal cures. The oldest, the Kahun Papyri, is a four-millennia-old text describing treatment for women's health, gynecological disease, and contraception.[1] Other papyri addressed a variety of ailments, ranging from everyday aches and pains to diabetes and eye diseases.

As civilizations expanded their worldly knowledge and ventured forth geographically, more and more plants (and occasionally animals and medicinal clays) were encountered; the collective knowledge expanded to include ever more remedies. As the sheer amount of information grew, full-time specialists were required to keep track of, recommend, prepare, and dispense medicines, essentially creating the need for what we would refer to today as apothecaries (a precursor of pharmacists), as well as primary and specialty care physicians. Apothecaries expanded around the world, each shop generally focused on the herbs and other remedies arising from locally sourced plants and animals. Many continue to thrive, especially in tradition-based societies such as purveyors of Chinese medicines in modern-day Asia. Most of these have been replaced by pharmacies in Europe and the Americas, but this is a comparatively recent phenomenon. Looking back and depending upon the size of a village, there might be one or more of these specialists available to address the aches and pains of daily life. For the purposes of this story, we will focus upon apothecaries: the individuals responsible for creating and dispensing medicines.

Apothecaries generally learned their trade by observation, discussions with elders, and reading the few written texts that might be available. As the profession became more formalized, apprenticeships came into being, which allowed seasoned professionals to train a new generation of practitioners in the art of sourcing the right ingredients and preparing and combining them into various elixirs and cures. As the profession developed, these apprenticeships grew more stringent and generally required intensive training for at least seven or eight years before a trainee could strike out on his own.[2] This long time period was necessary to allow apothecaries to transfer the key tools of the trade. Some of these tricks were what we would call trade secrets today, cherished confidences passed down orally from generation to generation (since writing these down might allow a secret recipe to fall into the hands of rivals; which also explains why texts were so rare). As the profession grew in prestige and importance, the apothecaries began to be regulated to prevent ancient hucksters from selling dangerous or ineffective products, a challenge that remains to the present day. Given these new and presumably unwanted constraints, the apothecaries began to organize (a response to regulation that we will see arising time and time again). The emergence of these guilds allowed apothecaries to share their expertise and experiences. For example, the Guild of Pepperers dates back to 1180 and was formed to create standards for spices sold in medieval England. It's interesting to note that many early seasonings were not deployed for purposes of improving taste, but rather to prevent food spoilage and aid digestion.

The First Brain Drain

Apothecaries played a vital role in the community. David Thomson, the first apothecary documented in the New England colonies, arrived there in 1623, just three years after the *Mayflower* landed near Plymouth Rock. Life in the New World was harsh, and Thomson died a mere five years later at the advanced age of thirty-seven. Two years later, John Winthrop, the future first governor of the Massachusetts Colony, arrived as part of an eleven-ship fleet of Puritan immigrants, who departed the Isle of Wight in search of a "City upon a Hill." This city was eventually founded in what is present-day Boston.

Winthrop was an amateur apothecary with a lifelong interest in medicinal herbs. As part of this side gig, Winthrop began importing herbs from Europe, but soon realized that he needed someone with more experience to help develop his business. After all, it was difficult to be both the primary drug dealer and titular leader of a burgeoning colony. Soon after his arrival, Winthrop attempted to recruit another Puritan, Robert Cooke, to establish an apothecary in Boston.

Cooke arrived in 1638, just ahead of another apothecary, John Johnstone, who immigrated from Scotland to the Swedish colony of Perth Amboy in modern-day New Jersey.[3] It was a bit of an unstable time, as the Swedish colony had just been taken over by the Dutch and in rapid succession would be forcibly acquired by the British. Although Johnstone remained in business, Cooke was not destined to remain in the colonies, as the early death of his father (also an apothecary) compelled Cooke to return to Britain to take over his father's business. By this time, Boston already had a second apothecary, William Davis, who would establish a more durable business in New England.

Trained in England, Davis did not have access to most of the native plants of his homeland and had to identify substitutes from plants native to New England. Thus, in these early days, Davis, like Winthrop before him, was compelled to dispense many medicines that had been prepared by fellow apothecaries in England. Such intershop trade was not particularly unusual, since an apothecary might intentionally make a larger batch of medicine than was required for his own use and then sell or barter the extra material to others in the profession. In this way, Davis was unknowingly helping pave the path for a new and more efficient industry that would ultimately render the apothecary profession utterly obsolete.

For most of the 18th century, most medicinal plants and their crude extracts were purchased from small distributors located in the United Kingdom, with the remainder grown and purified in the American colonies. A critical need for domestic sourcing arose with the break of the American colonies from the mother country. No less a historical figure than Benedict Arnold provides an example of the growing pains facing the nation. Arnold trained as an apothecary by apprenticing with a cousin. He set up shop in New Haven, Connecticut, before the war and would gain notoriety and later infamy for his valiant battlefield efforts and scurrilous defection, respectively.

British apothecary distributors, who had supplied colonial customers, were understandably concerned about working with the enemy. Of particular concern was that governments might accuse them of supplying their rebel customers with vital ingredients that would be used to heal the wounded, only to have them go and kill more British soldiers. Even after the American victory at Yorktown, the new nation's infrastructure was creaky, with the American government frequently teetering on the edge of bankruptcy. Consequently, creditors remained understandably hesitant to accept the risks of lending money to the former colonies in a period of acute uncertainty as the new nation worked out how it would introduce its own currency and develop its trade policies. There was also, in effect, a prominent brain drain from Great Britain to the Americas. Benedict Arnold again provides an interesting example as he, like other loyalist and British-trained apothecaries, left the nation forever.

Planting the Seeds for a New Nation

The newly formed United States was thus compelled to emphasize domestic sources of medicines. One of the early actions by the individual states, and later the nation as a whole, was the creation of a pharmacopeia. This mouthful of a word is essentially a list in book form of all medicines utilized in a particular territory, the intended (and sometimes unexpected) medicinal effects of these drugs, and directions for their preparation and storage. Perhaps most importantly, these pharmacopeias conveyed an agreed-upon standard for concocting these medicines, acting as a sort of cookbook for new drugs and providing detailed descriptions of the final products. To create these standards, it was common practice to gather the apothecaries from around a territory and gain agreement, both as to the essential medicines used and the means for producing them and ensuring their quality. One might suspect these to have been tense exchanges at times since the field was characterized by secret recipes, proprietary approaches, and even disagreements about the definition of measures, including something as fundamental as a pound or ounce. The pound was not officially defined in the United States until 1893.[4] Colonial pharmacopeias had been borrowing from Britain, but the newly independent states began to compile their own versions in the first years of the 19th century, with the first formally introduced by Massachusetts in 1808.[5]

Although the early American Federal government did not desire to control medicines at this early stage, the need for a national pharmacopeia was advocated by Samuel Latham Mitchill, a Long Island-born Quaker, who had earned a medical degree in Scotland. When he returned to New York, Mitchill served as a prominent physician and later represented the state in both the House of Representatives and Senate, advocating for medical causes.[6] Given his background and status, Mitchill advocated for the creation of a national pharmacopeia. To help facilitate a positive outcome, he made the still-new Senate chambers (now known as the Old Senate Chamber) available for an invitation-only convention to be attended by an elite society of American physicians and apothecaries. Mitchill himself was elected president of the convention.

The day-to-day activities for this prestigious meeting would be organized and led by Lyman Spalding, a precocious physician with a knack for being in the right place at the right time. Spalding had helped found a school of medicine at Dartmouth in the same year that he himself had graduated from Harvard.[7] Soon thereafter, Spalding began a correspondence with no less a personage than President Thomas Jefferson about the causes of disease and mortality in the early United States.[8] Jefferson, a known data junkie, encouraged Spalding's efforts, including his desire to compile a comprehensive document to convey all the legitimate remedies and medicinal plants discovered or utilized throughout the former colonies, a subject that aligned him with Mitchill.

On New Year's Day 1820, Spalding arrived at the Senate chambers to join Mitchill amid one of the coldest winters Washington, DC, had experienced in almost a decade.[9] Spalding arrived with an expectation of mingling with dozens of the nation's top medical intelligentsia. To his dismay, he instead encountered five colleagues, who would later be joined by six additional arrivals that trickled in over the following days. Despite a disappointing turnout, Spalding's small but focused team compiled all the different regional pharmacopeia from around the nation into a comprehensive pharmacopeia.

This was not an easy process, as much of the extant materials were based on hearsay or lacked solid experimental evidence (e.g., a demonstration that the treatment worked in people). Given these activities were taking place in what is considered "The Age of Reason," the results were intended to be based upon facts rather than superstition. Consequently, many of the remedies to be compiled in the national pharmacopeia were debated, sometimes quite fiercely. Indeed, the arguments often became sufficiently hot to require Mitchill's smooth touch, which had been developed by surviving years of congressional rancor. By the end of just a week, the convention had, in the mind of Mitchill at least, completed its work and would appoint a five-person commission, led again by Spalding, to polish and publish the findings. This commission would then identify printers for the publication of a book by the end of the year. In reality, the undertaking was far from simple polishing and required full-time effort and debate for months to come. Nonetheless, the commission met the timeline (barely), contracting with printers on December 22, 1820.[10]

In the months following the publication of the inaugural United States Pharmacopeia, another American first was achieved with the founding of a college of pharmacy in Philadelphia. This school is known today as the University of the Sciences. A second school, the Massachusetts School of Pharmacy, would follow in Boston two years later. This geography is significant as these cities have since, as we will see, played pivotal roles in shaping the American pharmaceutical industry.

The creation of a unified American pharmacopeia coincided with a transition from apothecaries, where the viability of whatever they were selling was left up to the discretion of the apothecary (and the consumer who would decide whether or not they trusted the apothecary's judgment or skill) into more standardized university programs meant to train pharmacists. These new pharmacist professionals would work to standardize the creation of new medicines, emphasizing the production and distribution of medicines with a higher quality than had ever been possible before. Likewise, the pharmacists would work to increase the quantity of new medicines that could be made to address the needs of a growing nation. Nonetheless, these improvements would come at a cost, as the credentialing of pharmacists might improve the quality of their work, but would necessarily limit their numbers. Even using standardized and presumably more efficient techniques catalogued in the pharmacopeia and taught in pharmacy schools, the average pharmacist could prepare only a handful of medicines per day. Given the fundamental law of supply and demand, these inefficiencies contributed to cost. To counter this trend, the pharmacists of the 19th century turned to a more efficient source of medicines than was possible when limited by creations made with their mortars and pestles. For this part of the story, we must leave the American shores and relocate for a time to Central Europe.

Making His Merck

A theme that runs throughout this book is the creation of new industries, all of which seek to maximize their profitability. Their development was quite rational and, indeed, intended to increase the efficiency of drug development or distribution. We will now meet the first example of this trend with the formation of what would become the modern pharmaceutical industry. While the transition to educated and licensed pharmacists was one trend that disrupted apothecaries, the coup de grâce was delivered by a pioneering innovator in a small Hessian pharmacy tucked into a corner of modern-day southwest Germany. Like most apothecaries of his day, Heinrich Emanuel Merck (he went by Emanuel) had learned his profession as an apprentice to his father. Indeed, the Engel-Apotheke (Angel Apothecary) had been the family business for six generations, having its roots in the founding of a modest shop in 1668.[11] Inheriting the business from his father in 1816, Merck had powerful entrepreneurial aspirations.

Rather than concocting relatively small batches of material, Emanuel Merck took the rather audacious approach of expanding his workforce to create vastly larger batches of medicines, a time- and money-saving approach adopted by other industry-disrupting innovators such as Eli Whitney and Henry Ford.[12] He would then sell his product in bulk to other apothecaries, saving his customers the need to manufacture their own medicines a batch at a time. Merck embarked upon a campaign to identify innovation in diverse ways, both to manufacture existing medicines at a larger scale and to identify emerging new medicines with which he might corner the market. A transformative moment came in 1827, by which time Emanuel changed the name of his business to E. Merck and purchased a recipe for the production of a seemingly mythical drug with extraordinary commercial potential.

Opium was a well-known remedy, having been harvested continuously from its earliest discovery by prehistoric cultures in the Middle East. The milk from the poppy, if harvested and prepared in just the right way, was known to relieve pain, but its potency (and safety) varied greatly from batch to batch. A young Prussian apprentice by the name of Friedrich Sertürner was determined to identify and consistently isolate the active ingredient within opium responsible for its analgesic (pain-relieving) properties.[13] After months of dedicated efforts, Sertürner had finally mastered a recipe for reliably purifying the pain-relieving ingredient from opium. He tested the outcome of his activities on local children, an unethical approach even by the standards of the day.

An attempt to share the discovery with the world, in the form of a scientific manuscript, was sidelined after an editor decided it was not important enough to warrant the space in his precious journal.[14] Sertürner gave up on his discovery in frustration until years later when a particularly painful toothache compelled him to make another batch of his maligned remedy.

Presumably reenergized and motivated by the intense pain relief, Sertürner decided again to convey the importance of his discovery.

In 1827, Sertürner had the luck to meet with Emanuel Merck, who was prospecting for unique products for his business where he manufactured bulk amounts of medicinal ingredients. Merck immediately saw the potential for Sertürner's product and purchased the recipe from Sertürner. Within months, Merck established one of the first mass-market pharmaceutical products that would create a major buzz: morphine. Still used today, morphine conveys a miraculous ability to alleviate excruciating pain (as it did for the grandfather of one of your authors, who at the end of his life suffered extreme bone pain from metastatic prostate cancer), but these benefits came at the cost of its addictive properties. Modern-day America remains all too familiar with such dependency issues with similar pain-relieving drugs, such as fentanyl and other opioids that led to a national crisis claiming thousands of lives and trapping millions more in the dependent powers of these pain-relieving drugs.

Wholesale Changes

Beyond morphine, Emanuel Merck had planted the seeds of an entire industry. In the years following the introduction of morphine, companies throughout the world built upon the approach pioneered by Merck, producing mass quantities of therapeutic molecules. Amid the industrialization mania that characterized the middle of the 19th century, the world witnessed a boom in the creation of other companies that produced pharmaceutical products. Names still recognizable today such as Pfizer (established 1849 in Brooklyn), Eli Lilly (established 1876 in Indianapolis), and Johnson and Johnson (established 1886 in New Brunswick, New Jersey), to name just a few, came into being during a transition to mass produce medically relevant chemicals. The active ingredients responsible for the efficacy of these medicines were initially chemicals isolated from plants. Later improvements in the chemical sciences would lead to some drugs to be produced not in plants, but in the laboratory, facilitating the scale-up to ever larger quantities in massive factories.

These changes portended doom for the apothecary profession, which had centered upon the accumulation of recipes that would be deployed on demand. The transition from one industry to another reflected a push for greater efficiency. We now see it as commonsensical that pharmacists should purchase ingredients from a wholesaler rather than create them by hand. However, this change was a significant disruption. The mortars and pestles that had been used for centuries to grind the leaves of medicinal herbs were increasingly shelved (though they would remain prominent symbols of the professions), while orders would be filled by pharmacists sourcing the medicines from wholesale distributors. Beyond the obvious efficiencies in cost, the average pharmacy could supply the community with a much larger array of medicines than their apothecary predecessors. Indeed, the local pharmacy quickly evolved to be a retail shop not merely for medicines but other staples of daily life. Indeed, the Merck & Co. drugstore on University Place in Manhattan soon became as well-known a place to purchase candy as it was to buy medicines.

A Prescription for Change

The rise of pharmaceutical wholesalers in the 19th century freed up time for pharmacists, allowing them to evolve their profession from producing the active ingredients of medicines to compounding, the process whereby medicinal ingredients were combined in a final form individualized for a patient's need. These products often took the form of pastes, pills, and elixirs (liquid-based medicinal mixtures). As the mechanized and mass-market factories of the pharmaceutical industry increased the availability of these final preparations, many pharmacies were left with unused fountains for soda water. This resource would soon find a new use to allow drugstores to become the perfect venue for a new generation of medicine-inspired products. Indeed, a medicinal cure produced in Atlanta, Georgia, would change the pharmacy profession forever.

On May 8, 1886, John Stith Pemberton, a physician and wounded veteran of the American Civil War, traveled from his home in rural Columbus, Georgia, a hundred miles north to the great city of Atlanta.[15] The reason for his trip was to test a new concoction he had developed to treat a widespread problem plaguing the nation since the cessation of hostilities two decades before. Like many veterans injured in combat, Pemberton had been given morphine to ease the pain and soon became addicted. By the time of this trip, Pemberton had developed a new means of treating opiate dependence by combining three substances, caffeine, alcohol, and cocaine, into a syrup meant to prevent the symptoms of addiction. The Pemberton's French Wine Coca was a commercial success in his hometown but could not be sold in Atlanta, which had succumbed to the temperance movement and become a dry town months before. Consequently, this new concoction lacked alcohol. It also did not have cocaine since alcohol was needed to liberate the powerful drug from the coca leaves used in the production of the syrup. An Atlanta pharmacist mistakenly diluted Pemberton's elixir with soda water and, in a remarkable twist of fate, Coca-Cola was born. As pharmacies were the primary sources of soda water in any given community, Coca-Cola allowed pharmacies to become a hub of social and commercial activity in communities around the United States.

Although born just a few years after the cola-driven peak of the neighborhood pharmacy, both authors have vivid early memories of the era of the small, independent corner pharmacy, with Dr. Kinch having a particular personal connection. His uncle was a licensed pharmacist and, as was the custom in many states, a pharmacist was required to be an owner of an independent pharmacy. This quaint pharmacy was located in the small college town of Oxford, Ohio, home to Miami University. For Dr. Kinch, memories abound of this authority figure, adorned in a white coat, standing on a dais at the back of the store, dispensing medicines into small plastic bottles. Indeed, this setup remains the general setup of the corner pharmacy, with retail purchases at the front of the business and shelves of medicines stored on a raised plinth at the back. By the final quarter of the 20th century, the pharmacy profession had again evolved, this time from compounding to dispensing to counting pills and measuring liquids. Moreover, the geography of this recollection, if not the timing, proved fateful for the future of the corner pharmacy due to the actions of a remarkable, yet little-known and underappreciated entrepreneur.

Markets and the Dow

Two dozen or so miles southeast of Oxford, Ohio, is the far larger river city of Cincinnati. The Cincinnati College of Pharmacy had formed in 1850, the first college dedicated to the training of pharmacists west of the Allegheny Mountains. In 1889, the college graduated one of its first female students, a twenty-one-year-old by the name of Margaret Cornelius Dow. Cora to her friends,[16] she was born on March 11, 1868, in Paterson, New Jersey. Cora moved with her family to Cincinnati at the age of two and was raised with a love and talent for music. At the age of seventeen, Cora was already listed as a piano teacher and had ambitions to be an operatic diva, aspiring to perform Wagner before adoring crowds.

Cora's plans changed when her father's health began deteriorating in 1878, the consequence of a long-standing battle against tuberculosis. Her father, Edwin Dow, had made his way as a wholesaler of medicines in Cincinnati and had purchased his own retail shop in 1885. In that same year, Cora began working with her father to help the family business as her father steadily deteriorated. He would die four years later. At the same time, Cora enrolled at the Cincinnati College of Pharmacy in 1886, passing the state board a year later, a particularly impressive feat as she had done so even before she graduated in 1888. The first female graduate from the Cincinnati College of Pharmacy had preceded Cora by only four years. Cora's age, rather than her gender, proved her first major hurdle as the precocious Dow was too young to work. Ohio law required a minimum age of twenty-one before one could be employed as a pharmacist and so she had to cool her heels a bit by working in her father's store.

Once allowed to do so and necessitated by the death of her father, Cora Dow soon took over the family business. Although the extant photographs of Dow convey her as a slight figure with what has been described as "large, soft, magnetic eyes," that was simply a stylistic bias of the late Victorian era.[17] Dow's solid actions belie such caricatures. Nonetheless, the Dow family business did indeed begin as a diminutive undertaking and Cora herself described the building at the corner of 5th and Vine Streets in Cincinnati as being a "shack" and "so small one could reach the pills with one hand, the striped sticks of candy on the opposite side of the store, with the other."[18]

The ambitious Dow soon shuttered this store, opening a larger successor on Race Street in 1890. Cora tirelessly devoted her waking hours to ensuring its success, with a particular emphasis on and talent for innovation. Taking a different approach from her male pharmacist counterparts, Dow adopted a strategy intent to create a shopping experience "with an eye to feminine desires and prejudices."[19] Her innovations included adopting a Greco-Italian architectural style ornamented with marble and onyx pillars decorated with gold leaf. As an early advocate of the commercial promises of the soda fountain, her custom-designed octagonal fountain attracted customers from far afield.

Dow soon opened a second store, not as a replacement, but as an expansion of a successful business strategy. The second store was strategically positioned near the railroad depot to attract travelers and commuters alike. Dow also took the virtually unprecedented approach of leaving the store open all day and night. By continuing to locate stores near commuter and transportation hubs, Dow grew her business into a large chain, triggering waves of envy and resentment by other pharmacists, who felt it unsavory to own "multiples." Dow drove customers into her successful "multiples" with newspaper advertisements to the general public and, in a daring move, extolled the virtues of her pharmacies in trade publications targeted at local doctors. She even offered discounts to physicians as a means of encouraging them to direct their patients to her stores; a smart and scandalous idea in a far more conservative time.

Beyond increasing the number of venues, Cora was also constantly testing and expanding the breadth of products that could be purchased at a Dow store. Soon, retail sales of nonpharmaceutical products drove customers to her stores, where they might also fill a prescription (the opposite business approach than traditional pharmacies). Using this approach, Dow's drugstores were soon filling over two thousand prescriptions per week, a remarkable number given the maturity of the industry and the limited availability of products as compared to conventional times. During her lifetime, Cora's empire consisted of eleven stores, strategically positioned at key transportation hubs that fully canvassed the greater Cincinnati community. Appreciating and enacting the concept of equal pay for equal work, Dow paid her male and female workers the same, adopting a gender-neutral approach that "a woman's work, like a man's work, is gauged by ability." This progressive view created loyal employees among both sexes and contributed to her businesses' success.

Beyond the keen entrepreneurial prowess as evidenced by her ever-expanding number of locations and offerings, Dow demonstrated an adept approach to drug pricing. The engine driving her business was the adoption of what is today known as "cut-rate" pricing policies. Rather than practicing the widely used approach of keeping prices and margins relatively high, Dow experimented with cutting the prices on medicines, the products that got customers in the doors. Her idea, which proved profitable, was that low margins on medicines would be offset by higher margins on consumer products in combination with an elevated volume of sales. Although such an approach is commonly practiced today, this strategy was a pioneering effort in the early days of the 20th century.

Dow's many audacious and impressive approaches would inevitably earn her the ire of both competitors and suppliers. Many suppliers and distributors mandated a minimum price, refusing to sell her their product and taking legal action when their preferences were ignored. Dow ignored the resistance and stared down a series of lawsuits from suppliers, who had been angered that a lower price at one store or city might force the producer to cut its prices everywhere else in that market. As Dow won case after case, her suppliers simply refused to work with her. Remaining undeterred, Cora Dow countered these actions by manufacturing her own line of pharmaceutical and consumer products.

By 1915, the seemingly indefatigable force of nature began to falter. Cora suffered a steep decline in health caused by the same disease that had plagued her father. Sadly, none of the innovative products sold in Dow drugstores were able to address tuberculosis any better than the far more limited arrays of drugs sold in her father's tiny shack years before. Tuberculosis's resistance to treatment in 1915 was every bit as stubborn as Cora Dow and was arguably the only obstacle she proved unable to overcome. As her health declined, Dow sold off her eleven stores, though they would retain the Dow name for generations to come. Upon her death later that year at the age of forty-seven, much of her inheritance was donated to the Cincinnati Symphony Orchestra, reflecting her lifelong love of music. She was such a dominant regional figure that her eulogy was given by none other than a former president and a Cincinnati center of gravity, William Howard Taft.

Chain Reaction

A new industry, one focused on "multiples" and cut-rate pricing, was indeed beginning to grow throughout the nation, pioneered by figures such as Cora

Dow. By the time of Dow's sale of her properties in 1915, she commanded more stores than the nine owned by Charles Walgreen, a distant competitor in far-off Chicago, Illinois. Walgreen had aped Dow's approach but was granted more time to live and extend his empire. By the time of Walgreen's death in 1939, the number of stores under Walgreen's control had expanded to 110. In doing so, Walgreen would usher in a new era of megachains that would eventually consume the concept and reality of independently owned local pharmacies.

The superchains of drugstores such as Walgreens deployed advertising to convey that their large buying power could allow them to provide medicines to consumers at a lower cost. Walgreen's was an expanded example of Dow's approach of local bulk discounting taken first to a state and then a national level. The massive volume achievable by marketing in hundreds of locations throughout the nation devastated most single-shop competitors. The pharmacy industry would soon change, as virtually all competitors were left to survive, if possible, by selling large amounts of medicines with tiny margins. For the consumer, this started off as a good thing, since they were able to access medicines at a lower cost for a time. However, the elimination of competition has the inevitable consequence of driving up prices over the long term, a fact that would prove prescient for this evolving industry.

A new era of pharmacies and pricing began with approaches that were similar to, but the polar opposite of, the pioneering strategy adopted by Dow. Cora had lured in customers to her drugstores who were lured in response to low drug prices and then purchased other products. The new entrants into the pharmaceutical world turned this rationale on its head, introducing pharmaceutical products as a new offering to consumers shopping for food. These grocery-store based pharmacies, including high-profile names such as Walmart and Kroger, would ultimately prove to be fatal for many local, independently owned pharmacies. Although the idea of the first supermarket pharmacies had been tested by another pioneering and ambitious Cincinnati company, Kroger, in 1961,[20] the concept did not take off for decades.

The advent of just-in-time inventory, a practice attributed to the pioneering retailer Sam Walton, would radically change the composition of a supermarket building. Prior to this revolution, roughly two-thirds of a market would be devoted to storing products, with the remaining third devoted to customer sales. The pioneering approach most aggressively deployed by Walton flipped the ratio, doubling the space available to customers and halving storage space.[21] Among the new products that could be displayed were first over-the-counter and later prescription medicines.

The emerging dominance of grocery-store pharmacies would prove to be short-lived as a new wave of competitors would soon enter and disrupt the field yet again. Likewise, this revolution would soon threaten even the largest chain drugstores, which quickly realized they would either have to adapt or be driven out of business. As we will soon see, these pressures compelled waves of industry consolidation via mergers and acquisitions, but for now we will focus upon this new and innovative threat.

As the large chain pharmacies grew and increased the breadth and depth of cut-rate pricing, smaller pharmacies increasingly faced a choice of either joining the consolidation boom or risking going out of business. The result was a shuttering of many independent pharmacies. Those that remained often were serving as contractors for larger networks and eventually for pharmacy benefit managers.

This new source of competition would arise and upend or dishearten even the most powerful of the chain store pharmacies as the 20th century drew to a close and a new millennium began. However, we can trace the roots of these competitors back to the remarkable Cora Dow herself and her chain of Cincinnati pharmacies at the beginning of the 20th century.

It seems that by 1913, Dow had successfully introduced the audacious concept of mail ordering medicines to customers any product that was available in her stores (a rare exception made for "poisons"). Certainly, the idea of mail ordering had been established for everything from trinkets to entire houses by the Sears catalog, but Dow was a pioneer in adding prescription medicines to the list of conveniences that could be accessed through the postal service. Most of these products could merely be requested, while a limited few, including cocaine and morphine, required a prescription from a "reputable" physician.[22] Moreover, Dow made these services available not merely to customers in the Cincinnati region, but well beyond. Although the shipments originated from Cincinnati, Dow's advertising reveals the service was available to any point east of St. Louis.

The first attempt at mail-order pharmaceuticals was pioneering but, as the saying goes, perhaps a bit too far ahead of its time. Mail order did not maintain a durable hold but would return again nearly a century later. As we will see, a new generation of mail-order (and later internet) entrants has been exceedingly controversial and implicated with accusations they are now major contributors to rising drug prices in the United States.

But let's not get ahead of ourselves quite yet. The increasingly widespread growth of new drugs and ways to obtain them would lead to an ever-increasing web of regulations needed to prevent abuses of the system and to ensure citizens had access to safe and effective medicines.

CHAPTER THREE

The More Things Change, the More They Stay the Same

T he modern pharmaceutical enterprise deals in arguably the most highly regulated commodities in the United States, perhaps the world. What led to this complex web of regulatory guidance that evolved to ensure that medicines prescribed in this nation are safe and effective? Contrary to popular assumption, in which heavy-handed regulation of medicines is frequently cited as a key reason for the escalating costs for developing new medicines, which in turn affect the ultimate price of the drugs, history will show that it is not so simple. As we will see, the organizations and enforcement mechanisms used by the federal government are a rational response to dramatic events, most of which took the form of high-profile national tragedies. We will see that each action taken by legislators or regulators has been well-reasoned and intended to improve the quality of new medicines. As our story progresses, we will find that an unintentional consequence of the collective buildup of such well-intended regulations has been the creation of an infrastructure that has often been accused (sometimes rightfully so) of impeding the speed of new medicine development.

According to its own history, the modern Food and Drug Administration (FDA) traces its birth back to Lyman Spalding, whom we met in Chapter Two as he compiled the first United States Pharmacopeia in 1820.[1] Although the document created was extra-governmental, its framework and approach proved pivotal in later years, when changing times and technologies necessitated government intervention. Specifically, the practice of huckster medicine and faith-based medical care have consistently been a problem, characterized by quick and easy, yet unproven (and often harmful), "cures." Keeping with the fundamental principles of the Age of Enlightenment, Spalding was an early proponent of what we today refer to as evidence-based medicine, a term that nicely defines itself. Consequently, he was driven to compile a list of safe, effective, and reliable remedies available to physicians and pharmacists in the United States.

The regulatory oversight tasked to the FDA is a consequence of Spalding's rational approach. More than two centuries later, we remain ever more dependent upon strong regulation, much of which has been cobbled together and compelled by extreme public outrage following tragedies. We will convey a few of these tragedies and the impact they continue to have on contemporary drug development and pricing.

Ginning Up Controversy

One of the lesser appreciated but pivotal events in the evolution of the United States was the Mexican-American War.[2] This 1846 conflict was a blatant land grab set in motion by one of America's least known but most impactful presidents, James K. Polk.[3] The international struggle nearly doubled the land area of the United States and would set the stage for the Civil War geographically by reopening vexatious questions about the expansion of slavery and militarily by serving as a training ground for the leadership of both the Union and Confederate armies. From the perspective of our story, the Mexican-American War also provides an entry point for understanding the need for federal regulation of pharmaceuticals.

The Mexican-American War would prove to be a rout and lead to the unnecessary slaughter of more than 25,000 Mexican troops. America only lost a total of 1,773 soldiers on the battlefield. However, nearly ten times more men died on the front from other causes: infectious diseases in general, and malaria in particular. The primary tonic used to prevent or treat malaria is quinine, a compound first isolated from the bark of the cinchona tree. Indeed, the bitter tang of the compound gives tonic water both its distinctive name and taste.[4] A few decades before the Mexican-American War, British officials posted to India imbibed tonic water as, well, a tonic, but soon realized that, when partnered with gin, the medicine imparted rather desirable side effects.

Although the American army in Mexico might have dreamed of the luxury of sipping gin and tonics, long supply lines and poor logistics limited access to even the most basic quinine pills. This defect proved to be the difference between life and death in the tropical climates south of the ever-expanding border. Most of the world's quinine was produced, unsurprisingly, by and for the British Empire.[5] The spike in demand from the United States military depleted domestic and international reserves (similar to the situation with toilet paper in the early weeks of 2020 as the country grappled with COVID-19), and costs soared.[6] These conditions created opportunities for parasitic manufacturers and distributors to adulterate, dilute, and even exclude the quinine in the medicines they sold. The consequence was that the very expensive and hoped-for remedies procured by the army were largely ineffective—and casualties from disease multiplied.

Public outrage at the unnecessary carnage compelled Congress to take action. As the war was winding down, President Polk signed into law the Drug Importation Act of 1848. This legislation charged the United States Customs Service with ensuring the purity of any foreign-made medicine that entered the country. Notably, domestic manufacturers were exempted from these rules, which would create problems with unsavory domestic manufacturers when a far bloodier war, this one Civil, would burst forward in years to come.

The importation law worked well at first, but the aforementioned loophole allowed domestic companies to evade inspection. As domestic abuses increased, the military became increasingly frustrated with their inability to procure reliable sources of quinine and other drugs. Consequently, they took the matter into their own hands. One example was former Navy physician and Mexican-American War veteran, Edward R. Squibb. During his time in the Navy, Squibb had witnessed the effects of the false and adulterated medicines provided by contractors. Before resigning from the Navy, Squibb had worked with that service to instead have the government produce their own medicines.[7]

In 1858 Squibb built upon his experiences and founded a company to supply quinine and other drugs to both military and civilian customers. Edward Squibb would soon find himself lobbying the Lincoln administration for stricter enforcement of the adulteration law as it became clear that the Civil War would be a protracted conflict rather than a quick victory over the secessionist states.[8] These actions coincidentally also helped his young company to emerge as a prominent wartime supplier of medicines.[9] Indeed, this company still thrives today in the form of Bristol Myers Squibb.

Fears of drug adulteration would remain a fixture of American pharmaceutical regulation for the remainder of the 19th century and into the 20th. Over this time, Squibb's desire to apply adulteration laws was realized as the government increasingly applied these rules to domestic manufacturers. A particularly strident enforcer of anti-adulteration laws was Harvey Washington Wiley, a zealot who ran a nascent agency known as the Bureau of Chemistry, a precursor that later evolved into the modern FDA.[10] Washington ruled with an iron fist and had a showman's penchant for captivating the attention of the press at a time when muckrakers ruled. Indeed, the public media during turn of the (20th) century America was filled with high-profile journalism conveying the need for greater control over the safety and efficacy of the foods eaten and the medicines meant to protect. These sentiments would eventually culminate in congressional passage of the Pure Food and Drugs Act, which was signed into law by Theodore Roosevelt in 1906.[11] This legislation prevented unscrupulous and nauseating practices such as watering down milk and then adding chalk or plaster to cover up this action.[12] Similarly, heavy metal lead was added to coffee, wine, and tea (along with dirt and sand).

Frowning upon Adultery

The Pure Food and Drugs Act was another knee-jerk response to public outrage, this time over macabre incidents revealing stomach-turning contamination of consumer foods and medicines. The most famous residue of this tainted age is arguably Upton Sinclair's novel *The Jungle*. Equally important (and nauseating) work exposing adulterated food and drugs was published in a series of widely read reports from the muckraking journalist Samuel Hopkins Adams in *Collier's* magazine.[13] At the same time, a pair of tragedies, each killing dozens of children treated with pioneering new vaccines, erupted in St. Louis and the Jersey suburbs of Philadelphia in late 1901.[14] [15] These calamities were persistently pushed to the top of the headlines and sensationalized by newspapers owned by another muckraker, Joseph Pulitzer, who coincidentally owned major newspapers in and around both the New York and St Louis metropolitan regions.[16]

The Pure Food and Drugs Act was designed to protect the public by preventing the adulteration of consumer products. The legislation invoked the United States Pharmacopeia, which has been periodically updated since 1820, as a source to define "pure" versus "adulterated." This act created the structure known today at the Food and Drug Administration but was short-sighted in that it failed to mandate the agency with the ability to refuse medicines deemed unsafe or ineffective. Rather, the law was restricted to the issue of the day, which was widespread concern about product contamination as revealed in so many sickening muckraking news stories.

As related in Dr. Kinch's prior book, *A Prescription for Change,* the 1906 law drove an already vociferous Harvey Washington Wiley to accuse Coca-Cola as an "adulterer." Wiley charged the product (not the company, but the actual bottles and cases of the sugary product) with, among other things, being deceptive because the carbonated product did not contain cocaine as might be implied by its name. Most of the charges were eventually dropped. Although Wiley won some minor points on a technicality,[17] his career in government had fizzled with the Coca-Cola fiasco. He left the FDA for *Good Housekeeping* magazine, where he cleaned up—both professionally and financially—after he created their "Seal of Approval" program.[18]

Throughout most of the first three decades of the 20th century after Wiley stepped down, federal regulation of medicines underwent some relatively minor and incremental revisions, remaining largely on the back burner in Congress. During this time, the most substantial regulation imposed on the pharmaceutical industry came from a nongovernmental source, the American Medical Association (AMA). In 1905, the leadership of this largest association of physicians and lobby used their considerable clout to compel pharmaceutical companies to demonstrate that their products were effective before they could advertise their products in widely read AMA journals.[19] This accreditation was left to outside experts, who would review information submitted by the drug companies. In a true sense of irony, many of these same huckster products were ferociously advertised in the same broadsheets that hosted muckraking stories about adulterated medicines. Consequently, the AMA's stance to verify the usefulness of advertised medical products proved invaluable to exposing the myriad bogus "snake oils" that had duped an unsuspecting public (and physicians).

A Serious Rodent Problem

Three decades after Theodore Roosevelt's administration, his distant cousin Franklin (FDR) was swept into office in 1933 amid the languor of the Great Depression. FDR had intended to launch a revision of the FDA, but this became bogged down in the Senate for five years. To help break the logjam, the FDA launched a road show in major American cities to advertise major flaws in the 1906 law that allowed for deceptive practices in everything from drug safety to false advertising and packaging. The exhibit was visited by the new First Lady, Eleanor Roosevelt, in 1933 and dubbed by one of the reporters in her press pool as "the American Chamber of Horrors."[20] This traveling creep show was accompanied by the publication of a book meant to educate the public about the dangers to the American consumer, aptly named *100,000,000 Guinea Pigs*.[21]

Despite the horrors conveyed in museums and the printed word, an even more compelling terror finally prompted legislators into action. In 1937, the S. E. Massengill company of Bristol, Tennessee, launched Elixir Sulfanilamide, a much-anticipated product.[22] Just months before, a new class of medicine, known as sulfa drugs, had been introduced. These products were among the first reliable means to treat infections, the greatest source of human suffering for virtually all of our species' history. Whereas most sulfa drugs came in the form of a pill, Massengill's goal was to target children. As any parent knows, ear infections are a common source of pain and misery in the pediatric population. To appeal to children, the drug was introduced as a sweet syrup with a raspberry flavor. The only problem was that the sweetness was not made by sugar but through the use of diethylene glycol, which along with its nearly identical cousin, ethylene glycol, is the primary component of radiator fluid.[23]

Within days of the product's introduction, a flood of poisoning cases were documented throughout the nation, but primarily in the American South, which has a particular preference for elixirs. The resulting destruction of the kidneys by ethylene glycol caused a particularly slow and agonizing death for more than one hundred children. News accounts of these tragic deaths filled the headlines and fueled outrage.[24] As the public steamed over the use of engine coolant in medicines, Congress finally acted upon Roosevelt's FDA legislation. The bill sailed through both houses with a simple voice vote and the act was immediately signed into law by FDR on June 25, 1938.[25]

With the passage of the 1938 Federal Food, Drug, and Cosmetic Act, we again encounter an example of lawmakers looking backward at a past tragedy rather than anticipating future ones.[26] The legislation empowered the FDA to ensure that all medicines are safe and to improve oversight into their manufacturing; both issues that were directly relevant and at the front of mind in the days following the Elixir Sulfanilamide disaster. However, the law failed to require that drugs be effective, merely safe. Attempting to rectify this deficiency, the FDA challenged the approval of certain high-profile drug applications of products they deemed useless. However, these battles proved to be unsuccessful uphill struggles as companies won one legal case after another on the claim that the 1938 law did not confer such powers upon the agency.

Yet again, a tragedy would be necessary to rectify the situation once and for all. This time, the tragedy largely spared the United States, though not quite as thoroughly as many Americans believe.

Making a Muck of Things

Penicillin was introduced to the world as part of a collaboration between the British and American governments during the Second World War. Penicillin was one of the most important, if least appreciated, articles of war, as it saved countless lives and limbs that might have been lost to infection. The nearly ten-to-one ratio of infections versus battlefield wounds experienced a century before during the Mexican-American War would remain just as prescient up to the moment that penicillin was introduced.[27]

The defeat of Germany led to its subdivision and political oversight by the Allied Control Council. In the West, the Franco-Anglo-American alliance undertook a concerted effort to restore the economic vibrancy of what became known as West Germany. Part of this was the awarding of a contract for the production of penicillin to a newly formed company known as Chemie Grünenthal.[28]

The selection of Grünenthal by the Allied Control was controversial and unfortunate for many reasons. First, the company had deep Nazi roots and its founding family, Alfred and Hermann Wirtz, remained loyal Nazi party members and directly benefitted from Hitler's maniacal plans when they gobbled up Jewish companies at fire sale prices.[29] Muddying their reputation even further, the researchers hired by the Wirtz family included many of the war's more notorious figures, who would collectively engineer another tragedy yet to come.[30]

Heinrich Mückter was born in Germany two months before the beginning of the First World War and would become one of the more controversial characters of the Second. Trained as a physician, Mückter joined the notorious Nazi "Brown Shirts" coincident with Hitler's rise to the chancellorship. In his professional life, Mückter specialized in infectious diseases, and these talents would prove tragically useful during the war as Mückter apparently practiced his profession to deadly effect in the concentration camps, experimenting on prisoners with infectious pathogens. Accused of war crimes by the Polish government in Krakow, Mückter escaped to the West and surrendered to American authorities in 1945, who decided not to prosecute him.[31] Within a year, Mückter had been hired by Grünenthal, where he joined a rogue's gallery that included Otto Ambros (who invented the nerve gas sarin and was convicted of mass murder and enslavement and yet released to work at Grünenthal), Heinz Baumkötter (the former medical head of the Sachsenhausen concentration camp, which conducted human experimentation), and Karl Brandt (the lead defendant in the Nuremburg war crime trials of doctors).[32]

Yet it would be inaccurate to presume that the reputation of these men had reached a nadir with Germany's surrender. Instead, history will also record that they were all involved in the development of another notorious killer.

Because the Allies' granted Grünenthal a license to produce penicillin, revenues skyrocketed and the company prudently invested much of its earnings into the development of new products. One of their pet projects was a by-product of the drug glutethimide, a sedative related to diazepam (better known as Valium).[33] This discovery led to the marketing of the drug in Germany and throughout Europe as Contergan. The product was an overnight wonder based on its demonstrated abilities not only to overcome insomnia, but also to prevent vomiting and other symptoms of influenza. Based on this latter property, the drug was also marketed as Grippex (a modification of the Franco-German word for flu, *grippe*). Beyond infection, vomiting and insomnia are also frequent symptoms experienced as a result of hormonal changes in early-stage pregnancy. Thus, Grünenthal established yet another base of customers for Contergan, convincing many investors that the drug could become the first ever to reach "blockbuster" status; a designation given to drugs that generate at least a billion dollars in annual sales. The blockbuster milestone had never been reached (not even by the extraordinarily popular drug Valium) but marketing experts predicted that Contergan could be the first to do so. For this to occur, Grünenthal needed to enter the American market. Like many European companies at the time, the company decided to partner its product with an established American pharmaceutical company and so partnered with the William S. Merrell Company in early 1959.

Merrell, a middling company in the middle of the country, headquartered in Cincinnati, was not the company's first choice of a partner. Grünenthal had wanted to partner with Smith, Kline, and French (SKF) to take advantage of its gravitas as an international behemoth. Lured by the potential for lucrative sales, SKF began working with Grünenthal in 1956, but after three years elected to pass on the opportunity. The reason for doing so was in part because SKF scientists became worried when a patient in a clinical trial delivered a child with severe birth defects.[34] They requested safety information from Grünenthal but their requests were all refused, informed instead that all the records had been burned in 1949.

You see, we forgot to mention the name of the drug, one you may have heard of: Thalidomide.

Merrell intended to launch the product in parallel with the performance of the necessary safety studies. Given its extensive history in Europe and Canada for the past few years, the company presumed it could file papers with the FDA, begin sales a month later, and then backfill any desired safety evidence once their small safety trial had concluded. Indeed, this was common practice at the time and the FDA itself assigned the Contergan application to be reviewed by a brand-new employee since this was thought to be an easy first assignment.[35]

American law also allowed the company to begin providing samples to doctors so long as they did not accept compensation for the product. Seizing the initiative, Merrell began handing out free samples, targeting obstetricians in particular given its ability to prevent morning sickness.

Much to the chagrin of executives at Merrell, the rookie FDA employee was a female physician by the name of Frances Oldham Kelsey. Kelsey was skeptical of the safety of thalidomide and kept demanding more information to assuage her concerns. Holding her ground despite increasing pressure from her bosses at the FDA and even in the face of remonstrances from angry senators, Kelsey was soon proven right as evidence swelled demonstrating that thalidomide caused severe birth malformations.

A generation of "thalidomide babies," often lacking arms, legs, or both, would be born in the 1950s and early 1960s. The drug also caused uncounted fetuses to be spontaneously aborted in utero as well. While the United States was largely spared, at least one hundred deformed children (and an unknown number of spontaneous abortions) were documented; the results of the practice of distributing free samples. Kelsey would receive many well-deserved accolades, a presidential medal from John F. Kennedy, and remain a fixture at the FDA for decades, retiring from the administration in 2005 at the age of ninety.

No More Free Lunches

The thalidomide tragedy was yet another example of a crisis that finally spurred Congress into action. The high-profile tragedy motivated a prominent lawmaker who was already skeptical of the growing power of the pharmaceutical industry. As a consequence of the tragic news reports of deformed babies, Estes Kefauver from Tennessee, arguably the most powerful senator in Congress, expanded the purview of his committee. Kefauver was already investigating potential concerns about collusion between the American

Medical Association and the pharmaceutical industry (a subject to which we will return) and expanded his mandate to address consumer protection from bad medicines such as thalidomide.[36] The resulting Kefauver-Harris Amendment to the Federal Food, Drug, and Cosmetic Act was quickly passed through both houses and was signed by President Kennedy on October 10, 1962 (while Frances Oldham Kelsey looked on over his shoulder).[37] The amendment empowered the FDA to demand extensive safety and efficacy data prior to approving a new medicine. This law also banned the practice of distributing free samples to physicians before a medicine has received an FDA approval. In the months after its adoption, these new powers were applied prospectively to new products. In 1969, the National Research Council had completed the first retrospective analysis of more than 3,000 medicines that had been marketed in the United States before 1962.[38] These analyses would continue through 1984. As a consequence of this Drug Efficacy Study Implementation (DESI), one third of these medicines were discontinued, either because they did not meet the necessary standards or because their manufacturers determined future revenues were insufficient to offset the costs of additional testing that would be needed to continue their sales.[39]

By the 1970s, the modern regulatory framework that governs drug development still today was largely in place. This timing was fortunate as it allowed the agency to assess all the conventional medicines, chemicals referred to in the parlance as "small molecules." As we will soon see, this bit of housekeeping was useful because the FDA would face a far greater challenge in the form of larger and more complex molecules that would arise as a result of the biotechnology revolution.

Before addressing this new era of medicines, it is important to return to our primary question about why medicines have become so expensive. All the while that the regulatory framework was being established to distinguish safe and effective medicines from less worthy drugs, the costs to develop new therapeutics had been quietly rising at an alarming rate. Many pharmaceutical companies and their defenders cite ever-increasing regulation as a reason why the price of medicines has been skyrocketing in recent years. Indeed, we will review these claims and evaluate their validity as part of our investigation as to the reasons for escalating costs, notably the cost to develop a new medicine, which we will examine next.

CHAPTER FOUR

I Fought the Law
(and the Law Won)

I t might seem that the FDA dominates every aspect of every pharmaceutical product marketed in the United States. However, two glaring exceptions betray this notion: the FDA does not track the expenses paid by companies to perform research and development necessary to gain an FDA approval nor the prices that these companies intend to charge to the consumers of these drugs. According to PhRMA (Pharmaceutical Research and Manufacturers of America), the member-funded trade association for the pharmaceutical industry that advocates and lobbies on behalf of its members in Washington, DC, and across the country, these two components are interlocked. Moreover, the former justifies the latter, a contention that we will challenge later in our story. To understand where all the money needed to develop a new medicine goes, what follows is a brief overview to convey how the FDA interacts with the biopharmaceutical industry, along with an exploration of the costs needed to gain a regulatory approval.

The development of a new medicine is a complex process that averages more than ten years. The expenses paid are invariably the highest just before and after a new product is granted permission from the FDA to be marketed. What follows is a rule-of-thumb characterization of an "average" medicine. It is important to note that there truly is no such thing as an "average" medicine because each campaign to develop a new drug is unique, with its own set of unexpected opportunities and challenges. Indeed, the fact that the word "campaign" is used so often to describe the efforts to develop a drug and should be interpreted not in the political use of the word so much as the military. Much as historians describe the Second World War in terms of the European and Pacific campaigns, a campaign to develop a single new medicine requires an immense amount of scientific, engineering, medical and business logistics, and strategy that involves thousands of people all around the world. These activities can cost many millions or billions of dollars to introduce one new medicine. Let us begin at the beginning: the discovery process to begin developing a new medicine.

The early costs to develop a new drug are undoubtedly the most risk-laden and vague. Basic research includes, but is not limited to, the types of studies conducted within universities and funded by federal and nonprofit organizations such as the National Institutes of Health (NIH) or the American Cancer Society. Basic research is just that: research on fundamental questions of science. As one discovers an interesting finding that could have implications for the foundation of a new medicine, it magically (and often unknowingly) progresses out of the world of basic science into applied (sometimes referred to as translational) research. This is not a well-demarcated transition rather one that meanders through the world of trial and error. It is only in retrospect, after a drug has advanced somewhat, that one might be able to divine a "Eureka!" moment (think Archimedes in a bathtub) that defined the path leading to a new medicine.

An often-cited example of a "Eureka!" moment came in 1928, when Alexander Fleming returned to work after a summer holiday. Fleming's specialty at the time was microbiology. He had a reputation for becoming engrossed in his work, so much so that he was working on a project studying staphylococcal bacteria up to the moment he left for a two-week trip with his wife.[1] Rather than cleaning up, Fleming rushed out of the laboratory. Upon his return, he found a stack of dirty labware, most of which were overgrown with the bacteria agar, a gelatin-like substance derived from seaweed. Legend states that Fleming noted one plate where a large circle of bacteria was utterly devoid. At the center of this circle was a cluster of mold, a common species known as *Penicillium notatum*. Fleming realized that the mold must be producing a substance that killed the bacteria.

Fleming claims he did not maniacally scream "Eureka!" but rather emitted a far more subdued and quintessentially English murmur under his breath of, "That's funny." Years later, and after an investment of many thousands of hours of labor and millions of dollars, the understated simple observation of Fleming had finally been translated into the "discovery" of penicillin. Later still, the mass production of the lifesaving antibiotic would be achieved, changing the lives of millions and the course of history.

As pointed out in *A Prescription for Change*, Fleming was not the first to discover the miraculous antibiotic properties of this fungi; that attribution has been lost to history as the disinfectant properties of the mold had been in use for thousands of years.[2] We can only reconstruct from Fleming's discovery forward because it makes for a convenient story. Likewise, the reconstruction of basic and applied science efforts that lead to a new medicine is comparably ambiguous and generally related in retrospect and usually with an overly clean story. This same tendency applies to assessments of the amount of time and dollars invested to enable the discovery of a new medicine. These facts alone are sufficient to justify the public monies that are invested into basic research. Yet from the standpoint of understanding costs, basic research is not quite so cut-and-dry.

Relatively little early-stage discovery research now takes place in private sector companies. As we will see, companies have increasingly abandoned these earliest basic scientific efforts, leaving them to be done by academic investigators. This was not always the case, and companies such as Pfizer, Merck, and Genentech used to lead the world with their discoveries. Instead, academic organizations tend to perform the earliest stages of research and as we will see when we discuss the Bayh-Dole Act, certain incentives have been created to prod these organizations into developing new medicines. Though on one hand, this outcome has had the desired effect (to promote innovation), it unexpectedly created yet another group seeking revenues (e.g., universities) to cover the costs of legal staffs conducting technology transfer activities and legal work focused on protecting the innovation and entrepreneurship. While we fully support such activities and believe that society has benefited in the form of faster and better cures, the infrastructure costs are not insignificant. This fact fits nicely into our central thesis about the ever-expanding and exponentially costly pharmaceutical enterprise.

What (and Who) Drives Drug Discovery?

Returning to the private sector, most companies involved in the pharmaceutical enterprise continuum function at the mercy of their owners, which are primarily Wall Street investors who demand a quarter-to-quarter report on profitability. The fiduciary responsibility of corporate management to maximize return to shareholders has resulted in fewer and fewer organizations venturing into pure scientific activities. And those that do are small, venture-capital-funded entities whose goal is to capitalize on selling to the larger fish in the pond. In fact, the term "serial entrepreneur" is the overly generous term used to describe pharma and biotech executives who run this particular gamut over and over, reaping immense personal financial gain without ever seeing a drug successfully developed or used to treat patients. Consistent again with our central thesis, the specialization of early-stage drug discovery activities has created a sub-industry focused upon the earliest activities, which are companies intended to be "lambs to the slaughter" that are formed to develop one drug and are then consumed and dismantled. One can certainly argue that a constant churn in these discovery-based sub-industry organizations is not a terribly efficient approach as teams that developed a drug are usually disbanded, which limits institutional learning and capabilities of once-successful teams.

To better understand the reason this rapid disbanding is so disruptive, we must first account for the costs needed to develop a new drug from the point a new target has been established or a lead candidate for a new drug has been isolated. We might be comforted in a strange sense by knowing that while many later-stage research activities involve chemical improvements needed to optimize the construction of a drug (or biology in the case of recombinant DNA products), these expenses tend to be nothing more than rounding errors as compared to the expenditures involved in clinical investigation.

When a potential new experimental drug has been identified, the development campaign begins in the laboratory. Parallel activities must be performed. Answers to key questions about the molecule must be found: Is the drug safe? Efficacious? Amenable to being delivered to the right place in the body and at the right time? Can its manufacturing be accomplished at a large scale? Likewise, a developer must figure out how to manufacture the drug at sufficient levels for further investigation and with sufficient reproducibility that will prevent variations from batch to batch. These activities are broadly labeled as "preclinical development" but do not stop there.

Once enough of the candidate drug has been produced, it is subjected to an intensive bank of studies to ensure that the drug is safe for use in humans. These analyses include assessments of potential risks to the heart, lungs, and other vital organs (known collectively as safety pharmacology), as well as evaluation of the safety of the drug in living creatures over time (toxicology). In general, the drug candidate must be evaluated in two different mammalian species, with one usually being a rabbit or rodent, such as a mouse or rat. This avoids the potential that an overreliance upon one species might fail to identify a potential risk relevant to humans.

As a brief aside, no one in the drug development world particularly likes the fact that animals must be used for testing. The reader should rest assured that industry good-practice standards require that every effort is made to minimize both the number of animals needed as well as the risks or discomfort imparted upon them. As our understanding of diseases and drug side effects has grown, technological improvements have been invoked whenever possible to perform laboratory testing in cultured cell systems or even in silico (using a computer to predict outcomes) and avoid (or at least reduce) the need for testing in animals. Nonetheless, testing of a new medicine in animals remains a necessity, required by regulations, to identify potential side effects before testing in humans can begin.

The dosing of these animals must reflect the intended use in humans, with compensations made for differences in the metabolism and other biological features that distinguish humans from our animal cousins. For example, a drug tested for a chronic indication, such as hypertension, must be tested for longer than drugs intended for an acute application, such as an antibiotic. Likewise, intensive investigation must ask where the drug goes in the body, how long it stays there, whether and how it changes as a result of metabolism, and how it is eliminated from the body. Altogether, these complicated assessments are known as toxicology and ADME, the latter being an acronym representing analyses of absorption, distribution, metabolism, and elimination.

The animals dosed for toxicology studies are closely observed for gross changes in health, but this is not generally the primary indicator of a problem. Were a drug to cause a macroscopic effect, such as a seizure or other suggestion of distress, then the drug likely is quite toxic. Thankfully, such outcomes are relatively rare. Instead, far more subtle potential evidence of distress is analyzed by collecting tissues from the experimental subjects treated with the drug at different times and at many different doses. These tissues are dissected in fine detail under a microscope and are intensively analyzed by veterinary pathologists in an attempt to identify the telltale signs of a potential toxicity.

As our experience in evaluating medicines has increased over time, so have the clues that might suggest a potential problem. For example, we know the reason why the anti-inflammatory drug Vioxx caused heart attacks, which necessitated its withdrawal from the market. All potential experimental drugs are now routinely tested to avoid a potential repeat of this same problem.[3] Given that our knowledge of adverse events, and their causes, has grown, so too has the need for additional testing and hence, additional costs.

During these analyses, particular emphasis is placed upon vital organs and tissues, including the heart, lungs, liver, kidneys, and brain. All of these studies are performed in specialized laboratories staffed by trained individuals, who detail their every action with extensive notes in a process known as good laboratory practice or GLP. This detail-intensive GLP investigation is not inexpensive and commonly requires between one and five million dollars and at least six to twelve months to complete. The broad range of costs cited reflects again the types of studies performed (e.g., acute versus chronic dosing) and the outcomes of these tests. For example, a potential red flag identified in one assay might necessitate additional follow-on investigation to assess whether this might be a showstopper for an experimental drug candidate and how any potential side effects might be avoided.

As the battery of preclinical tests are compiled and analyzed, the results are discussed internally and eventually shared with regulators at the Food and Drug Administration. In an attempt to be more responsive, FDA staff have become ever more open to interaction (either in person or electronically) to converse about ongoing investigation prior to the official submission of what is known as an investigational new medicine application (IND).

An IND is a rather intense document, providing aspects about every detail regarding the potential safety and risk of a drug, its intended use (both the types of patients who might benefit from it, as well as how the experimental medicine would be dosed), and the means by which the drug will be safely and reproducibly manufactured, stored, and assessed in volunteer subjects. This brief overview of an IND application summarizes a document that, if printed out, would require quite a sturdy table to hold its weight. The time and financial costs required to compile and error-check the information in this document often entail hundreds of hours of focused work by specialized experts in an obscure field known as "regulatory scientists." Unsurprisingly, these regulatory scientists have often worked for the FDA and can bring their extensive experience to anticipate the questions and potential concerns that the regulatory agency might find in analyzing the IND application. Such expertise comes at a cost, of course, as the comparative rarity of such experience translates into pricey salaries or, as increasingly is the case for an industry ever more dependent upon outsourcing, high fees paid to regulatory consultants.

Once received, the FDA has a mere thirty days to digest and come to conclusions based upon their review of this massive amount of information, dissecting each and every experimental detail with the intent to minimize risks to the brave volunteers who will be the first to be treated using an experimental medicine. These professionals are specifically tasked with determining whether a clinical trial should begin or not. More often than might be expected (given the considerable monies and expertise invested into preclinical drug activities), the FDA will refuse to allow the investigation to proceed or will require follow-up studies before allowing a clinical trial (meaning a study in humans) to begin. Again, the primary concern nearly always centers upon safety and this remains a focus of regulatory actions throughout the life of a medicine.

Evaluating Drug Candidates in Human Studies

Avoiding an elaborate recitation of the many reasons why the FDA might reject an IND application (a subject that could fill endless volumes), the clinical testing of a new medicine begins with Phase I clinical trials. The goal of this early investigation is twofold. First, it is crucial to ensure that the dose levels of the experimental drug are safe. This concern is addressed by starting with a dose level deemed to be safe based upon the animal data. A typical trial will then begin with volunteers being dosed with a small fraction of an equivalent dose that displayed no evidence, even on a microscopic level, of drug toxicity. The drug is administered to each volunteer (usually fewer than a dozen) as a single dose. These results are then closely scrutinized to ensure that level is safe (and as verified by an independent set of safety advisors) before the amount of drug can be increased. Even then, the dose escalation can only occur under conditions that have been agreed upon with FDA regulators.

Importantly, the clinical findings are reviewed by an independent medical and ethical board for each dose level before progressing to the next level. This board is created by and paid for by the developer and is composed of experts who are not associated with the company nor the FDA. If objective evidence of toxicity is encountered at a particular dose, then the trial will be suspended and the maximum dose that can be tested in future trials is at least one level below the dose that caused the toxicity (in other words, the safest, highest dose). This level is defined as the maximum tolerated dose (MTD) and the toxicity that forced a halt to the trial is known by drug development professionals as a dose-limiting toxicity (DLT). Such a trial is known as a single-ascending dose (or SAD) trial. Continuing with another emotion-linked acronym, a SAD trial is often followed by a MAD trial, which analyzes patients that have received repeated dosing (MAD standing for multiple ascending dose) to assess the safety of many doses and to assess if and where the drug might accumulate in the body over time.

Beyond monitoring for safety concerns, Phase I studies determine the pharmacokinetics of an experimental medicine. Although the word may sound intimidating, pharmacokinetics is the science of understanding where a drug goes in the body and how quickly it becomes distributed, modified, and eliminated over time. This information is gleaned by assessing the amount of drug in the blood and, whenever possible, relevant fluids or sites in the body.[4] Such studies also might ask if the drug is metabolized in the body (changed by exposure to various chemicals and enzymes in organs like the liver) and if these metabolites (modifications to the drug by natural processes in the body) remain at safe levels throughout the investigation. This can be a rather controversial subject within the wonkish scientific community as the volunteers in a Phase I clinical trial are often college students and other young people seeking side money that can be earned through participation in a clinical trial. As nearly everyone over the age of thirty knows, the metabolism of an early twenty-something differs greatly from older generations.[5]

Phase I clinical investigation is comparatively inexpensive, but not by any means cheap, clocking in generally at a few million dollars per trial. For one thing, volunteers must be compensated for their time and efforts. These activities can be substantial, not merely serving as docile human guinea pigs but often donating various bodily fluids at defined intervals and being required to fill out regular surveys and interviews inquiring as to how they feel, including any strange sensations or issues encountered. Such surveys might continue for weeks or even months after the end of the trial. In addition, these subjects are generally hooked up to wires and many types of instruments that are not only invasive, but each requires additional costs to gather the data and analyze each individual measurement. Altogether, these expenses can quickly add up to rather impressive figures.

The real cost of Phase I trials varies depending on the number of patients tested, the number of dose levels to be tested, the tests to be performed and many other factors. These expenditures now routinely add up to tens or hundreds of thousands of dollars per patient and this cost doubles roughly every decade.[6]

As we have already mentioned, a Phase I clinical trial is intended merely to gain information about the safety and the pharmacology of an experimental medicine. As the investigation progresses, an obvious question is whether the drug displays any evidence of its intended function (i.e., to treat or prevent a disease). Some developers, who are most commonly referred to as a drug's sponsor, might try to gather hints of efficacy in their Phase I investigation and are not formally prevented from doing so, but this curiosity might add considerably more costs and time to the trial.

Before advancing into the next stage of development, the sponsor of an experimental medicine must present all findings from all patients to regulators at the FDA. The goal is to make sure that the data were gathered and interpreted accurately and objectively, with a particularly important endpoint in mind: identifying a safe dose of the drug that will be carried forward for future trials to assess its usefulness. This dose must be below the maximum tolerated dose (MTD) and special emphasis must be placed in future investigation to detect the dose-limiting toxicity (DLT).

Often a Phase II clinical trial is performed to test different dose levels (each of which must have been shown to be safe), with an eye to seeing if the hoped-for benefits of treatment will relate to the dose of drug given. Such studies can involve hundreds of subjects and, rather than healthy college students, generally involve the intended patient population. Beyond the fact that the same safety parameters are often measured as in Phase I (and perhaps even more vigilant safety monitoring if the FDA review of the data suggested a particularly worrying DLT), a Phase II trial sponsor seeks to gather evidence of whether and how the drug is mediating its beneficial effects. In addition, the sponsor of the clinical trial is generally tasked with underwriting the costs of patient care during the trial and for a period beyond the trial. Both activities inevitably entail even more clinical testing and support. Consequently, the costs of a Phase II clinical trial can scale upward at a disproportionate rate, perhaps costing tens or hundreds of millions of dollars. Compounding the situation, a sponsor might decide to test their drug in multiple settings. For example, a cancer drug might be investigated to assess its utility against different patient populations or types of cancer, which can quickly multiply the rate of resource expenditure.

Yet even these Phase II expenses will pale in comparison with outlays made in Phase III clinical trials. By this stage of development, a single dose of the drug to be administered has been selected and is compared with the current standard of medical care. These studies are conducted using a statistical design to ensure that any therapeutic benefit can be reproducibly and unequivocally defined. The final study design will vary from drug to drug and among different diseases, but often entails thousands of patients and often depends on the number of people who suffer from the disease in the general public. For example, a drug that treats a rare genetic disorder may require only a relatively small number of participants, while a drug to treat hypertension may involve thousands of patients. For vaccines, tens of thousands of volunteers might need to be monitored since both the need for safety and the ability to demonstrate a decreased disease incidence or severity of disease can be more challenging for vaccines than for drugs. For example, the Phase III studies for first COVID-19 vaccines were initially tested on at least 30,000 participants, with many companies scrambling to complete their enrollment as quickly as possible. All of these factors affect the cost of a Phase III trial.

The sponsor of a clinical trial is generally required to pay for the costs of patients receiving the standard of care comparator, as well as those given the experimental treatment. Given the rising costs of drugs, the cost of a comparator drug alone might involve tens or hundreds of thousands of dollars per patient. (Ironically, leading pharmaceutical companies complain about the rising costs of drugs in this very context.) In the US, but only in some cases, the Affordable Care Act was supposed to transfer the costs of routine care back to insurance companies. Yet in practice, many expenses, including the comparator drug, remain with the sponsor.[7] An insider with information about drug development surprised us by stating their company calculated one to one-and-a-half million dollars are required for each patient enrolled in a clinical trial for cancer. The costs of clinical investigation of an experimental medicine therefore can be breathtaking.

The results of a successful Phase III clinical trial are then exhaustively reviewed by the FDA, often entailing a fee of a few additional hundreds of thousands of dollars (known as a PDUFA fee, a subject to which we will return). The FDA will then pass judgment as to whether the experimental medicine has achieved its desired endpoints and thus is worthy to be marketed to the American public. As we saw with Eli Lilly and other companies developing late-stage Alzheimer's drugs, a disappointing clinical trial or FDA readout can mean the loss of billions of dollars and might even force a change in company leadership.

Increasingly, the costs of clinical trials do not end with a simple nod from the FDA. An additional set of clinical trials were envisioned to address lingering questions about safety or the long-term consequences of an approved product. Although intended to be an exception, the number of Phase IV trials have increased dramatically in recent years. Dr. Kinch's team at Washington University has found an increasing prevalence of post-approval Phase IV trials. Whereas 2001 witnessed the listing of 129 Phase IV clinical trials, the number of Phase IV trials had increased tenfold by 2008 and has remained at that level ever since. Some of this dramatic increase reflected

Phase IV trials conducted with drugs that had been originally approved for orphan diseases or other expedited FDA approval practices. Regardless, one pharmaceutical executive informed us during a casual conversation that Phase IV commitments rival and now often exceed the costs of Phase III trials. They continued that a combination of Phase III and IV clinical trial costs, divided roughly equally between these two requirements, obligates more than 90 percent of pharmaceutical research and development budget.

Beyond the fact that the numbers cited are enough to bring a tear to the eye of even the boldest gambler, planning for the costs of such trials is often outdated even before a trial can be initiated. Moreover, the increasing frequency of Phase IV trials raises questions about whether such costs fall into development or marketing expenses.

Efficiency Insufficiency

Research and development costs have consistently accelerated since the 1950s. This fact is one indication of the declining efficiency (or rising costs, depending on your perspective) of drug development. In a way, these trends might be viewed as a reflection of both success and failure.

Bernard Munos and Steven Paul, senior researchers at the Lilly Research Laboratories in Indianapolis, provided early evidence of declining research and development efficiency.[8][9] Building upon this work, Jack Scannell, a financial analyst employed at an investment brokerage firm, penned a highly insightful yet playful overview that appeared in the scientific literature in early 2012. His article, titled "Diagnosing the decline in pharmaceutical efficiency," nearly instantly became a landmark for the field of drug development.[10] In this article, Scannell contrasted pharmaceutical efficiency with Moore's Law, the well-known fact that computer processing speed (to be accurate: transistor density) has been increasing at an exponential rate since the end of the Second World War. The fact that pharmaceutical efficiency has been moving backward caused Scannell to cleverly invert the name of this eponymous computer genius, introducing the concept of "Eroom's Law" to describe the situation with drug development.

Scannell stated that Eroom's Law largely reflects four factors that have consistently increased the costs to develop new medicines. The "Better than the Beatles" phenomenon reflects a somewhat unique situation for pharmaceuticals, where a new medicine can gain regulatory approval only if it were at least as good (both in terms of safety and effectiveness) as existing market alternatives.

Were such rules to apply to the music industry, it is difficult to imagine how sparse a selection of music would be available should all albums be at least as good as *Abbey Road*. This concept also addresses a much-discussed idea that "low hanging fruit" (i.e., conditions easily addressed by earlier medicines) have been picked. Thus, future drugs must be better than the comparatively easy pickings of the past.

Let us use the war against infectious disease as an example. A desperate need for medicines to counter deadly contagions meant that the first sulfa drugs were eagerly embraced despite considerable dangers associated with their use and their limited efficacy. Starting with the widespread adoption of penicillin, a far more effective and safer antibacterial agent, the bar had been raised to a degree that considerably more time and money were required to discover superior medicines that could compete in the market. These costs required ever more investment to identify novel antibiotics that were at least as good, and preferably better, than penicillin. As penicillin set a very high bar indeed, the costs needed to both discover a new drug and to test that the drug is at least as good as penicillin required more subjects to provide statistical proof.

An alternative approach for developing a new antibiotic would be to develop a drug that could be used after penicillin fails. However, this approach would necessarily take longer as the developer of the drug would have to exert considerable patience given the slow accrual of patients in a clinical trial for a drug that is used as a fallback option. The developer of this experimental medicine must also accept that these patients are likely to be far more ill, which raises the bar needed to gain an approval even further, since a sick person is generally more sensitive to side effects and suffers from a more severe form of infection. Again, the clinical trials meant to address this population will necessarily be longer, larger, and more expensive.

Hubristic notions have been floated that humanity has won the war against microorganisms.[11] Unfortunately, no one seems to have informed the bacteria, fungi, or viruses of their humiliating defeat. Drug-resistant bacteria, HIV, and influenza viruses abound, not to mention new plagues caused by Ebola, SARS-CoV-2, and other emerging diseases, which provide evidence that the natural world will never halt its attempts to check the spread of humanity. Instead, our tiny enemies have devotedly continued exploiting their extraordinary command over evolution to render into obsolescence entire classes of antibiotics and antivirals. Our letting up of the pressure (i.e., the failure to introduce different and better antibiotics and antivirals due to escalating costs and return) now leaves us vulnerable to drug-resistant infections, with many experts of the field referring to our present age as the "post-antibiotic era."

This example is by no means unique to antibiotics or infectious diseases. The same challenges confront drugs meant to treat cancer, heart disease, and every other unmet medical need. And yet antibiotics provide a unique, important, and relatable insight into a growing trend in the pharmaceutical industry thinking. Many companies, especially those that have historically been the leaders in developing innovative antibiotics, have actively decided to surrender all efforts to develop a better drug to fight bacteria (a subject to which we will return). This trend might be extending to other therapeutic needs and, in an extreme, could presage the end of all pharmaceutical research and development. An astonishing claim to make, but if current trends continue, one that could be the most dire of unintended consequences.

The rising hurdles and costs required to discover and develop new medicines is exacerbated by another factor that Scannell referred to as the "cautious regulator." We would take a slight exception and suggest the tendency might be more accurately described as the "inconsistent regulator." The overarching idea here is that experience has taught us innumerable ways that an unwanted side effect might arise. There are many molecules in the human body, whose functions might be unintentionally perturbed by a drug and manifest themselves as a drug toxicity (also known as an "adverse event"). The accumulation of information about drug dangers is generally a good thing because it can prevent future tragedies such as disasters associated with Elixir Sulfanilamide, thalidomide, and other "bad drugs." A more recent situation involves Vioxx, an anti-inflammatory agent introduced and then pulled off the market in the early 2000s.[12] Indeed, Vioxx is a textbook example of the tendency of a regulator to become more cautious.

The specific damage attributed to Vioxx was a change in heart rhythms experienced by an unfortunate few (contributing to more than 60,000 deaths, including a parent of one of the authors). After the high-visibility disaster that left strong negative impressions of regulators following its pro-filing in headlines and courtrooms around the world, the FDA mandated a higher level of cardiac monitoring for experimental medicines.

On one hand, this was a logical and defensible response because the damage caused by Vioxx could be detected by the required tests. At the other end of the spectrum, the additional testing was broadly applied to virtually all medicines subject to clinical investigation, even those unlikely to ever trigger any untoward effects on the heart, such as most monoclonal antibodies. Consequently, while the number of patients needed to participate in a clinical trial had been increasing (due to the need to have enough data for a trial to convey statistically meaningful data), the cost per patient was simultaneously escalating (due to the need to monitor an ever-larger number of potential toxicities or, in some cases, new ways to define effectiveness). The additional expenditures required for clinical trials raised the costs to develop a new medicine, but did not necessarily improve the safety of new medicines in a proportionate way.

While the Vioxx example is but one consistent with a "cautious regulator," we prefer the descriptor "inconsistent" because there are not infrequent situations where organizations such as the FDA find themselves pushing forward the pharmaceutical industry, rather than curtailing it. A classic example is the situation in the late 1980s and 1990s with the HIV/AIDS crisis, where the FDA expedited the review of medicines in response to growing political pressure. Likewise, the agency has experienced other bouts of exuberance such as the approval of a controversial medication for Duchenne's muscular dystrophy, which got a nod from the FDA despite a paucity of data to support claims of its effectiveness.[13] In this case, the regulator was again ahead of the mainstream and approved the drug despite considerable criticism and indeed, this decision led to the resignation of a senior official in protest against what he perceived as an overly hasty decision.

Most recently and egregiously, the FDA seemed to have forgotten its own history when it authorized the emergency use of hydroxychloroquine during the COVID-19 pandemic.[14] This action was both regrettable (due to the fact that the drug conveyed no meaningful benefit) but also tragic as hydroxychloroquine causes the same cardiac Q-T prolongation as Vioxx. Indeed, evidence would soon emerge that patients taking this drug were dying at a faster rate than patients without.[15]

In many ways, the behavior of regulators such as the FDA is analogous to a timeless critique of military leaders, who are always fighting the last war and thus are doomed to be caught flat-footed when confronted by entirely different strategies. Despite being the primary regulator of products encompassing one-quarter of all American consumer spending (yes, you read that right), the FDA is one of the smaller agencies in the federal government; employing fewer than 15,000 total staff, according to a study conducted by the Pew Charitable Trusts.[16]

Although we believe sincerely that the FDA strives to provide a high-quality service to ensure the introduction of safe and effective medicines, the agency is insufficiently funded. These shortages render the FDA incapable of anticipating the opportunities and complications of new medicines. Exacerbating the problem, a new generation of experimental medicines represents a wave of challenges as they utilize new cell and gene-based therapies with little or no precedent. Consequently, the adoption of their benefits and inevitable side effects will have to be learned "on the fly," perhaps resulting in unnecessary deaths and triggering future controversies. If so, then even more time and resources will be needed to allow regulators to catch up and cope with the consequences of a new generation of medicines.

Self-Inflicted Wounds

Although one could argue that the "better than the Beatles" and "cautious regulator" challenges have external causes, the pharmaceutical industry itself has committed considerable self-harm and in rather creative ways that have escalated the costs of drug development. It suffices to say that poor decision-making and a desire both to keep pace with its competition and embrace new technologies have led to a situation summarized by Scannell as tendencies to "throw money at it" and the "basic-research brute force bias."

The early 2000s was a period dominated by the catch phrase "shots on goal," a sports analogy meaning that the likelihood of gaining an FDA approval would be increased by having a robust pipeline of experimental products. The prevailing presumption was that one of these shots would certainly land in the goal and become a blockbuster. Within such an atmosphere, the CEO of MedImmune, the large biotech company where both authors were at one point employed, announced during one particular early-morning quarterly investor call that the company would begin clinical testing of four new compounds over the upcoming four quarters. This pronouncement would later be whispered in the hallways as "four in four." Three months later, the next quarterly investor call revised this number upward to eight new experimental medicines in the next eight quarters (eight in eight). A third pronouncement, three months hence, committed us to twelve in twelve, suggesting an arithmetic rather than logarithmic rate of rising expectations (it is important to look on the bright side of things).

Those impressive "stretch goals" were not achieved, and this led to an inevitable confrontation with top management. All the department heads in research and development had met to discuss how to achieve "twelve in twelve" and concluded it to be a fool's errand. To achieve this, we would need to advance incomplete or suboptimal drug candidates into clinical trials that would be destined to fail. One Friday afternoon, the R&D team leads were called into the board room and grilled over why the company was not on track for twelve in twelve.

Not being the brightest bulb in the socket, Dr. Kinch found himself representing the collective view that the goal was both not achievable and not desirable. Using a Socratic approach, it was queried, "Were we not in a business where revenue is generated by a drug that is approved for sale, not merely by the number of investigational medicines being tested?" Although all R&D colleagues had wholeheartedly agreed with this sentiment, not a peep was to be heard from the dozen or so people too intimidated to confront the CEO.

Dr. Kinch recalled informing his wife (who also worked at the company) that the events of the following Monday morning would be disturbingly predictable. He would be called up to the CEO's office, dressed down and dismissed. Sure enough, the phone rang in his office within seconds of sitting down and he embarked upon an exceeding lonely and dejected trudge up the stairs to the fifth floor, which housed the executives.

The encounter began predictably enough, with the CEO asking whether Dr. Kinch still believed in the points he had defended so vigorously just a few days before. With a nod, Dr. Kinch conveyed that his views represented those of other peers as well. If so, the CEO countered, why had no one else spoken up? This was presumed to be an indictment, but fear turned into shock as the conversation suddenly shifted. The CEO revealed he had likewise talked to many of the coconspirators, who conveyed that "twelve in twelve" was both unachievable and undesirable. Dr. Kinch's conversation with the CEO then pivoted to questions about the corporate culture that accounted for this trepidation. Within weeks, the company had contracted with an external consulting agency, which dispelled the notion of "twelve in twelve" and thus ensured Dr. Kinch would keep his job a bit longer.

Beyond this humorous (though only in retrospect) story, the need to "keep up with the Joneses" in combination with "shots on goal" was shared by numerous biopharmaceutical companies as the approach was widely embraced by the industry. There was simply not enough opposition in most places to overcome this glib approach. Consequently, enormous amounts of monies were invested into products that had little chance of gaining an FDA approval. Such pressures undoubtedly lowered morale throughout the industry and contributed to the futile outlay of millions, indeed billions, of research and development dollars. Too many of us, it seems, had stayed silent when pushed too hard.

Far worse was the fact that the "shots on goal" strategy meant that many patients had been deprived of a better experimental medicine than they had received. Although many of the specific actors and motivations responsible for shots on goal have left the business or learned from their experiences, similar self-destructive tendencies have remained. One of these is a herd mentality that reveals itself as companies race to match their competitors in embracing new technologies. For example, word that a particular target or disease has attracted attention from one prominent organization might compel others to dive in as part of a race (as we will soon see, a race that many companies would prefer to lose). A present-day example is the frenzy that currently surrounds immune oncology, the idea of reprogramming the immune system to target cancer. While the results have revolutionized the treatment and survival of cancer and are a favorite topic of the authors (and the subject of *The End of the Beginning*), our studies have revealed that a large number of companies continue to perform duplicative work on a surprisingly narrow set of overused cancer immunotherapy targets. Similarly, the flock of Alzheimer's disease drugs that failed with great fanfare in August 2012 were almost all focused upon a single target; and all delivered the same disappointing outcome.

This phenomenon is nothing new and is often driven by the desires and reactions of investors on Wall Street. Oftentimes, good news of a new breakthrough, even at early stages of development, can send a stock soaring for a small or midsized biotech company. Immediately after that, investors will scour the universe for companies that may have similar technologies or products in their pipelines and begin gobbling up shares of those companies as well speculating that they will also benefit from this breakthrough news. Any company who had technology on the shelf that could be used for COVID-19 experienced the frenzy such investor behavior can lead to. In fact, many companies take advantage of such opportunities and issue press releases highlighting their technology to ensure they won't be overlooked during such financially beneficial times. Ms. Weiman recalls her first exposure to this behavior just months after taking her first job with a biotech company. She'd left for a regular lunch break on a nondescript normal workday, only to return to her desk to find that her company's stock had tripled based solely on speculation because they were a small company with oncology products in their pipeline. This being the time before the internet, it took a few well-placed calls to figure out what was responsible for the sudden interest. Apparently, an industry bigwig (who had nothing to do with Ms. Weiman's company) made the claim at an industry luncheon that his and other biotech companies were on the verge of curing cancer. A journalist in attendance at said luncheon picked up the story and ran with it. Ms. Weiman's stock, and that of many other oncology biotech companies, were swept up in the hubbub, even if only for a short while, because as fast as her company's stock rose, it stayed true to the old adage that "what goes up, must come down."

While this activity did lead to new opportunities for Ms. Weiman's company at the time, primarily being greater exposure to new investors that had never heard of them before or had not given their pipeline any real consideration, there were downsides, too, mostly related to the desire of these new investors for the company to embrace a more aggressive stance on making projections and the growing undercurrent of "keeping up with the Joneses."

Unfortunately, this need to be bold and stake a bigger claim to success than deserved would continue to evolve in the biotech industry as management from small companies tried to gain the interest of prominent investors. Ms. Weiman remembers the story of how an analyst for a large investment bank organized an investor trip in the early 2000s to visit MedImmune and Human Genome Sciences, two prominent biotech companies in suburban Maryland at the time. While their market capitalization levels were comparable and both were regarded at the time as "large cap biotechs," only one had significant revenues from a breakthrough product it had launched a few years prior. Human Genome Sciences had no approved products at the time, but was not shy about making big promises. They also had built what was jokingly referred to as the Taj Mahal of biotech headquarters, with art adorning the walls and a massive manufacturing facility constructed upon the speculation that it would eventually be deployed to mass-produce all the successful products they would introduce. The bus tour of investors was awed by the lavish Taj Mahal during their morning meetings but not so much impressed by the lackluster accommodations provided by their afternoon sojourn at the local Marriott. MedImmune at the time lacked a stylish headquarters or even the capacity to accommodate a busload of investors. Instead, the company was domiciled in what might be generously regarded as a nondescript strip mall setting indistinguishable from comparable structures of the time that were populated primarily by discount record shops and yogurt vendors. One analyst jokingly pointed out to Ms. Weiman as they were loading their plates at the hotel buffet that the scenario seemed somewhat "backwards." One might have expected the company banking revenues from a successful, breakthrough product would be the one with the more elaborate digs. MedImmune would later go on to build its own large and impressive new headquarters, but was primarily motivated to do so in response for a need for additional laboratory space. Its new lodgings, while quite nice and clean, still did not compare with the Taj Mahal.[17]

Bernard Munos reenters our story to convey what may be the largest contributor to the ever-rising costs of drug development. Munos's recent work has emphasized what he cleverly refers to as "costs of scale." The concept of "economies of scale" is well-known, reflecting the idea that the costs to develop and market a product generally decrease with the growing size of an organization and the breadth of sales. For example, common sense dictates that McDonald's can invoke just a bit more leverage in negotiating the prices of beef and buns than a competing mom-and-pop hamburger joint. Munos has identified the opposite situation when looking at pharmaceutical companies. His work suggests that the larger a pharmaceutical company becomes, the larger the cost to develop and maintain a new medicine becomes. This declining efficiency is what led Munos to coin the term "costs of scale."

What is going on here?

This seeming paradox begins to resolve when you consider the life cycle of a medicine. After a new drug is approved, the costs do not end. Not including the costs of the aforementioned Phase IV clinical trials, the research and development costs devoted to support the sales and marketing of a drug are not insignificant. Indeed, these may even exceed the costs needed to develop the drug in the first place. One cost arises from a need to update basic information about safety and effectiveness, information periodically submitted to the FDA to keep the drug (and its sponsor) in the good graces of the regulatory agency, which is of obvious value for the organization as a whole.

Other costs are certainly less defensible. For example, a sales representative might interact with one or more physicians who recommend that a clinical trial be conducted on a different or more specific population of patients (preferably to be conducted by that physician, for a fee of course). These studies would not necessarily be required or even sought by the FDA but simply conducted to "flip" the views of an influencer. For example, a specialist who is regarded as a key opinion leader (KOL) might receive a large amount of funding to conduct a clinical study at their center (and also might be paid to consult for the organization). The fact that such a luminary embraces a particular product might compel more junior colleagues to similarly adopt the new medicine. Indeed, a former executive at one major pharmaceutical company conveyed disbelief that some of these activities could even be legal (although they are). This same executive maintained that post-approval studies are driven not by science but sales, a view shared by numerous current and former biopharmaceutical executives, who say such costs are growing and challenging to track.

As the breadth of different products sold by a company increases, these legacy costs increase proportionally. Worse still, as a product ages and loses its sparkle, the sales force representing it will increasingly seek a quick remedy in the form of a high-profile partnership or a moonshot study. Sales and marketing expenditures will increasingly be funneled to KOLs and their academic organizations to underwrite additional studies and, in many cases, the research and development teams, and indeed, upper management, may remain oblivious to the amount of money being spent to conduct clinical investigation. Ironically, some of the highest expenditures on research and development may be realized just as the drug reaches the end of its patent life and succumbs to generic competition. As one begins to appreciate these tendencies, Munos's wisdom in defining "costs of scale" comes into greater focus as a large and aging pipeline evolves from a reliable revenue generator to a source of destructive legacy costs.

Although we are certainly aware of these costs, if nothing else than as a reason that industry leaders have used to justify rising drug prices, the precise impact of rising costs remains quite speculative, which is a result of the near-complete opacity surrounding the costs of the core of the entire business: drug development.

CHAPTER FIVE

The Man behind the Curtain:
Wizard of Odds

———————

Pharmaceutical companies frequently cite rising escalating expenditures for research and development as a reason for why the price of new drugs rise.[1] Such claims are difficult to evaluate because there is a dearth of publicly available information about the monies actually spent to introduce a new medicine to the market. The opacity of this critical factor is fiercely debated and protected by individual companies and the industry at large and is the subject to be addressed in this chapter. We therefore seek to shed a bit of light on the interests of promoting transparency, with the ultimate goal of helping to alleviate this problem.

A team led by Dr. Kinch at Washington University has been researching the questions of biopharmaceutical innovation and efficiency for years and have consistently been surprised at the lack of reliable sources to assess these questions. One approach could begin with a presumption that public financial records as required by the Securities Exchange Commission might provide objective information relating to research and development costs of individual companies with information about drugs that have been given a nod by the FDA. We reasoned this approach would rely upon the regular reports submitted by pharmaceutical companies and allow us to tally up research and development costs. For example, we know from a July 2018 release that Pfizer had announced their intention to increase the amount of research and development spending from $7.7 to $8.1 billion for that calendar year. Pfizer would in fact report $8.0 billion in research and development for 2018, which was 23.8 percent of Pfizer's overall expenses for that year. In theory, one could simply ask how many drugs were approved in a given year and divide by the research expenditure and arrive at an average number of what it cost to develop a drug.

However, any conclusion arising from such an exercise would be rendered useless by manifold problems. First, most established pharmaceutical companies have extensive pipelines of experimental drugs and many of these are intentionally kept below water for fear of alerting the competition as to their intended markets. The odds are that many of these drugs will fail, prompting the needs for write-offs of millions or billions of dollars. Such opacity complicates a full understanding of the activities being performed, even at the most transparent public company. Worst of all, at private companies, whose shares are not traded on the market, such information is utterly unknowable because they are not compelled by any law to disclose their financial status. Consequently, we and others have approached the question from a different angle, utilizing our training as data-driven basic scientists to address this question.

Unknown Knowns

Science is hard and applying scientific knowledge to develop safe and effective medicines even more so. Many ambitious campaigns to develop a new drug will wash out completely, often zeroing out the considerable dollars and years of effort invested into their research and development. One of us, Ms. Weiman, remembers vividly early in her career as the head of investor relations for a small Minneapolis-based biotech company, where a Phase III clinical study for a new cancer product was stopped midtrial due to issues that had not shown up in previous studies. As this study was being conducted by a small, not-yet-established (meaning not-yet-profitable) company, announcing the demise of the trial, and eventually the product itself, was devastating for the company, including a precipitous drop in the company's stock value. Even at much larger companies, corporate management is understandably shy about admitting high-profile failures to shareholders (although they are required by law to do so if they are material to the company's financial outlook). As such, failures may be consciously or unconsciously buried or forgotten (sometimes accompanied by a reassignment or turnover of staff and, hence, a loss of institutional memory). Compounding the problem, a successful campaign to develop a new medicine can take more than a decade. For a vaccine, it is often double the investment in time and dollars.

Corporate memory is surprisingly short. There is an old adage in the pharmaceutical industry with two parts: First, a new head of research and development will sincerely believe that the portfolio developed by their predecessor is ridiculous (the clean version) while they convince themselves of the brilliance of the portfolio that they are building. The second part of the problem is that the tenure of the average head of R&D is generally ranging from seven to nine years, considerably less than the time needed to develop a drug from beginning to end.[2] Consequently, research and development activities at large companies are often in a constant state of flux, both in terms of the projects being performed and at all levels of staffing. This high turnover rate breeds inefficiency.

However, this rule of thumb does not address the key question: How much money does the pharmaceutical industry spend to develop new medicines?

Lasagna's Secret Sauce

Recognizing an opportunity to address the need for transparency, a pivotal but largely unsung hero (despite having arguably the greatest name ever) enters into our abbreviated history of drug development. Louis Lasagna was born into an immigrant family in Queens, New York, and grew up in New Brunswick, New Jersey.[3] A gifted student from a family with modest means, Louis nonetheless graduated from Rutgers University and obtained medical training from Columbia before landing a job as a professor at Johns Hopkins.[4] His academic expertise was in clinical pharmacology, the science of understanding how medicines work in the body, including where they go and how long they stay there.

Lasagna was also an early explorer and advocate of the "placebo effect." Along with dark energy and quantum gravity, the placebo effect is one of the most studied and yet intriguing phenomena ever to bewilder our species. A very real occurrence arises when a patient is given an utterly inactive substance (most famously, a sugar pill). Despite being part of a "control" group that should not differ from an untreated volunteer, the individual given a placebo often responds just as well as someone administered with a highly active substance. In an extreme version, even if the person is told that the drug they are receiving is a placebo (as opposed to the experimental medicine), they may continue to demonstrate a positive outcome.[5] The response is quite real and can be durable (in some cases, leading to cures). Though widely misunderstood, the placebo effect is presumed to entail a mysterious role for the brain to facilitate self-healing.

Rather than simply discounting the placebo effect, Lasagna published respected manuscripts in the scientific literature on the placebo effect starting in the 1950s and maintained that a placebo must be factored into clinical trials.[6] His advocacy for the proper design of clinical trials, including the need to improve design studies that test the safety of new medicines, came at a crucial time; just as the thalidomide crisis began to come into sharp focus. He also pioneered the rollout of informed consent, the concept of sharing with the volunteer in a clinical trial not merely the potential benefits of an experimental treatment, but the risks as well. In this manner, Lasagna found himself in the right place and time, playing a key role in congressional testimonies before Estes Kefauver's committee.[7] Lasagna shared the powerful senator's suspicions about false claims and irresponsible use of medicines by the pharmaceutical industry. His efforts would help guide the core structure of the 1962 Kefauver-Harris Amendment, emphasizing the need for transparency and safety in the evaluation of new medicines. Lasagna also frequently criticized the pharmaceutical industry for its opacity, particularly its reticence to discuss the details of its research and development activities, the "secret sauce" whose recipes are held quite close to the chest.

Lasagna would seek to force transparency by establishing a center for the study of drug development; first in upstate New York at the University of Rochester and later relocating the center to Tufts University outside of Boston. This center was intended upon shedding light upon the activities of the pharmaceutical industry. As part of his efforts, Lasagna would pen a series of updates, which identified and evaluated trends in the research and development patterns underpinning the FDA approval of new medicines. In doing so, Louis Lasagna would devote more than five decades of his professional career to help guide the FDA in its efforts to develop a framework to help convey a steady flow of new cures while assuring new medicines remained safe and effective.[8]

In an effort to assess the costs needed to develop a new medicine, Lasagna and his colleagues at Tufts began to solicit information in the form of surveys sent to pharmaceutical companies. These questionnaires sought to assess the efficiency of private sector interactions with the FDA. The questions asked ranged from queries about the time needed to develop a new medicine, monies, and time spent on their research and development activities, as well as assessments of the quality of the interactions the company had with regulators at the FDA. The goal of these studies was to provide a report card that could shed light upon the efficiency of drug development, both in terms of time and dollars. Over the years, Tufts developed a questionnaire that was increasingly acted upon by many willing pharmaceutical companies. The information gathered included the types of projects (admittedly a sensitive issue), the costs expended on research, and the time required to progress an experimental drug from one stage of development to another. Such efforts were well-intended and meant to provide a framework to optimize the processes and resources required to develop a new medicine.

The costs to develop drugs, as revealed by Tufts, were truly breathtaking. The average cost to develop a new medicine, as of 2014, was estimated to be nearly $2.6 billion.[9] This average includes drugs developed for diseases that are life-threatening as well as those that, while important to those suffering from them, are more cosmetic or medically inconvenient in nature (e.g., hair loss, psoriasis, constipation). However, some of the most complicated indications (such as cancer and Alzheimer's disease) presumably cost disproportionately more, depending of course on the size of the patient population, though the sheer opacity of the data has precluded accurate analyses. A similar analysis by the Deloitte UK Center for Health Solutions, an auditing agency, suggested a lower average price tag of $1.4 billion later that same year.[10] However, the Deloitte study was limited to a dozen publicly traded companies and included new formulations (means of delivering medicines) and other incremental changes that are less relevant than the Tufts data, which focused upon new medicines. Clearly, some companies were more efficient than others. A study from Reutlingen University revealed that AbbVie (a spin-off of Abbott Pharmaceuticals) spent an astonishing average of more than $31 billion to develop each new medicine, not a particularly inspiring number for many shareholders of that stock.[11]

Although these headline numbers were truly impressive, further inspection raised important questions about the findings. The approaches used by Tufts and Deloitte revealed that these reported expenditures did not simply reflect a high price tag to discover and advance a single molecule, but instead included many additional factors, including development failures, which are, more often than not, the end result of drug development initiatives. For example, the current estimate is that roughly one drug of ten that enters clinical trials in the United States will ultimately be approved for use by the FDA.[12] Consequently, the late-stage failures of five programs that had cost a billion dollars each but never received an FDA approval might be included in estimates of the efficiency of an organization that had received only one FDA approval for a medicine that cost "only" $100 million to develop. As a result, that single and comparatively inexpensive drug would have accrued a cost of $5.1 billion to develop.

These numbers have come under intense scrutiny. Critics have claimed that the formulas used by the Tufts investigators are inaccurate, but even this is generous as the data is almost entirely kept secret. Other concerns about what is conveyed in these reports surrounds the use of "opportunity costs," which refer to the loss of revenues that might have been generated had research and development dollars been invested elsewhere in the business. Even more suspicion arose from the fact that the results were obtained as part of a voluntary survey and completed by organizations who might benefit by artificially inflating the costs of their research and development activities (as a means of eliciting public sympathy or justifying high prices). Moreover, the ubiquitous thought leader Bernard Munos points out that the

Tufts data seems to have excluded "outliers" such as companies that were particularly efficient or lucky in getting a drug to market.[13]

Such criticisms could not be easily dismissed by the Tufts team because their data could not be independently verified by others, a major faux pas for academics, who adhere to the basic tenets of peer review. Moreover, the results of the 2016 study were protested by Tufts's own medical students, joined by student colleagues from Harvard, who claimed the Tufts center was too biased in favor of the pharmaceutical industry.[14] This particular concern, one pertaining to the fundamentals of conflict of interest, was prompted by yet another unintended consequence.

Hitting the Paywall

The costs expended by Tufts to compile and analyze the results of drug development could themselves become rather expensive, including the need to hire experts to collect, monitor, and analyze data provided by participating pharmaceutical companies. As the center at Tufts expanded its mandate to include analyses of many aspects of drug development in the years after Louis Lasagna's 2003 death, its need for funding burgeoned. The settled-on solution was for Tufts to share the details of its findings with pharmaceutical companies and others through a subscription model. The monies collected from interested sponsors, rumored to cost each company tens to hundreds of thousands of dollars per year, could then be used to offset the costs of collecting and analyzing the information. This practice might seem benign enough until one considers accusations that the information was being used to create a climate that was sympathetic to biopharmaceutical companies. Specifically, the retention of the data behind a paid firewall meant it was not available for outside scrutiny by third-party analysts. This opacity fueled conspiratorial notions that the data might be manipulated to serve the needs of the corporate sponsors. Thus, an organization created to combat opacity had itself become opaque.

Although it is our impression that the trends identified by Tufts are probably somewhere in the right ballpark, an inability to verify the findings does fly in the face of the most basic scientific tenets associated with peer review and validation. Sadly, this view is a bit more generous than many, who entirely dismiss the idea of escalating drug costs as being an apologist view for an abusive pharmaceutical industry as it pertains to drug pricing.

Consequently, after all of this lead-up, a critic can accurately claim we are nowhere closer to knowing how much it costs to develop a new medicine. To get another perspective on this question, we will introduce a unique feature that distinguishes the biopharmaceutical industry from most other business sectors and meet one of the major players in the field. This story will also set the scene for understanding the perils of the industry as a whole and the bedeviling question of how much it really costs to develop a new medicine.

Seeking a Colonel of Truth

A key feature that distinguishes the pharmaceutical industry from many other enterprises is incredible dependence upon patents to fend off competition, a subject that we will interweave throughout the rest of our story. A decade of hard work and huge numbers of dollars needed for research and development, will, for a fortunate few, generate a blockbuster drug and lucrative revenues (and in many cases huge stock windfalls for corporate executives and investors). Yet, today's billion-dollar revenue generator will invariably and quite suddenly be snuffed out as generic competitors cannibalize the market. Indeed, the lifeblood of even the most highly capitalized companies may be dependent upon a frighteningly small number of products, each of which is inevitably fated to succumb to generic pressure. Far-sighted executives must therefore ensure that a new generation of replacement products will be available by the time today's cash cow stops giving milk. This sudden stop is referred to as a "patent cliff," the place where revenues suddenly drop off.

One can view the entire pharmaceutical industry with an analogy of a type of sadistic treadmill in which even standing still requires constant replenishment with innovative new products. The problem is that the pace exerted by this treadmill is constantly accelerating.

A real-world example of the problem was very publicly experienced by one of the most venerated pharmaceutical innovators, Eli Lilly & Co. Since the formation of the Indianapolis company in 1876, its eponymous founder, a practicing pharmacist who took some time off to become a Civil

War colonel, emphasized innovation to support the production of "ethical medicines" (as opposed to snake oils). Since that time, Eli Lilly has maintained a niche for pioneering new ideas and technologies into the marketplace. Work from Dr. Kinch's team at Washington University in St. Louis has demonstrated that despite the fact that Eli Lilly has generally tended to remain one of the smaller pharmaceutical companies, it has introduced more novel therapies than any other company in each decade from the 1940s through 2000, coming in second only once during the 1960s. Among its accomplishments, Lilly pioneered the development of gelatin-coated and flavored medicines, was the first to introduce the Salk vaccine for polio, and marketed the first insulin products (both animal-derived as well as material created using recombinant DNA technology). However, the Lilly product to which we will turn our attention was a breakthrough in the field of neuroscience and psychiatry.

A Sad Antidepressant Side Effect

In 1987, the company scored a blockbuster in the form of fluoxetine (Prozac), the first selective serotonin reuptake inhibitor (SSRI), a new type of antidepressant that is ubiquitous today. According to Andrew Dahlem, the former chief operations officer of Lilly Research Laboratories, the discovery of Prozac was the culmination of nearly two decades of investment.[15] Work had begun in the 1970s as a collaboration between two Lilly scientists who had found that diphenhydramine (better known as Benadryl) had the unintended consequence of easing the debilitating effects of depression in some patients.[16] With this as a starting point, investigators began to create and test various chemical versions of the drug, eventually demonstrating that the drugs worked by preventing the reabsorption of a key neurotransmitter (a molecule that delivers signals in the brain), which is often lacking in depressed individuals.

Given the paucity of information available at the time about depression, serotonin, and nervous system biology in general, the company had to develop many activities from scratch. The breakthrough required new animal models to test drug candidates, the discovery and optimization of the intended drug, and its testing in human clinical trials as necessary to gain

FDA approval. Each of these activities required a close partnership between the company's research scientists and business leaders as the discovery efforts of a new drug entailed sustained and expensive research and development campaigns. As with all experimental medicines, the intended new type of medicine was certainly not guaranteed to deliver the hoped-for outcome, either medically or in terms of revenue generation. Nonetheless, a feeling of shared trust and cooperation meant both scientists and corporate executives were willing to throw the dice and share the consequences.

Fortunately for the company and for society, the coordinated business, scientific, and medical efforts at Eli Lilly did not go unrewarded. The resulting product, trade name Prozac, was the first of a new class of SSRI drugs that would revolutionize mental health. Indeed, it is now estimated that more than one in eight Americans (12.7 percent) are currently prescribed an antidepressant pioneered by the types of new science enabled at Eli Lilly.[17] The company likewise did quite well for itself as the annual sales of Prozac peaked worldwide in 2001 in excess of $2.6 billion, a huge number for the time (and still rather impressive today). Indeed, Prozac sales quickly became a disproportionately large source of Lilly's revenues.

Despite the good times facilitated by Prozac, the prospect of the new millennium was looking quite depressing in parts of Indianapolis in the early 1990s. The issue was not Y2K, the worldwide angst gripping the planet in the final decade of the 20th century, but a much more localized fear. The primary patent for fluoxetine was scheduled to expire early in the first year of the new millennium after ten fruitful years, exposing Eli Lilly to a sudden loss of its primary revenue generator. The company mobilized in preparation, declaring 2001 to be "Year X."[18] Corporate management then embarked upon a series of radical efforts, determined to offset the losses with a new generation of medicines. An ambitious, company-wide program was launched, both to maximize the efficiency of corporate activities (in an effort to avoid layoffs, a source of pride since the company had never laid off employees in the century and a quarter of its existence; not even during the Great Depression). Everyone at Eli Lilly was inculcated with the need to become more efficient and to replace Prozac with new and even more lucrative products.

The strategy proved successful, as fluoxetine's outgoing sales paled in comparison with newly launched drugs. These new revenues were anchored by the cancer drug gemcitabine (Gemzar; approved in 1996), the osteoporosis drug raloxifene (Evista; launched in 1997), and two antipsychotics, olanzapine (Zyprexa; 1996) and duloxetine (Cymbalta; 2004). This impressive burst of drug development innovation not only offset the revenue loss from Prozac, but was celebrated internally as it would ultimately generate annual revenues in excess of ten billion dollars. However, the company now faced a new problem: This new generation of blockbuster drugs were slated to expire in a decade, just like Prozac had done. The company was desperately trying to keep pace on the treadmill, with a hidden figure constantly pressing the "accelerate" button.

Returning to a strategy that had worked once, company insiders, led by its chief executive, John Lechleiter, began whispering that a period starting in 2011 would be termed "Year Y/Z."[19] Once again, the company emphasized bolstering its pipeline of experimental medicines, taking the rare step (for Eli Lilly, at least) of acquiring a few small biotechnology companies to bolster its pipeline of products through corporate acquisitions.[20] Unlike other companies, which had embraced large mergers to create ever-larger pharmaceutical behemoths, Lechleiter remained adamant that Lilly would not contemplate a merger with a comparably sized partner, much less serve as prey for a larger competitor seeking to consolidate Eli Lilly. This fact reflected in large part a corporate ethos, the same pride that had kept the company from laying off employees in challenging economic times.[21]

As is so often the case in the biopharmaceutical industry, the company experienced unexpected failures of high-profile, late-stage developmental products, many of which included what had been widely regarded both within and outside the company as promising and costly Phase III candidates. Given its emphasis upon neurosciences (the same expertise that pioneered Prozac), the company ventured forth into Alzheimer's, a neurodegenerative disease whose prevalence (and thus revenue potential) has been projected to increase as the nation's, and indeed the world's, population grows progressively older.

Lilly was not alone in this quest to develop drugs to address neurodegenerative diseases: Pfizer, Johnson and Johnson, and other pharmaceutical companies were looking to address this massive market. Yet, Alzheimer's disease proved too great a challenge. All three of the companies—Lilly, Pfizer, and Johnson and Johnson—announced a series of failures, nearly in unison, during August 2012. None of these experimental medicines would receive a nod from the FDA and, collectively, billions of dollars invested into research and development were not able to be recouped through the sales of products to consumers.

Compounding the pain of its Alzheimer's debacle, Eli Lilly was forced to halt the development of a new drug for schizophrenia and had to report disappointing news about prasugrel (Effient), a blood thinner that proved no better than its competitor (Plavix). The company seemed doomed to be acquired by a larger competitor or worse still, to fade out altogether.

Despite these setbacks, Lilly would double down on its investment in research and development. This diligence would eventually be rewarded with a basket of approvals in 2014 and 2015 for the oncology drug ramucirumab (Cyramza) as well as the diabetes drug dulaglutide (Trulicity). Because of these new products, the company would survive the storm of "Year Y/Z," but it ultimately had to fall back upon a corporate strategy that had been used far more liberally in other companies: slashing jobs. The fears caused by Year Y/Z would force management to cut deeply in 2017, eliminating five thousand positions (8 percent of its total workforce), with many of these in research and development.[22] Looking further, the little engine that had delivered the company through both Year X and Y/Z crises had been heavily culled, raising serious questions as to whether it had hobbled the ability to survive future crises or whether, like the alphabetic letters of its most recent crisis, the company was nearing its conclusion.

Beyond its research and development capabilities, a key reason why Lilly had been able to remain competitive and survive both Year X and Year Y/Z was a keen interest in competitive intelligence, the science of reading the tea leaves to anticipate how your industry has and will change over time. Lilly intended to utilize such efforts to remain at the razor's edge without being cut to pieces. This emphasis allowed the comparatively small company to identify niche opportunities where it could most efficiently deploy its more limited resources to perform out-sized efforts relative to its larger rivals.

Among its competitive intelligence activities, the company had been tracking the costs to develop new medicines and determining how these trends changed over time. Steven Paul and Bernard Munos, two Lilly executives, analyzed the sources and costs of innovation that included and expanded upon results shared by Tufts University. Not content to analyze current trends, Munos assessed how the cost to develop a new drug had changed over time; from the 1950s onward.[23] The outcomes of this study were circulated internally and eventually made public in a scientific article penned in late 2009. The outcomes made for quite troubling reading.

Even after correcting for the impact of inflation, Munos found the expenditures required to develop a single new medicine had increased exponentially, equating to a compounded annual rate of more than 13 percent. Another interesting tidbit, to be expanded upon later in our story, is the identification of a positive economic "spillover effect," which grew in prominence during the mid-1990s and persisted for much of the following decade. For the many noneconomists reading this story, a positive spillover effect can be thought of as a type of "wisdom of the crowd." Benefits arise when the number of companies in an industry grows, imparting an industry-wide benefit that allows each company within that industry to be more productive.[24] In terms of the number of companies within an industry, more is better, presumably because this equates to a larger breadth and depth of innovative ideas and products. And yet despite that positive spillover, the costs to develop a new drug kept escalating. Stated differently, the efficiency of the biopharmaceutical industry has been steadily *declining* for more than fifty years.

Before discussing the reasons for the increasing costs of research and development, it is important to introduce a phenomenon that will hereafter play a crucial role in all aspects of our current story. All attempts to assess the factors contributing to the costs of developing, or prices assigned, to medicines were either stymied or made more challenging by an utter lack of transparency. As we will see, this opacity pervades virtually all aspects pertaining to the pharmaceutical life cycle, including the costs needed to discover new medicines, to conduct laboratory or clinical research, or the expenses needed for manufacturing. Most of all, these companies often state that the rationale underpinning pricing decisions are based upon these numbers. Numbers no one can account for or verify. Therefore, it is essential to demand greater transparency with the goal of making medicines affordable and available to those who need them.

As we will soon see, even after a drug leaves the pharmaceutical company and wends its way through an increasing number of waypoints involving pharmacies and payers before it reaches the patient, the financial details surrounding the reimbursement and distribution practices of many pharmacy managers and insurance companies are almost entirely, and purposefully, opaque. Indeed, at times these latter problems and practices of said players can make the pharmaceutical industry look positively transparent in comparison.

What forces are responsible for this opacity? Given the tight regulation of medicines and the regular documentation required by the FDA and another regulator, the US Securities and Exchange Commission (SEC), one could understandably presume that objective information about research and development costs must be known. Sadly, this is generally not the case as revealed by the results conveyed in regularly required SEC reports (known as 10-Q and 10-K reports) are sufficiently sporadic and vague as to confound broad conclusions. For example, although most publicly traded companies must cite their research expenses on a quarterly and annual basis, any attempts to decipher how much is spent developing or supporting one product versus another can quickly evolve into a master class on the subject of futility. This is true even though the SEC has a specific regulation addressing certain aspects of fairness and transparency and reporting of material information called "Regulation Full Disclosure," which was promulgated in August 2000. The regulation was codified as 17 CFR243.

The reasons for this lack of clarity are manifold and not necessarily nefarious. For example, one company might decide that proceeds spent purchasing another company to gain access to a product or technology is a research expense whereas another might book this as a business expense. Likewise, the monies spent on a clinical trial to expand the market for a drug that has already been approved by the FDA might be considered a research cost for one organization but as a sales and marketing cost by another. The frustration in realizing there is no unambiguous way for accounting for all of the costs of drug development became a passion and frustration that we came to share with Munos.

Returning back to our story, we spoke with Bernard Munos to discuss the planning for this book and shared experiences dealing with the opacity of all things associated with drug costs and pricing. Munos is exceedingly sharp-minded and savvy, a passionate data wonk and thus a kindred spirit. He indicated early in our conversation that he had interacted indirectly with investigators from Tufts while penning his landmark paper. At that time, he was concerned that some of the sources might have been less than objective and that the overall study data was by no means systematic. In particular, this information tended to exclude outliers, such as small or nimble organizations that were particularly adept or lucky. Instead the data were heavily skewed toward larger companies, which tend to have large pipelines and thus a higher likelihood of experiencing costly, late-stage product failures. As imperfect as it was, the Tufts data were the only available information to inform a frustratingly opaque subject. However, Munos was not content to settle and instead devised a new way to estimate the costs of drug development.

The approach Munos has taken in recent years has been to work on another comparably skewed but more accessible set of data; information originating from smaller companies. His work is focused upon smaller publicly traded companies with a single drug development project. This approach simplified analyses considerably because these companies tend to be more transparent in conveying research and development costs to their shareholders and because they are necessarily hunkered down to advance their one and only product. Based on this strategy, Munos estimated that the costs needed to develop a new drug range from roughly fifty to three hundred million dollars. Even at the highest point in the range, this is one-tenth the estimate arising from Tufts.

As we will soon see, trends identified using information gleaned from these small, nimble companies is also imperfect. Munos would be the first to agree that his estimate is an underestimation. Specifically, this approach tends to exclude failed projects from small companies that never went public and from large pharmaceutical companies that may not have disclosed failed efforts. Moreover, smaller companies tend to partner with, or be acquired by, larger companies seeking to gain access to a potential blockbuster drug (a subject to which we will repeatedly return). Consequently, many of the late-stage costs of failure are borne by the larger and more established company rather than by the upstart company.

Despite the consequence of the challenges presented in this chapter, the pharmaceutical industry has remained frustratingly adherent to the letter of the law—Eroom's Law, that is. We will now take an adrenaline-filled ride to review the many (yet futile) attempts to break this law and the consequences. Some of these attempts to break the law—done in the name of creating new medicines—might instead actually preclude our ability to continue enjoying the benefits arising from the introduction of new medicines.

CHAPTER SIX

Finding a New Purpose in Life

A s we have seen, the costs to discover and develop new medicines have grown ever more expensive as the pharmaceutical industry has sought ways to circumvent Eroom's Law. As the magnitude of concern about the rising costs to develop new medicines increased over the years, some of the cleverer individuals began to ask, "Why should we create new drugs at all?" They reasoned, quite accurately in retrospect, that existing medicines could be substantially improved, and this is the subject of our present chapter.

It would be reasonable to presume that making new and better uses of existing medicines would deliver less expensive cures. However, the old saying about common sense being neither common nor sensical would seem to apply here. We will explore three different ways that revamping existing medicines have surprisingly contributed to the costs of healthcare. Although much of this part of our story could be presented and received with considerable cynicism, we would ask that you suspend that natural inclination for a time as many of these efforts were undertaken with real sincerity. The work below will convey real benefits that have been invested into old medicines to make them better or expand their use. We will also see that such activities indeed deserve to be rewarded, though perhaps not as much as they are. Under the presumption that a conventional risk-to-reward balance is at play, a question that will pervade this entire story is whether the rewards are proportionate to the risks taken. This decision will be left to the reader, but is an important question to consider throughout.

Overtly Formulaic

To start at the very beginning, we will turn to a drug that virtually all of us have used and that many of us imbibe on a daily basis. Found among the oldest known clay tablets from Ur, the capital of ancient Sumer, are references to medicinal plants that contain what we today refer to as salicylates.[1] Salicylates are quite important molecules from the perspective of a tree or plant as they evolved as a sort of botanical immune response, chemicals meant to keep pesky insects and other potential damaging invaders at bay. Independent of these benefits, salicylates also tend to have remarkably useful properties for humans.

A prominent salicylate-bearing plant is the willow tree. The bark of the willow has been known for millennia to decrease discomfort as evidenced by the Ebers Papyrus, an ancient medical text from 1550 BCE and the even older Sumerian clay tablets. For those suffering from pain or fever, from ancient times until surprisingly recently, apothecaries would grind up some tree bark, mix it with water, and provide it as an elixir. This practice remained routine for decades after the end of the American Civil War.

As our understanding of chemistry evolved, scientists became interested in isolating the chemical responsible for the beneficial effects of willow bark. The pain-relieving activity of willow tree bark was attributed by German chemists in 1828 to a molecule known as salicylic acid. Soon thereafter, the molecule could be produced in the laboratory and scaled up so that the new drug could be marketed to the masses.

Salicylic acid was a hit and can still be readily found in virtually every pharmacy and is on the World Health Organization's List of Essential

Medicines.[2] However, the beneficial effects of salicylic acid were tempered by its tendency to be highly caustic. Ingesting salicylic acid can cause terrible ulcers and other erosions of the esophagus and intestine and, when placed on the skin, the purified compound can cause rather painful burns. Indeed, the primary use today for salicylic acid is as part of wart-removing medications or to exfoliate skin as a means to treat acne and other skin maladies.

The opportunity to develop a better product compelled early pharmaceutical companies to develop newer and better ways to maximize the benefit of salicylic acid while minimizing its corrosive side effects. In the late 1890s, a young scientist by the name of Arthur Eichengrün had chemically modified salicylic acid by adding an acetyl group (two extra carbons and an oxygen atom along with some accompanying hydrogen atoms) to create a drug known today as aspirin.[3] [4]

Aspirin has rightfully earned the moniker of "the wonder drug." Although originally developed to treat fever and pain, the drug has also saved the lives of countless individuals given its ability to block platelets and prevent or even treat heart attacks. The drug also has shown promise to treat or prevent a wide range of ailments. The health benefits of aspirin are so wide that it could rightfully take its place along with fluoridated water or iodized salt as a required human supplement except for a nagging problem: the drug shares with salicylic acid a tendency to irritate the various linings of the gastrointestinal system. Some people are particularly sensitive and can suffer quite serious internal bleeding. The esophagus and stomach are particularly sensitive to this unwanted burning side effect.

This problem was partially solved by happenstance. William D. Paul, known to his friends as "Shorty," was a young physician specializing in orthopedics, but his lifelong passion was devoted to chemistry.[5] Amid the carnage of the Second World War, Paul started an academic career as a sports medicine doctor for the University of Iowa. Shortly after Shorty's arrival, he was having a casual conversation with the chair of the department of nutrition, Kate Daum, when she complained of a headache.[6] Paul offered her an aspirin, but she declined, stating that aspirin upset her stomach.

This polite refusal catalyzed a revelation when Paul and a colleague, Joseph Routh, realized that acids such as aspirin could be contained with specialized chemicals known as buffers. The two went on to develop a remedy in which aspirin was not changed, but instead packaged with a buffer that would prevent stomach irritation. This new product, later known as Bufferin, was sold to the Bristol-Myers company and has remained a commercial hit for decades.[7]

Bufferin is a classic example of a reformulated product. This category reflects products where the active ingredient itself is not fundamentally changed, but rather is administered in a way that is different or improved. The benefits of Bufferin as compared to nonbuffered aspirin are obvious and warrant a higher price. But how high is reasonable for a repurposed product? In this example a tablet of Bufferin will set you back an average of eleven cents whereas the store-brand cost of aspirin is less than a penny. This is not an unreasonable markup for those who would gladly pay the extra dime to avoid a night with an upset stomach. Would you, however, be willing to pay seven dollars for the drug?

Critics of the FDA can often be heard to comment something to the effect of, "If aspirin were to be submitted as a new drug today, the overly conservative FDA would surely reject it." If ever you find yourself on the quiz show *Jeopardy!*, don't worry if confronted by the following: "The year aspirin was formally approved by FDA." The answer would be, using proper wording, "What is 2015?" This response would likely be met with another question such as, "Seriously?" But indeed, that is accurate.

Although introduced in 1899, aspirin was among a small number of products exempted by certain small print found in the 1962 Kefauver-Harris Amendment (you may recall this as the legislation we discussed in Chapter Two that required existing products to be tested to ensure their safety and efficacy in the days following thalidomide). The argument for "grandfathering" aspirin was that the drug was so widely used that it did not need to undergo additional testing to prove its effectiveness.

On September 8, 2015, a New Haven, Connecticut, pharmaceutical company with the rather inspired name of New Haven Pharmaceuticals was awarded an FDA approval for aspirin. Their product, Durlaza, was a reformulation of baby aspirin that extended the release of the drug for a full twenty-four hours. This modification was developed to provide continual support for high-risk patients who had suffered a previous heart attack or stroke.

Again, this new formulation, like Bufferin, deserved to be rewarded. What was the price of Durlaza? According to New Haven Pharmaceuticals, the product would cost $200 per month, $2,400 a year. That price is roughly 600 times the price of a regular aspirin (or 1,200 times the price if you cut the aspirin in half, which is the equivalent of one day's worth of Durlaza).

Although it is worth repeating that an improved formulation does indeed warrant a bump in price, a twelve-hundred-fold increase seems a bit extreme. New Haven Pharmaceuticals faced enormous criticism, but countered that the price reflects the costs of research and development. The company drew a line in the sand, staking its reputation and indeed entire business upon the assumption that people would be willing to pay the Durlaza premium. The product failed and the company shuttered its doors in 2016, suggesting that perhaps we are now reaching a point where drug prices can be too high (at least for a revamped drug). This is a point we will visit again in future chapters: that consumers have reached the point where they have had enough and are simply refusing to accept higher prices and are demanding changes by either refusing to purchase certain drugs and/or encouraging legislative measures to curtail prices.

Nonetheless, billions of dollars in annual premiums are expended for medicines, which have long existed and been sold as generics (and even over the counter). Often, these improvements are well worth the cost. For example, long-acting forms of insulin or a prostate cancer drug known as leuprolide have provided clear benefits over the original dosage forms of these drugs.[8][9] The unresolved question is, "What is a reasonable price?" Whereas we as consumers (and our insurance plans) have merely accepted these increases in the past, the experience with Durlarza suggests the answer to that simple question is currently changing.

Compounding Interest

An ancient art passed down among apothecaries is still in use today, or at least a form of it. Certain patients are unable to take a medicine in its original manufactured form and require an alternative version. Such needs might arise from an inability to swallow pills, for example, or if existing preparations contain allergens, gluten (for patients with celiac disease), or if the patient requires a specialized dose not provided by traditional manufacturers.

Such needs can be addressed by individual pharmacists, who gain experience in the art known as compounding. This practice entails the isolation of active ingredients from conventional medicines and individualized reformulation into a product amenable to the patient. Compounding pharmacies that specialize in small batches often do not come under FDA scrutiny. As the practice of compounding grew, so did the problems.

By definition, compounding is supposed to occur in small batches to meet the needs of individual patients, a true form of "personalized medicine." Over time, some compounding pharmacies grew both in the number of patients served but also in the size of batches of drugs prepared. Their rationale, which is understandable at one level, relied upon the fact that it is far more efficient to anticipate needs and have a drug readily at hand when the need arises than to begin compounding after an order is received. However, this practice raises questions about if or when a compounding pharmacy crosses the line to become a pharmaceutical company, the latter of which is generally subject to more rigorous regulation by the FDA.

Muddying the waters further, the mandate of the FDA, as a federal agency, is limited to regulating interstate drug transport. Within a state, the powers of the FDA are more limited. A prominent example is the ongoing situation with medical cannabis. As individual states legalize medical marijuana, the FDA has no jurisdiction as the product will not (legally) cross state lines. A similar situation arises with compounding pharmacies, which can create medicines for patients within a state and thus are not subject to FDA oversight.

The fundamental fact that federal agencies have limited or no control over certain activities within states has been the impetus for many disagreements and has proven to be a recipe for disaster. Restricting ourselves to questions surrounding compounding, the headlines ring every few years with stories of tragic mistakes. Arguably, the most famous of these in recent years centered upon a 2012 outbreak of fungal meningitis caused by a contaminated batch of epidural steroids produced by the New England Compounding Center (NECC).[10] More than a hundred patients died. Although NECC would declare bankruptcy and dissolve by the end of that year, more than a dozen employees were later arrested, one as he was trying to board a flight to Hong Kong. Four employees in total would be convicted, including the CEO of NECC, with charges ranging from mail fraud to racketeering (a second-degree murder charge was sought by pros-ecutors but turned down by the jury). This particular incident did happen to fall under federal regulation because the contaminated material was dispersed among twenty-three states. Many compounding pharmacies are small-scale operations that operate solely within a given state. One example is a Kansas City pharmacist, who adulterated dozens of drugs by watering them down to maximize profits.[11] In such cases, the FDA is restricted to providing "guidance" or "concern."

Beyond safety concerns, compounding has contributed to the rising costs of new medicines. For example, a 2016 study concluded that for services managed by Express Scripts, a large pharmacy benefit manager (we will meet this industry in a later chapter), the price of compounded medicines increased by 130 percent from 2012 to 2013. By comparison, the price of noncompounded ingredients had increased by 7.7 percent. This translated into a total cost of $710.36 per patient for compounded drugs versus $160.20 for noncompounded equivalents. As a consequence, Express Scripts announced that more than a thousand ingredients used for compounding would no longer qualify for reimbursement.[12]

The situation with compounding pharmacies is exceedingly complex given questions about states' rights, safety, and cost. However, what can be stated rather unambiguously is that the costs of compounding are rising at a rate higher than inflation and even higher than the costs of conventional pharmaceuticals—a rather remarkable feat, if not admirable.

Old Dogs with New Tricks

Despite what you might have felt in high school, chemistry can be a terribly exciting and whimsical subject. For proof, look no further than your medi-cine cabinet. Despite the fact most of the drugs we take fall into the category known as "small molecules," nature provides extraordinary flexibility to these molecules. Rather than the stodgy two-dimensional lines and letters on paper (or wooden pegs for those acquainted with 1950s-style molecular models), the embraces exchanged among carbon, oxygen, hydrogen and other atoms are exceedingly dynamic. Electrons dance back and forth, while large sections of molecules are constantly flexing and bending.

All of these molecular gymnastics therefore make it possible for one molecule to behave in many different ways. This dynamism is one reason that propels continued interest in drug repurposing (also known as drug repositioning). For example, the different changes in the chemical character of a molecule as it flexes and bends might allow it to engage with something utterly different than expected (anthropomorphically defined as its "intended target"). Such chemical behavior can have negative consequences if, for example, the drug perturbs a molecule that is essential for good health, and such negative interactions might contribute to the unintended side effects that we all dread. For the purposes of concluding this chapter, we will focus upon those happy accidents that arise and provide opportunities for expanding the usefulness of a medicine.

In some cases, a molecule can impact a target in a way that is utterly distinct from the manner for which it was intended. As an example, Dr. Kinch's team at Yale in 2011 helped reveal a new purpose for an old antibiotic. It turns out that an antibiotic, which had not been marketed for years, happened to have the surprisingly beneficial effect of blocking a protein that contributed to the growth of certain cancers. With growing understanding of the microbiome, the collection of bacteria and other microorganisms within us all, Dr. Kinch presumed that the antibiotic was exerting its effects by changing the resident bacteria in the body. Although this was a very trendy hypothesis, it was utterly wrong. The answer was that a part of the antibiotic that had nothing to do with the antibacterial properties, junk atoms we had utterly ignored, happened to disrupt the function of a key molecule in the tumor cells. As is so often the case in science, it was luck, not hypothesis, that facilitated the fortunate discovery.

Perhaps the most compelling example of the repurposing of a drug that had been utterly (and quite understandably) demonized is thalidomide. We have already seen how and why thalidomide earned its dismal reputation by causing innumerable spontaneous abortions and causing far too many children to be born with pronounced birth defects. However, as the late radio announcer Paul Harvey used to say, now it is time for "the rest of the story."

In the wake of the tragedy, much research was conducted to uncover the reasons why thalidomide had proven so dangerous for pregnant women. The answer, it turns out, was that thalidomide was a particularly powerful inhibitor of a process known as angiogenesis. Taking apart this word, the term *angio* is derived from a Greek term referring to "vessels" and *genesis* refers to the English terms for "origin." The vessels referred to in angiogenesis are blood vessels and without a proper supply of blood vessels, a developing fetus will not be able to create vital structures such as limbs. Hence the fact that thalidomide blocked angiogenesis explains why so many children (from those fetuses fortunate to survive at all) had been born without arms and/or legs.

While understanding of the biology of human development was being uncovered, a Harvard professor by the name of Judah Folkman was studying cancer. In 1971, Folkman published a groundbreaking study in the *New England Journal of Medicine*, which demonstrated that a growing tumor required the constant creation of a new blood supply—and thus new blood vessels.[13] This created a new opportunity for thalidomide as it worked to the strengths of this old killer. In 1998, the drug Thalomid was approved for sale in the United States. Learning from the past, this reintroduction of thalidomide was tightly regulated such that patients had to undergo extensive counseling and security procedures to ensure that women who were, or might become, pregnant would have no unintended exposure to the drug. Consequently, a drug that had killed or disfigured so many was able to be rehabilitated as a lifesaving treatment for cancer.

Other repurposing examples are neither so dramatic nor impactful. Indeed, many repurposing opportunities are actively ignored by the pharmaceutical industry. The reason for this relates back to patents. Once the intellectual property behind a medicine has expired, there remains little incentive for the innovator to conduct the very expensive clinical investigation to widen its use. Indeed, the innovator may no longer even market the medicine, having abandoned it to generic competitors.

The manufacturers of generic medicines often do not conduct experimental research, particularly for medicines that are the least expensive (and hence with small margins). While there are other types of patents (known as "use" patents) that can help carve out and protect intellectual property for particular uses of a drug, these tend to be viewed rather skeptically, both by established companies and venture investors alike. Consequently, some of the best opportunities for repurposing may be lost or ignored.

Arising from such experiences, the scientific and business worlds have embraced a form of repurposing that can generate novel intellectual property—and thus be used to increase the price of medicines even though the research and development costs, as well as the risk, are considerably lower than for completely new medicines. Another subindustry of the pharmaceutical enterprise centers upon "specialty pharmaceutical companies." Much as we saw with aspirin, these companies identify ways to improve existing drugs, often by allowing them to be delivered in new or improved ways. Oftentimes, these products can also create new "methods of use" or even "composition of matter" by attaching or modifying existing drugs to improve how these medicines are absorbed, distributed, or metabolized in the body. These improvements come at a cost as the companies understandably seek to be rewarded for the improvements. These specialty pharmaceuticals are invariably more expensive and the improvements are often incremental, rather than transformative. Consistent with the theme of our story, the creation of the specialty pharmaceuticals subindustry has increased both the number of mouths to feed and a new cast of characters bent upon maximizing their profits—and sometimes in breathtaking ways—and thereby contributing to the price of health.

We will return to these lost opportunities and their potential ability to finally circumvent Eroom's Law, but now we must look at how this quest to maximize profit has led the industry to try to break actual laws.

CHAPTER SEVEN

Self-Inflicted Wounds

n recalling the cluster of fascinating studies published by Bernard Munos and Jack Scannell in or around 2010, their motivations were driven by recognition of the rising costs to develop a new medicine, which had been expanding at an exponential rate since the 1950s. Munos in particular has emphasized a positive "spillover effect" in drug development. This economic principle suggests an increase in the overall number of companies involved in drug development should enhance the productivity of the individual companies within the industry. Based on a greater number of new medicines approved by the FDA than might have been otherwise expected in the 1990s, Munos suggested this higher rate of productivity may "spill over" into the following decade and this positive influence would likely counter much of the havoc wrought by Eroom's Law. In this chapter, we will suggest not merely that the benefits of a spillover effect have already or may soon end, but that we may soon experience the opposite: an inability to keep up with the need for new medicines in a rapidly changing world.

Consistent with our theme of unintended consequences, failed attempts to tame Eroom's Law by the pharmaceutical industry have degraded its ability to develop new medicines, threatening the future of public health and a vital sector of the American economy. The responsibility for these activities must necessarily lie at the top. In advising the authors, Bernard Munos pointed out that the fundamentals of pharmaceutical research are widely misunderstood, even by many of its most prominent leaders.[1] Unlike most process-driven industries, he conveyed that the pharmaceutical research is a creative industry, aligned more closely with entertainment, publishing, and fashion industries, which are often subject to seemingly whimsical changes in business operations and strategies as well as perception of demand. Not long ago, most publishing houses were dismissive of the idea that children would have the attention span to digest books that were many hundreds of pages long. Yet, a more creative-minded executive at Scholastic believed in this new thinking and green-lighted an unknown author by the name of J. K. Rowling.

Scientific and medical breakthroughs can be comparably unanticipated (and seemingly magical at times) and, as the saying goes, chance favors the prepared mind. In a conversation with Charles Muscoplat, who has an extraordinary track record leading research and development activities in both biotechnology companies and academia, he said, "One successful drug developed six levels below can make a CEO look brilliant."[2] The key to the CEO looking brilliant is therefore the ability to create a culture that favors orthogonal thinking and to recognize and seize upon these rare opportunities.

The training of scientists is not merely attuned to this type of thinking but fully embraces the idea of disrupting paradigms and emphasizing creative ideas. When confronted with the question of whether scientific training was necessary to be a pharmaceutical company CEO, Bernard Munos responded, "It is not necessary, but it helps."[3] He then qualified the statement that a successful pharmaceutical leader needs to understand unique dynamics of science or to surround themselves with people who do. In an industry where decisions can have ramifications easily reaching the billions of dollars, it thus seems sensible to have scientists at or at least near the helm. Yet, this is the opposite of recent trends. Whereas scientists tended to dominate pharmaceutical industry leadership in the 20th century, leadership is increasingly handed off to attorneys, MBAs, accountants, and other fields that might be best described by Munos as process-driven or further away from the creative.

Little Consolation in Consolidation

Given the importance of the industry, Dr. Kinch's team at Washington University in St. Louis began analyzing the innovative sources responsible for the waves of miraculous medicines introduced into the American market since the Second World War. By focusing on a set of organizations that had conducted the research and development of new medicines, the investigators hoped to determine if there were any trends that might be instructive for identifying factors responsible for Eroom's Law or the responses to it.

By looking backward at history, the findings from the Washington University team have suggested the pharmaceutical industry began to recognize the impact of Eroom's Law as early as the 1970s.[4] They based this conclusion upon an uptick in the frequency of mergers and acquisitions within this time period. This tendency accelerated in later years, particularly among large pharmaceutical partners. Arguably the highest profile and most prolific player in this process was the biopharmaceutical giant known today as Pfizer.

Charles Pfizer & Co. started in Brooklyn, New York, named after its founder, who had emigrated from Germany in October 1848 (one of many Germanic speakers who left Europe amid the revolutionary fervor of that year).[5] Within a year, Pfizer had established a partnership with his cousin, Karl F. Erhardt, to found a firm that would manufacture a drug discovered in Germany only a few years earlier. Santonin was a compound isolated from a seed plant native to the area now known as Turkmenistan.[6] When combined with the laxative castor oil, the extract from the seeds of this plant proved to be a useful means to expel worms. Indeed, *Artemisia cina* is more commonly known as "wormseed." Just a few years before Pfizer's emigration to the United States, German chemists had isolated santonin from wormseed and the product would soon be marketed to a citizenry squirming to get a medicine for parasites that were all too prevalent. Back in the United States, Charles Pfizer, a chemist, learned about santonin and began purifying the compound. His cousin, a confectioner, then created a candy-based form of the drug. The sugar-coated pill was a huge hit in their adopted land.

From these humble beginnings, Pfizer (the company) spent most of the following century and a half as a modestly sized business. The company was roughly the same size as Eli Lilly & Co but far less productive in terms of introducing innovative new medicines into the marketplace. Indeed, Pfizer was not even among the top ten companies in terms of introducing new products, lagging behind more established companies such as Wyeth, Parke-Davis, and Upjohn. All of this changed starting in 1999, when Pfizer announced its intention to purchase Warner-Lambert, the parent company of Parke-Davis.

Warner-Lambert had been developing a new drug since the early 1990s. This molecule, atorvastatin, was the fifth and otherwise unremarkable cholesterol-lowering drug to enter the market. As a late entry, it was generally presumed this drug would be unremarkable, hence a decision by Warner-Lambert to do a deal with Pfizer and allow the smaller company to capture much of the royalties. Yet, Pfizer executives had a plan. They developed a scheme to use a saturation campaign of direct-to-consumer advertising to accompany the launch of atorvastatin, whose trade name, Lipitor, would soon become a household fixture.

This would not be the only time that Pfizer emphasized direct-to-consumer advertising. The list of drugs in the late 1990s backed by Pfizer's aggressive marketing approach includes celecoxib (Celebrex), sildenafil (Viagra®), and donepezil (Aricept®).[7] Working with a rising guru of Madison Avenue advertising, a young Donny Deutsch, Pfizer launched one successful campaign after another, dramatically bolstering its revenues. This masterful emphasis upon advertising (a subject soon to be addressed in our story) increased Pfizer revenues so suddenly and thoroughly that it allowed the otherwise unremarkable company to pull off the $90.2 billion buyout of its larger and more prominent rival and erstwhile collaborator, Warner-Lambert.[8]

The argument made by Pfizer to justify its takeover of Warner-Lambert was quite rational. Executives confidently stated the efficiency of their business, and thus shareholder value, would benefit from new ideas and economies at scale. The bottom line would be further bolstered by reducing management and administrative positions. Indeed, it seems obvious that overlapping activities, such as sales or manufacturing, could be performed with greater efficiency and fewer people. Driven by this rationale and tempted by the ever-escalating bounties and market valuation of both the hunter and prey, such mergers were cheered by investors.

Buoyed by the sales and vigorous marketing, Pfizer continued its buying spree, acquiring Pharmacia in 2002 (itself a megamerger company that included the companies formerly known as Upjohn, Pharmacia, and Searle), Wyeth in 2009, and King Pharmaceuticals a year later. Indeed, these are merely the largest examples of an acquisition frenzy that would entail twenty-nine different mergers or acquisitions conducted between 1999 and 2019. If you count the organizations that these other companies had executed prior to their being devoured by Pfizer, an additional thirty-seven companies were introduced into the Pfizer network. Altogether this consolidation activity represented sixty-six different companies were brought under the Pfizer umbrella over two decades.

All the while, Pfizer's competition was not sitting idle, particularly in Europe. Indeed, one might argue Pfizer was simply aping an approach that had begun with the first European pharmaceutical megamerger. In 1970, two Swiss-based companies, CIBA and Geigy, had come together and formed a powerful company that would later undertake even more rounds of consolidation that resulted in the creation of a company today known as Novartis.

Even with this overseas competition, Pfizer soon found itself at the top of the league charts, both in terms of sales and the number of innovative products introduced in the first decade of the 21st century. Pfizer was followed by Merck (which had undergone a megamerger with Schering Plough in 2009) and three European giants: Novartis, Sanofi-Aventis, and Glaxo-SmithKline, the hyphenated or run-on names of the latter two companies bearing witness to the many mergers that occurred in the 1990s and early years of the 2000s.

By this time, Eli Lilly & Co was no longer included in the rolls of the companies delivering the most innovative drugs. The company that had so clearly dominated innovation in research and development for most of the 20th century would largely ignore the innovation in business practices that swept away many of its peers.

The feverish waves of mergers and acquisitions were a reflection of, and driven by, waves of entrepreneurship that had begun in the 1970s. This period marked the creation of the first biotechnology endeavors, companies whose drug candidates were largely based on recent understanding of DNA and protein engineering rather than traditional chemistry. In a phenomenon that blossomed on both coasts of the United States, waves of innovation and entrepreneurship brought forth a generation of biotechnology companies that would revolutionize the medicine, business, and science of healthcare. We will return again to the more elaborate, complicated, and expensive medicines introduced by these organizations later in our story. For now, it suffices to say that these products provided both new opportunities for therapeutic breakthrough as well as lucrative opportunities for investors.

After a relatively short period of autonomy lasting until the early days of a new millennium, biotechnology companies began to disappear. Long gone are pioneering companies with prominent names, including Alza, Millennium, Chiron, Genzyme, and MedImmune. Each has been swept away and merged into an established pharmaceutical company. Even the dominant princess of biotechnology, California-based Genentech, was fated to be subsumed by the Swiss company Roche and its name will eventually fade just as these others have done. This new wave of acquisitions, which ruled over the first decade of the new millennium, arose as pharmaceutical companies dwindled and the insatiable companies like Pfizer and the European megapharma companies were compelled to dine upon smaller and smaller fish, an early indication that this trend would not be sustainable. Indeed, Dr. Kinch's work at Washington University reveals that the overall number of organizations that have contributed to the research or development of a new medicine has nearly halved since 2003 (from 250 to 130 companies in the span of fifteen years). The remaining companies can be broadly divided into a small number (roughly twenty or so) of hungry sharks surrounded by comparatively small minnows, whose consumption is unlikely to satiate the needs of the top predators that need to keep up this acquisitive momentum in order to survive and thrive. Each of these companies harkens back to Eli Lilly during its scramble to replace Prozac in Year X and a bevy of resulting medicines in anticipation of Year Y/Z. Eventually, this wild ride, ever accelerating, reaches a point where the company is both unable to stop and comparably incapable of keeping up.

Another unintended consequence of the feeding frenzy that has dominated the pharmaceutical industry is the impact of the premiums required to pay for the mergers and acquisitions. One justification used throughout the years has been that economies of scale would translate into savings. The rationale was that, for example, two sales forces (one from each company) could be consolidated into a single, more efficient team. Indeed, cuts were inevitably made to eliminate overlapping activities, starting with the sales forces but not stopping there. Eventually, these cuts would extend beyond the perceived "fat" of the companies and venture into muscle and then the structural bones needed for future performance.

To pay off these debts and satisfy investor demands, these companies would soon need to begin chopping away at the research and development teams that were responsible for delivering the new products needed to keep apace on the ever-accelerating pharmaceutical treadmill. Willfully ignorant of the medium- and long-term implication of such a strategy, even companies that should have known better, such as Eli Lilly, began to lop away substantial portions of the same research and development activities that had allowed them to survive Years X and Y/Z.

Accelerating the depth of the peril, these companies would continue to suffer an expanded form of what Bernard Munos referred to as the "costs of scale." Unlike the positive outcomes associated with economies of scale these costs of scale continued to mount and worsen as mergers merely increased the breadth of the causes of declining efficiency. The resulting shortfalls in profitability would demand further cuts to the workforce, eventually causing companies to cut ever deeper into the most fundamental sinews and bones of these organizations.

This already-grim situation compounded a related trend associated with industry consolidation. Soon after a merger, the product pipelines of the newly conjoined companies would be scrutinized, with a goal of pruning those projects less relevant to the long-term aspirations of the new company or deemed too far over the time horizon to be maintained, regardless of future potential. As the cuts deepened with each additional merger or patent expiry, the muscle of these organizations became progressively more denuded or atrophied.

Particular gusto has been devoted to slashing earlier and earlier stages of research and development activities. Such actions were justified by an assumption that research and discovery efforts are too far distant from revenue generation. One bit of evidence supporting this contention is the scramble that accompanied the recent COVID-19 outbreak. Many companies had dismantled their own abilities to develop vaccines and instead were forced to do last-minute deals with start-up companies, often with inflated prices and outsized risks, in an effort to simply be perceived as playing a role in the emergency.[9] A cynic might question how much of this activity was performed in an effort to address the problem versus managing their images before a public that had an increasingly negative view of the pharmaceutical industry.[10]

Moreover, such actions reflected an assumption built over the years that large companies could simply rely upon purchase, as needed, to acquire products developed by a seemingly endless number of small start-up companies. We will probe that assumption in a later chapter but for now, it must be stated that these deals are never cheap, as they include the millions of dollars paid to investment bankers, lawyers, and specialty PR and IR firms. Further, these deals drain resources needed to back the acquisitions. Such penalties can only be paid by raising the prices charged for the resulting products, thereby contributing to the rising prices of medicines.

The pruning of research and development activities also had the perverse effect of excising much of the internal scientific and medical institutional memory and expertise that had propelled large, established companies for decades, with a gross analogy being that the industry had voluntarily lobotomized itself. A destructive consequence of this strategy is an understandable breakdown of the intimate business-science partnerships that had enabled investment into breakthrough medicines like Prozac. In the interests of maintaining a focus on quarterly profits, many corporate executives have pruned or entirely eliminated research capabilities, thereby virtually guaranteeing future crises. Worse still, the elimination of internal scientific capabilities left many companies without the breadth of talent needed to evaluate the risks and merits of potential merger or licensing deals. These are dangerous practices as such short-term thinking has increasingly threatened the ability of individual companies to respond to future patent expiries and loss of products to generic competitors.

Compounding the decline in the size of the industry was an increasingly entrenched mindset that Munos characterized in an interview with the catchphrase, "Failure is not an option." As we have already seen, a mere one in ten experimental medicines tested in the clinic (meaning they survived to the human stage of testing) will ultimately succeed to become a marketed product. It seems these failures tend to occur at a relatively late stage, perhaps a lingering consequence of advancing products begun during the "shots of goal" era, when subpar products were rushed into clinical development, warts and all, and thus being an even greater cost drain than they would have been if they had just been written off as busts, pretrial. At these later stages, millions, and perhaps even billions, of dollars have been sunk into the program. To counter such high-profile debacles, more and more established companies took an approach of tackling less risky projects with a higher likelihood of success.

A pattern of risk aversion was particularly obvious in the activities immediately following the period characterized by waves of mergers and acquisitions. The management of a newly renovated company might immediately be confronted with harmonizing the pipelines and priorities of what had been two separate organizations, each with its own appetite for risk. Beyond shedding duplicative programs (as might be required by financial regulators to avoid trade monopolies), key decisions must be made to prioritize projects based on their likelihood for success. Given concerns about risk exposure, the most ambitious and innovative programs often found themselves on the chopping block of an organization under pressure to cut costs and appeal to Wall Street.

In what Munos refers to as a "death spiral," executive boardrooms have been increasingly reluctant to initiate or maintain the most innovative projects or address the most widely applicable needs. Research and development activities have increasingly become regimented and discourage outside-the-box thinking. Alzheimer's is a prominent example. The past two decades are replete with examples of failed clinical-stage programs, which destroyed or set back both novel scientific hypotheses and wasted billions of dollars. In the early days, failures in Alzheimer's research were to be expected as the disease target was relatively new and scientists had much to learn. However, as the number of high-profile drug failures mounted, corporate executives, pressured by anxious Wall Street investors, increasingly shied away from pursuing new research projects in the Alzheimer's field. As a consequence, the amount of pharmaceutical development activity directed at Alzheimer's disease has dwindled since the terrible summer of 2012.

Another example of the tendency to avoid risk has taken the form of what historically has been known as a "me-too" drug (a label that should quickly be relegated to the dustbin given the more recent and far more serious connotations of the term "me-too" associated with harassment and abuse of women). Also known as a fast-follower drug, the lower risk profile drugs generally entail chemical or formulation improvements upon existing medicines. High profile examples include Lipitor, which was the fifth cholesterol-lowering statin to get a nod from the FDA, and Viibryd, being the seventh SSRI (the first being Prozac) approved for use in the United States.

Fast-follower drugs are attractive to drug companies because they tend to be more predictable in terms of their science, medicine, and business. The heavy lifting needed to develop an entirely new type of medicine, from gaining regulatory approval to marketing it to physicians and patients can be relegated to predecessor drugs, while a fast-follower can capitalize upon all of these pioneering efforts. As demonstrated by the growing revenues garnered by each new generation of fast-follower drugs, many corporate boardrooms have clearly taken to heart a lesson that innovation in the pharmaceutical industry is something to be avoided, not cherished. Earlier generations of drugs have to convince a skeptical marketplace of their utility and may not catch on until they have succumbed to generic competition. In contrast, a late arrival will benefit from the increasing recognition of its potential value and, paradoxically, be able to command a higher price, even when it works no better than the original drug.[11]

Yet the public health benefits of fast-follower drugs, if any, tend to be incremental. One side effect of this approach is that an increasing emphasis upon fast-follower drugs necessarily comes at the expense of discovering and deploying truly innovative new medicines, those with the ability to convey orthogonal benefits to society. As evinced by Munos, an emphasis upon fast-follower drugs starts a company down a path on which revenues will invariably disappoint investors as they enter a competitive marketplace. At the same time, a tendency to prefer second, third, or even seventh prizes serves to demoralize the companies' research and development teams. The groups are individuals who became scientists to pioneer new work rather than remain merely tweaking an existing drug.

The resulting impact of layoffs and fast-follow emphasis also had deleterious consequences for the innovation culture, both in mindset and action. After the announcement of a merger, one will often hear that the best and brightest will voluntarily leave to seek new opportunities, the lowest performers will be laid off, and the company will be left with an uninspired workforce. Such changes tend to reinforce a culture already susceptible to risk-avoiding mediocrity and may even convey a coup de grâce for a struggling organization. Indeed, Munos and others have projected a rather bleak future for many of the largest pharmaceutical companies absent a dramatic reshuffling of their business strategies. Roughly half of the dozen or so pharmaceutical giants are helmed by low-quality leadership; a feature that may have already sealed their fate.[12]

For an industry facing such dire straits, Wall Street has been unexpectedly kind. Pharmaceutical earnings and industry stock values have done remarkably well for an industry where patent cliffs shave billions of dollars in revenues each year. When challenged on this fact, Munos countered that even sophisticated institutional investors tend toward a relatively short-term horizon, with a maximum of perhaps three years in their investment horizon. Consequently, the views of most established companies are based solely upon the most mature (generally what is known as Phase III clinical-stage) programs. Within this relatively small window and mindset, the sky is unlikely to fall. Indeed, champagne corks continue to pop with announcements of initial public offerings (IPOs) and a seemingly never-ending string of mergers and acquisition.

One particularly alarming trend in investor perceptions of research and development was conveyed by Andrew Dahlem, a former executive at Eli Lilly. Prior to the current emphasis upon industry consolidation, a report of increased R&D expenditures was broadly perceived as a sign to expect strong future revenues and would therefore buoy the price of a pharmaceutical stock. In the wake of scar tissue deepened by decades of Eroom's Law and high-profile, late-stage drug failures, that view changed. Dahlem maintains that expenditures on experimental medicines are now viewed as inefficient and more likely to be interpreted as contributions into a money pit rather than as a promise of future returns. Toward this, one of our authors has had the unfortunate experience of being derided by analysts and investors when announcing an increase in expected R&D expenses, with said analysts and investors demanding to know how and when the investment will be realized. In fact, in her career as head of investor relations for biotech companies, Ms. Weiman was lobbied by investors and analysts to ask management to not develop a product, even as the company presented what it believed was positive results at a scientific conference. The general opinion was that that the return on the investment would be outside the preferred investment time horizon. When the opinion was shared and discussed with the CEO, he was stunned, especially since the analyst was from one of the largest investment banks and well-respected as being thoughtful, informed, and supportive of the company's initiatives. Even with the positive mid-stage study results and internal enthusiasm for continuing the project, the product was eventually killed.

Such negative views of research and development drove what might seem like a rather crazy approach to drug development. Although many pharmaceutical companies increasingly shun the earliest stages of drug development (known as discovery efforts), a brave few have remained devoted to the subject. These exceptions must constantly assure investors that they remain devoted to discovering new and lucrative medical breakthroughs. With a closer look, though, some of these companies were not quite as courageous as it might seem. Indeed, fear drove them to be quite wasteful and thus contributed further to Eroom's Law. For example, an early-stage project within a large company might soon prove itself so promising that the company just had to get rid of it. Yes, you read that correctly.

The idea here is that a really promising discovery would be cut away from the parent company and used as a seed for a new biotechnology company. The former owner would license away their rights and keep a fraction of ownership (at or just under 20 percent, a crucial number because any greater ownership would require the parent company to report any gains or losses in their own financial statements). The established companies would then negotiate a right to make the first bid to reacquire the new company at a future date. The fledgling organization would then raise investor monies to develop the project further, which usually means conducting clinical trials to assess the safety and effectiveness of the new experimental medicine. As the hoped-for positive results accumulate, the parent would then practice its first right of refusal and reacquire the asset it had shed years before.

Perhaps, you are thinking, "What is so wrong with this idea?" After all, the parent company sheds the risk that the product will not work, and the fledgling company gets a nice dividend. The issue, however, comes down to efficiency. First, the dollars invested by venture capitalists are not free, but come with the presumption that they and the founders will receive a sizable premium on the risks they have taken with their monies, time, and careers. These same venture capital financiers themselves have a portfolio of products, many of which will fail, and thus the premiums they receive on their successful products must be outsized to pay for these losses (just as they historically had to be paid for by large portfolio-based pharmaceutical companies in bygone years). Essentially then, this "release and catch" approach equates to the fact that the parent company will effectively pay considerably more to shed the products and reacquire them than they would have if they had simply developed the products internally.

Why then, you must be thinking, would an organization be so foolish as to undertake such a thing? The answer is reflected by a blend of short-term thinking by corporate executives and Wall Street investors motivated in large part by fears of risk. Executives are often more troubled about how an increased perception of risk will cause their stock price to be punished by investors than the premium that might have to be paid at a future date. And, frankly, many of the executives understand that the future premiums to be paid will be someone else's problem. On Wall Street, there is a constant drumbeat of "What have you done for me lately (meaning this quarter)?" The life cycle of a drug that takes ten years or more is of little interest to them.

Worse than even the "voodoo economics" of this strategy of "release and catch," the damage done to the parent company is compounded by the fact that the best and brightest of their researchers will necessarily have been shed to populate the new fledgling company. Once successful, these newly enriched individuals are highly unlikely to return to "the mothership." Over time, such outcomes diminish the excellence of the parent company, generally resulting in an enrichment for mediocrity and low morale for those remaining in the parent organization. Despite the apparent self-immolation of this strategy, the approach continues to be aped. Yet, it seems inevitable that the release and catch trend, like shots on goal before it, is destined to be short-lived as the quality and quantity of talent, not to mention the number of parent companies, will invariably diminish as the futility of this short-termism becomes apparent and takes its toll.

In retrospect, "release and catch" combined with "repurposing" was received with open arms and high expectations. The laying off of pharmaceutical projects and staff, either as a consequence of mergers and acquisitions or catch-and-release approaches, created a temporary bubble in the creation of new biotechnology companies in the early years of the new millennium. Many investors and entrepreneurial founders exuberantly took stakes in a myriad of companies that were birthed simply to act as "lambs to the slaughter," created in order to be quickly acquired, albeit with a high premium.

As is generally the case, smart money begat dumb money. Stated another way, years of experience, backed by generous financing, increases the likelihood of success, even in a business as volatile and fickle as pharmaceuticals. We define dumb money to be that offered by less sophisticated investors and entrepreneurs simply seeking to make a quick buck rather than those willing and able to objectively assess the merits and risks of ventures and industry knowledge that may require many years of nurturing and millions of dollars before a payoff can be achieved.

The consequence of an influx of dumb money is often the creation of a bubble, which will inevitably burst. As we will soon see, Dr. Kinch's work at Washington University revealed one sign of a problem with a change in new biopharmaceutical company formation. The rate of founding of a new biopharmaceutical company peaked in the first decade of the 21st century. Never mind that many of these companies were virtual (with few or no permanent employees) or were created to advance a single product that had been shed by another risk-averse company who did so to keep their research and development expenses to a minimum. Or that only a limited number of experienced repeat entrepreneurs were responsible for a disproportionate amount of the valuation generation (eventually, allowing them to retire). The mere creation of these companies, combined with the shots-on-goal mindset, generating much wealth for a relative few, and high expectations.

Another troubling sign of future problems showed itself in the ashes of the 2008 global financial crisis. A sharp reduction in interest rates might have provided an opportunity to invest cheap money into the research and development of new products or even the creation of new subsidiaries (lambs to the slaughter) to develop much-needed products for corporate pipelines. Instead, most large pharmaceutical companies elected to buy back shares, with thirteen of the largest companies alone returning over fifty billion dollars using this mechanism.[13] This was a further sign, if needed, that the mainstays of pharmaceutical research and development, established pharmaceutical companies, had lost confidence in their own ability to conduct research and development, a dire outcome of decades of Eroom's Law.

However, not all the news was bad. There was some cause for optimism: a handful of organizations were bucking the trend toward mediocrity and embracing innovation. One bold experiment was conducted by Johnson and Johnson, a giant in the pharmaceutical and medical device world. The inspiration for a new way of thinking about innovation occurred when a leader in the field was bitten by a bug to do so.

Shaking the Cradle

Melinda Richter was born to a poor family in rural Saskatchewan.[14] After graduating with a bachelor's degree from the local provincial school and an MBA from INSEAD (a business graduate school in Fontainebleau, France), she was recruited by Nortel, a high-flying international telecommunications company, and soon was on a fast-track to become a senior executive, which included frequent travel all across the world.[15] During one visit to Beijing in 1996, Richter was walking through the woods when she was bitten by an insect. Although she was a vibrant young woman of twenty-six, she quickly found her health to be in rapid tailspin, and she started to suffer from debilitating fever and pain. She was diagnosed with an unknown form of meningitis and informed that it was unlikely she would survive. Not willing to just curl up and die, she used her little remaining energy to get second opinions, but each delivered the same verdict.

All but one.

A London-based physician commissioned by Nortel helped identify her disease as a form of scarlet fever and this diagnosis allowed physicians to intervene and save Richter's life. With a new lease on life, Richter, though not trained as a scientist, decided she wanted healthcare to be "as sexy as telecommunications."[16]

Upon looking into the pharmaceutical industry, Richter appreciated the absurdity of requiring a company to raise millions of dollars to outfit laboratory space and billions more to bring a drug to the market. Inspired by a desire to promote research into new medicine, she established Prescience

International, a management firm that could provide the infrastructure for aspiring drug developers.[17] Her initial efforts resulted in the creation of forty-thousand square feet of research space located in the San Francisco Bay area, a hotbed of biotechnology activity. Unlike other realty firms, Prescience International offered budding scientific entrepreneurs rental space and equipment at as little as five hundred dollars a month. Recognizing that specialists trained in science often lack business experience or acumen, Prescience also offered courses in entrepreneurship and fundraising, which were complemented by Richter's recruitment of investors, nonprofit foundations, and established pharmaceutical companies to coinhabit the same space, thereby facilitating interactions among these individuals.

This model proved successful and by the beginning of 2012, Richter allowed her company to be taken over by an old pharmaceutical industry war horse, Johnson and Johnson. This relationship allowed Richter to expand to the region around San Diego and La Jolla, another biotechnology center of gravity. Prescience International was renamed JLabs and offered rents considerably below market rates. Richter's approach has proven highly successful for her clients and for Johnson and Johnson, which does not receive any preferred rights to companies incubating within JLabs, but does receive an opportunity for J&J to monitor the progress of innovative companies up close. J&J maintains this model, allows it to more than break even, and has expanded JLabs to eight sites around the world, with affiliates found in an additional five locations. This innovative approach offers a glimpse at how an entrepreneurial culture has begun to grow, if not within, then nearby, the largest and most established pharmaceutical companies. However, the question remains as to whether the model presented by JLabs will be sufficient to staunch the flow of damage caused by excessive industry consolidation and cuts to research and development.

This need to adapt exhibited by industry giants such as Johnson and Johnson reflects a larger and widely misunderstood trend that has overtaken the biopharmaceutical industry in the past few decades. As we have already seen, a wave of entrepreneurial activity began to flourish in the 1970s with the advent of the biotechnology revolution.

It is broadly assumed that we remain in the midst of a durable period of biotechnology entrepreneurship. However, we will soon review recent work from Dr. Kinch's team at Washington University that has revealed potential problems with such an assumption. Before doing so, we need to focus upon another major transition that has dramatically changed the activities of both established and start-up biopharmaceutical companies: the rise of contract research organizations.

Snap, CROckle, Pop!

As you may recall, an analysis of the industry reveals that we have lost nearly half of the companies developing new medicines since 2003, due almost entirely to industry consolidation. The remaining predator companies in this food chain financed these mergers and acquisitions in part by cutting internal programs and staff (the self-lobotomy as graphically detailed above). Recalling the "food chain" concept where the large sharks are increasingly compelled to reinvigorate themselves with a steady diet of ever-smaller fish, we now invoke the idea of additional prey to this thought experiment: tiny fish and microscopic krill.

Consistent with this micro-sizing of many companies, "capital efficient" and "lean" have become buzzwords in the biotechnology industry. Such ideas reflect a tendency for new companies to maintain a skeleton staff meant solely to guide an idea through to FDA licensure or, more likely, to seal the acquisition of the small fledgling company by a larger one. In the extreme (which is no longer regarded as such due to its commonality), many companies are utterly virtual, lacking physical headquarters, and retaining no full-time staff. These smallest organizations may indeed act solely as shell companies for investors. Nonetheless, these companies satisfy a need, given the dearth of feed material for established companies, and a symbol of the changing form of entrepreneurship that had been the mainstay of drug development for the past half century.

These virtual organizations accomplish their missions through outsourcing to a cadre of contract research organizations (CROs). Many of these contract-centered organizations have been created and staffed by former pharmaceutical employees who banded together to sell their services. For example, a St. Louis-based CRO named itself Seventh Wave to reflect the fact that its founding staff were former Pfizer employees, all of whom had been laid off in the seventh wave of Pfizer cutbacks. Although these CROs unquestionably have relevant experience, they work on a fee-for-service basis and generally lack control over or interest in the grand strategic vision of the projects they advance but instead participate as is required and affordable to their clients.

The trend toward CROs has been embraced by even the largest pharmaceutical giants. For example, Pfizer announced the disbanding of much of its clinical research infrastructure more than a decade ago, replacing it with a partnership with prominent CROs.[18] Sensing a trend (and presumably suffering from a fear of missing out), other pharmaceutical companies followed suit. However, one must wonder at the disillusionment that has undoubtedly taken over the boardrooms as executives failed to appreciate that the disbanding of their own teams created a major vulnerability. The disbanding of internal capabilities created a dependence upon CROs, which allows the contractor to increase the cost of their services ad libitum. Indeed, discussions with colleagues at many of these same companies reveal a desire to break free from CROs but these emotions are countered by a recognition that the expenses needed to reestablish such activities internally would be cost-prohibitive. Worse still, these executives realize that their past talent has since dispersed and that they would be unlikely to find, much less lure, potential replacements. The escalating costs to perform research with CROs instead of internally has guaranteed further conformity to Eroom's Law for at least the foreseeable future.

Nonetheless, the question arises whether capabilities and "efficiencies" enabled by CROs have enhanced entrepreneurship or are taking place at sufficient levels to counter the destructive consolidation tendencies that have characterized the biopharmaceutical industry over the past few decades.

To test this idea, Dr. Kinch's team in St. Louis compiled a list of all campaigns to develop new medicines that have ever been tested on people in those countries that keep records, including the United States, Canada, Australia, Japan, China, and most European nations. The fact that the fundamental information needed to gain approval for a new medicine is widely shared by different nations, means national borders have become irrelevant for most medicines. The Washington University study examined both approved and experimental drugs and aggregated information about the organizations (both private and public sector) that had contributed to the research and development of these medicines. This was not an easy undertaking and entailed a review of more than 160,000 different clinical trials, ultimately yielding information about tens of thousands of investigational medicines (most of which have not yet or will never be approved). We identified tens of thousands of experimental drugs that have been sponsored by a large number of private sector companies (more than twenty thousand companies), that span everything from the top predator sharks through the lowliest krill, many of which are entirely virtual, as previously pointed out.

Much to our surprise, this effort to catalog clinical trials was particularly challenging as much of the information provided to the government organizations, such as the National Institutes of Health (NIH) and the Food and Drug Administration (FDA), was error-prone and otherwise ambiguous. For example, our experience suggests that roughly one in five pieces of even the most fundamental information, such as the name of the drug or company sponsoring it, is inaccurate or confusing.[19] The cumulative outcome of these mistakes, intentional and otherwise, created an opacity that confounded a clear analysis. We therefore decided to address these ambiguities and, years after beginning, were finally able to start shedding light upon trends in pharmaceutical entrepreneurship.

When looking over the long run (from the 17th century onward), the formation of new companies that participated in drug discovery was a rare phenomenon until the years after the American Civil War. By 1865, there were a total of three hundred and fifty different organizations involved in pharmaceutical research, most of which were universities. Only sixty private sector companies were included among these innovators and most of this limited subset were involved in developing food, vitamins, and other products that can be obtained today without a prescription at your neighborhood pharmacy or nutrition store.

The century following the Civil War witnessed a steady rise of pharmaceutical companies. During the period from 1865 to 1965, 575 total companies were formed to create new medicines, largely in the United States. Of this number, 501 were still extant and conducting research and development in 1965. Stated another way, if one looks back to the earliest beginnings of the pharmaceutical industry (defined in our studies as the foundation of Merck in 1668), more than 87 percent of these organizations were still active and pursuing the investigation of new medicines as of 1965. This might sound like a large number but again, consider that most were primarily involved in retail sales (of vitamins and such) and that this number reflects a global census (not merely American companies).

Our findings also showed the impact of the biotechnology revolution. The period from 1970 through 2000 witnessed an extraordinary wave of biopharmaceutical entrepreneurship. At the beginning of the new millennium, the number of biotech companies anywhere in the world that had created at least one experimental medicine stood at 2,344, of which 78 percent were dedicated to new drug development. In this time period, an average of nearly sixty new companies were founded each year. In 2000 alone, 184 companies were created. Even in the carnage created by the bursting of the dot-com bubble, this rate had increased to just over 200 new companies founded in 2007. In short, the robust creation of new companies made the biopharmaceutical company seem like an enterprise still on the rise. But beneath the surface, it was a different story.

As we have already seen, the creation of these companies was occurring at a time when established pharmaceutical companies were already appreciating the effects of Eroom's Law and pulling back from the earliest and riskiest stages of drug discovery. This creates a bit of a chicken-and-egg phenomenon blending the rise of entrepreneurship with opportunities created by pharmaceutical industry recognition of their growing inefficiency. Consistent with our theme of the ever-growing pharmaceutical enterprise, these activities came with the creation of not one, but two entire industries, encompassing discovery-stage companies and the venture capital industry backing them. Understandably, both sets of institutions sought to maximize their revenues and profitability, and this contributed both to further adherence to Eroom's Law and to increasing drug prices.

Looking back, an unintended consequence of industry cutbacks helped to propel entrepreneurship, albeit temporarily. As we have already seen, a seemingly inevitable consequence of the consolidation trend was that the bringing together of two large companies compelled the shedding of both research programs and staff. In many cases, the detritus from one financial event created the feed material for another. Specifically, bands of scientists that had worked on a program sometimes came together to champion a forlorn project. They might raise venture capital and begin anew as an entrepreneurial spinout. Such opportunities could provide a temporary reprieve for an industry that would become increasingly hungry, searching for new opportunities to sustain the ever-growing industry giants arising from the ashes of consolidation. Likewise, the human genome project of the 1990s brought to the fore scores of opportunities to identify potential new medicines, especially for a spate of rare genetic diseases, a subject to which we will soon return.

Notwithstanding these temporary respites, a sudden retraction of financial resources compounded by steady adherence to Eroom's Law seemed to become increasingly apparent in the days following the 2008 recession. The number of companies established to develop new medicines has dropped by nearly a third since 2007. Unlike the situation in the days following the dot-com debacle, the rate of new company formation did not bounce back for at least a dozen years thereafter (and still had not as of the writing of this book in the year 2020).

Although a decline in the creation of new research companies may not sound particularly ominous, it must be considered in the context of two other trends. The financial risks associated with Eroom's Law contrasted with a burgeoning low-risk generics medicine industry. Indeed, one-third of the more than seven thousand pharmaceutical companies created since the 1980s were devoted solely to generics medicines or to technologies meant to deliver known medicines in new ways (e.g., extended release to decrease the frequency a medicine must be taken, or delivery to specialized sites in the body, such as the eye). Nonetheless, the remaining five thousand or so companies committed to drug research might be presumed to be more than sufficient to meet the insatiable public desires for new and better medicines.

Unfortunately, even this number of five thousand is a bit deceptive as it does not reflect the impact of industry consolidation. Recent studies conducted by Dr. Kinch's team at Washington University have revealed that nearly two-thirds of these pharmaceutical research companies have already been purchased or disbanded (figure 1). This figure reflects all pharmaceutical companies ever created over the past three-and-a-half centuries, from 1668 (with the foundation of Merck) through 2020. Even more troubling is that half of this total has been lost since 2013 alone. Putting this into perspective, the number of companies that either fail outright or are subject to consolidation has exceeded two hundred in each year since 2015 and surpassed 300 in 2019.

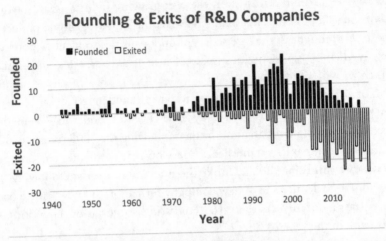

Figure 1. Rise of the Pharma Industry Consolidation
Declining number of companies with experience in the research and development of an FDA-approved drug. The positive axis indicates companies founded each year whereas the negative axis shows when a company exited (out of business or purchased; reproduced from data provided by the Center for Research Innovation in Biotechnology (CRIB) at Washington University in St. Louis).

Compounded by a drop in the formation of new organizations, our findings suggest a net loss of one hundred fifty companies per year. You may recall the concept of the "spillover effect" as defined by Bernard Munos. This concept suggests that the efficiency of the pharmaceutical industry has widely benefited from the rise in the ever-increasing number of organizations involved in research and development that predominated from the end of the American Civil War through the 2008 recession. Given the rapid loss of companies over the past few decades, it seems reasonable to assume that, at a minimum, the benefits of the "spillover effect" are likely to evaporate, if they have not done so already.

Worse still, the rate of net loss of companies (i.e., the number created minus those dissolved) has been accelerating and now stands at an annual loss of 300 companies worldwide (though the majority are located in the United States). Even were we to freeze this rate of loss at its five-year average, a decline of only 150 companies per year would be sufficient to deplete the total number of extant companies within fifteen years.

The situation is worse still if one limits themselves to companies that have achieved the lofty goal of scoring an FDA approval. This is a rarified subset of companies, totaling just over 550. As indicated in figure 2, most of these "successful" organizations have succumbed (almost entirely to mergers and acquisitions), leaving just over 150 still extant.

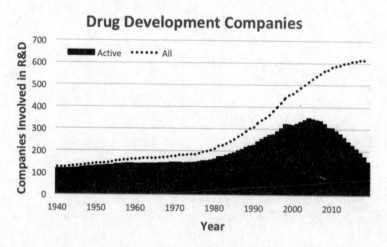

Figure 2. Impact of Industry Consolidation Graph
The dotted line shows the total number of pharmaceutical R&D companies over time. The solid line reveals the number of extant companies, revealing a dramatic loss of companies in the new century. (Results reproduced from data provided by CRIB).

We return to the idea of the pharmaceutical industry as a food chain. Using this analogy, all but a handful of the current nineteen hundred pharmaceutical companies would be regarded as small fish or krill, and this number, which has already shrunk by one-third since 2013, seems insufficient to maintain the larger fish and sharks, presumably dooming the top predators to extinction, or, using another analogy based on biology, to a period of dramatic, punctuated evolution, characterized by disruptive change.

It might seem logical to presume that the combination of the "pharmaceutical treadmill" and Eroom's Law is responsible for the escalating costs of new medicines. But it is just one facet of the price balloon. Converging information reveals that research costs by the biopharmaceutical industry, as exorbitant and flawed as they are, especially when coupled with the feeding frenzy of mergers and acquisitions (M&As) in the past decade, may have now been eclipsed by expenditures on sales and marketing alone.

CHAPTER EIGHT

As Seen on TV

I t seems impossible to avoid the ceaseless array of advertisements for the latest pharmaceutical products. The airwaves ring with commercials touting new medicines for diabetes, heart disease, and arthritis, along with the requisite and rapid listing of potential side effects. Not only is it rare to encounter a commercial break free of pharmaceutical advertisements, but one can craft a game by counting strings of competing commercials for a single clinical indication, such as psoriasis.

The saturation of pharmaceutical advertisements has fomented rather vigorous debates in both the workplace and homestead. Among industry professionals, a point of contention is whether a typical company expends more resources on research and development or sales and marketing (aptly referred to in many companies as its S&M).[1] As with most parts of the pharmaceutical pricing story, and consistent with the themes running throughout this book, an objective conclusion is not possible given that available data are so frustratingly opaque. For example, we witnessed earlier in our story that some studies are done solely to expand sales rather than make a significant public health contribution. Hence, it seems that an objective analysis reveals that sales and marketing expenses have indeed surpassed new product research and development spending. Distractive finger-pointing about which activity encumbers more resources nonetheless shadows the greater truth that medical marketing costs have been skyrocketing.

From a consumer standpoint, the arguments can be even more vigorous than the professional jousting between scientists and salespeople. In many households, including Dr. Kinch's, a rolling fight frequently dominates the dinner table as to relative value (or damage) caused by direct-to-consumer (DTC) advertising. Such arguments have triggered considerable indigestion, compelling repeated trips to the medicine cabinet (and thus working in a way to benefit the pharmaceutical industry). A common argument in support of direct-to-consumer pharmaceutical promotion maintains that television and print advertising makes the endpoint consumer aware of new treatment options. This contention states that a limited amount of quality time spent with a personal physician often does not provide ample opportunity for patients to learn about potential therapies. Consequently, a consumer must be their own advocate and be ready to use their limited time with their physicians to pepper them with requests for prescriptions and thereby to gain access to the newest pill or treatment of their choice. Of course, the opportunity for the average consumer to be misled is staggering, considering how advertising can subconsciously influence literally every facet of our lives, from love to health to politics.

This view is countered by a more rational response that only the collective experience gained through years or decades of education and experience can suitably allow physicians to appropriately recommend the best treatment from a growing armamentarium of available medicines. Moreover, the ongoing opioid and antibiotic-resistance crises are largely a consequence of inappropriate self-prescriptive advocacy from patients (and relatives) demanding remedies, along with, as a June 21, 2020, *60 Minutes* episode pointed out, the willingness of certain unethical doctors to rake in extra dollars at the expense of their patients misinformed (or malintent) insistence.[2] This argument concludes with the understanding that consumption of too many pills can cause unexpected interactions with the potential to confer considerable harm.

Though the authors might have made their own views on this clear, this is a debate that has occurred in households throughout the nation. In fact, Ms. Weiman can confirm this by reflecting on many heated debates about the pros and cons of DTC advertising with her now-deceased father, who thought such practices were another example of the fall of American morality into a den of greed, self-interest, and iniquity. For so long as pharmaceutical advertisement remains a part of popular culture, arguments will rage about their relative value or harm. Like many impassioned subjects, this one is fated to resemble contemporary and highly polarized politics or more accurately, a skit from the 1970s version of *Saturday Night Live*'s "Point/Counterpoint" with Dan Aykroyd and Jane Curtain. Specifically, such arguments inevitably become entrenched into a discussion of good (my view of the world) versus evil (everyone else's).

To suggest that such arguments are new or different from those fought by prior generations would be a mistake. Indeed, medical advertisement has been around for centuries and yet there is something markedly different about what is occurring today. To better understand this progression, and how it contributes to the rising cost of medicine, we first need to understand the history of pharmaceutical advertising, beginning with its unregulated, halcyon days.

Peppering Your Doctor

The advertising of new remedies is as old as media or indeed communication itself (recalling that the earliest discussions of medicines could be simplified as advertisements for "Eat This, Not That"). Prior to the creation of modern regulation of medicinal advertising, the propaganda utilized to market products went essentially unchecked. A prominent example was the rage to implement chain-smoking of cigarettes as a treatment for asthma.[3] No less a personage than the French novelist Marcel Proust, a lifelong asthmatic, adopted and advocated for this approach.[4] In a 1901 letter to his mother, he remarks with sincere wonder that, "Yesterday after I wrote to you I had an attack of asthma and incessant running at the nose, which obliged me to walk all doubled up and light anti-asthma cigarettes at every tobacconist's I passed, etc. And what's worse, I haven't been able to go to bed till midnight, after endless fumigations, and it's three or four hours after a real summer attack, an unheard of thing for me."[5] Some of the more cynical readers might even conclude from this statement that cigarettes might have perhaps worsened his respiratory distress (cough, cough).

Indeed, the practice of cigarette therapy for asthma persisted for a hundred years from the mid-18th century onward, driven largely by advertisement from tobacco companies. In some cases, the tobacco was cut with leaves from the stramonium plant (AKA devil's snare, a name that couldn't possibly be associated with harm). This medicine product was eventually removed from the shelves of pharmacies, not because it caused active harm but because Canadian teenagers in the 1960s were mixing crushed stramonium-laced cigarettes with water as a cheap means to induce out-of-body hallucinatory experiences.[6][7]

A less dangerous and even less effective medicinal outcome was achieved by another consumer product with an impressive-sounding name. In 1885, a Brooklyn-born pharmacist by the name of Charles Alderton had set up a practice in Waco, Texas. His business, Morrison's Old Corner Drug Store (named for its owner, Wade Morrison), was known for its soda fountain. It seems Alderton felt his adopted home was in need of a bit more pizazz and so created a "brain tonic" meant to stimulate the nervous system and promote memory.[8] The resulting concoction consisted of no fewer than twenty-three herbs and spices mixed with phosphoric acid into a secret formula. Texans could receive this mysterious remedy by walking up to an employee at Morrison's and asking them to "shoot me a Waco." The product became a hit and Morrison sensed great opportunity at a scale well beyond Waco or even Texas. The resulting product, Dr Pepper,[9] was patented and would thrive well beyond its creators, succeeding largely as a result of intensive advertising of its "brain tonic" properties.

Despite its supposed claims and names, Dr Pepper is not a medicine. Nor is Coca-Cola, a product created a year after Dr Pepper as a remedy for morphine addiction. These products and others were eventually called out for their lack of medicinal properties and would even be subject to federal lawsuits in the months following passage of the 1906 Pure Food and Drug

Act. The authors of that landmark legislation failed to include language to prevent companies from making "false therapeutic claims" in their advertising, a verdict that was brought to the fore by the United States Supreme Court in their 1911 judgment of the *United States v. Johnson.*[10] Consequently, the claims made to support various "snake oil" products would go unchallenged for a bit longer.

The situation had seemed to change for the better in 1912 with passage of the so-called Sherley Amendments, so named to recognize the sponsor of the key legislation, Kentucky Democrat, Joseph Swagar Sherley.[11] The much-needed modifications to the 1906 Pure Food and Drug Act outlawed false therapeutic claims but left a loophole that the law could only be enforced if the accused had intended to defraud the public. In practical terms, this loophole was a massive tunnel, and false claims continued to abound until these legislative defects were corrected with the passage of the 1938 Federal Food Drug and Cosmetic Act.

In what would be a surprise to most consumers today, the decision as to whether a drug could be obtained solely by those with a prescription or what we would recognize today as over-the-counter (OTC) was largely determined by pharmaceutical manufacturers and distributors.[12] Indeed, the ability of Americans to self-medicate had been labeled a "sacred right" up through the time of the Second World War.[13] This approach created obvious conflicts of interest and opportunities for disaster. The highs and lows of this imperfect solution included advertisements for pediatric cocaine or morphine-based toothache drops and soothing syrups that were simultaneously marketed to help both teething babies and their exhausted mothers.

Such oversights persisted until 1951, when two former pharmacists-turned-legislators, Hubert Horatio Humphrey Jr. of Minnesota and Carl Durham of North Carolina, ushered through legislation to distinguish medicines that could be dispensed with or without a doctor's prescription.[14] Pharmaceutical advertisement would now bifurcate, with medicines deemed safe enough for OTC sales supported by direct-to-consumer advertisements while prescription drug awareness targeted only medical practitioners. Indeed, a contemporaneous study revealed that in 1958 alone, the pharmaceutical industry had commissioned nearly 4 billion pages of advertising in medical journals, not to mention almost 800 million pieces of direct mail to doctors and 20 million on-site visits to physician offices.[15]

An unintended consequence of the well-intended Humphrey-Durham legislation was that the prices of OTC and prescription drugs began to trend differently, with higher prices for prescription medicines being justified by the assertion that these latter products had a more limited clientele. The industry could also contend their need for reimbursement for the additional costs to support the publication, mailings, and physician visits.

The split between the pricing of OTC and prescription drugs also triggered a second unexpected outcome. Whereas advertisements of OTC drugs were older than the United States itself, prescription medicines were held to be more sacrosanct. Pharmaceutical companies found themselves reluctant to initiate direct-to-consumer advertisements for fear of alienating themselves from medical professionals, whose participation would be needed to write prescriptions. These doctors and their supporting professional organizations were themselves fearful of loosening their grip and ceding power to a consumer, who might demand a particular medicine that might have no efficacy or worse still, cause unwanted side effects. Indeed, the American Medical Association has repeatedly voiced its opposition to direct-to-consumer advertisement, the most recent being a blunt call for a ban in late 2015 (inspired perhaps by comparable limitations on advertisements for cigarettes and alcohol that had been previously put in place).[16]

We have already seen how the thalidomide disaster triggered public outrage and vigorous action by Congress in the form of the Kefauver-Harris Amendments. The rapid response was due in part to the fact that the nation was already outraged at the perceived less-than-honorable practices by the pharmaceutical industry. A famous example was a 1958 claim by Pfizer in its advertising to physicians that Diabinese, its new medicine for diabetes, conveyed an "almost complete absence of unfavorable side effects."[17] The company stood by this claim in 1960 congressional hearings, even in light of evidence that more than quarter of patients prescribed the medicine had shown signs of severe liver damage.[18]

All the while, advertisements for new prescription medicines continued to be solely directed at medical practitioners, which reflected the prevailing concept that only health professionals had sufficient training and experience to recommend new medicines. However, a consumer culture that had relentlessly accelerated since the end of the Second World War militated against such control and pushed back. In particular, the battle cry of this movement centered upon patients' rights, the idea that a patient should have access to as much information as their prescribing physician.

In the immediate wake of thalidomide, the push for direct-to-consumer advertisement suffered a temporary setback with the passage of the Kefauver-Harris Amendment. This legislation included language discouraging DTC advertising by drug companies. As memories of the thalidomide tragedy faded, support for drug advertising regained momentum, emphasizing the fundamentally American notion that individuals had both a right to know and to take control of vital decisions regarding their health and livelihood. Although many consumer groups were opposed to DTC advertising, the FDA was bombarded with information that consumers wanted more information about the prescription medicines they had been ingesting at ever greater quantities since the Second World War.[19]

To offset growing rancor, the Food and Drug Administration put forward in 1969 a new set of regulations for pharmaceutical advertising, which opened the door a bit while still protecting consumers.[20] Although the advertising of prescription medicines were still limited to medical journals, largely due to industry reluctance to step on the toes of either the FDA or healthcare providers themselves, all professional advertisements were required to entail a "true statement of information to describe side effects, contraindications (i.e., circumstances when the medicine should not be used) and effectiveness." In particular, the regulators insisted that all potential side effects should be communicated to physicians, not merely the most common. These advertisements also required companies to provide a balanced view of the risks and benefits of medicines and include a summary of the risks in the labeling of the drug. This regulation might be regarded as the genesis of the fast-talking list of potential dangers rapidly conveyed in many television advertisements. As of the time these changes were enacted, the average consumer still did not have access to advertisements or commercials as the FDA continued to discourage direct-to-consumer advertisements. This stance, however, was about to change.

The Better to See You with, My Dear

A few short years after the 1969 FDA guidance, the first crack in the advertising ban on medical products came into focus and from a rather unusual source. Bausch and Lomb had developed the first soft contact lens and began a full direct-to-consumer advertising campaign. Despite the fact that the advertisements were found in mainstream newspapers and magazines, Bausch and Lomb maintained this campaign was merely targeting optometrists. As advertisements began appearing in local newspapers, their viewing triggered public outrage and inevitable congressional hearings to look into the practice. In testimony before the Senate Select Committee of Small Business on July 7, 1972, the president of the Soflens division of Bausch and Lomb touted the company's product and stated Bausch and Lomb had no control over whether these advertisements would cause physicians, in turn, to advocate for the Bausch and Lomb brand to consumers.[21] The committee seemed satisfied with this answer and the outrage over advertisement slowly faded, relegating the question of direct-to-consumer advertising to return to the back burner for another decade.

As too often seems to be the case, vaccines provided a source of controversy in the early 1980s. Many of us unwittingly walk around with a potential killer in our head. This is not a judgment on the mental health of our culture but rather the fact that a swab of the nose and throat reveals the presence of a bacterium known as *Streptococcus (Strep) pneumoniae.*[22] This bacterium makes it a life's work to test the effectiveness of our immune systems, making its way around the warm, wet environs of our throat and lungs, seeking a weakness in our body's defenses. The bacterium frequently falls down into the lungs but is eliminated and swept away by our powerful immune responses. However, these defenses might buckle or fail in the face of age or infection with another pathogen such as the influenza virus (or SARS-CoV-2). This damage or distraction could allow *S. pneumoniae* to take hold of the lung and, as its name suggests, to cause a dangerous form of pneumonia.

In aging adults, *S. pneumoniae* outbreaks can be quite deadly indeed. Each year, the bacterium manages to cause disease in nearly a million elderly Americans. When allowed to do so, the disease quickly overwhelms the lung, consolidates its hold and causes a form of pneumonia sufficiently dangerous to require the hospitalization of nearly half of those infected. Sadly, roughly one in sixteen of the hospitalized victims of *S. pneumoniae* will succumb to the disease. The situation is far worse if the victim's lungs are compromised by disease, immunological weakness, or age. Indeed, *S. pneumoniae* in 1918 conveyed the coup de grâce for millions of people around the world whose lungs had been weakened by infection with so-called Spanish influenza.[23]

To combat the disease, Merck developed a vaccine in the early 1980s to bolster the body's defenses against *S. pneumoniae*.[24] Beyond the ground-breaking research and extraordinary public health implications of this breakthrough, the story of Pneumovax impacts our story because of a fateful decision made not in the Merck's laboratories, but its boardroom.

In late 1981, the company decided to initiate a direct-to-consumer campaign to advertise Pneumovax to the general public.[25] The rationale of the company was that the elderly, who might benefit the most from their new product, should be aware that the vaccine was eligible for reimbursement from Medicare. To convey information to this population, the company began a six-month experiment, a print advertising campaign in *Reader's Digest*, a publication favored by older consumers. The company then monitored consumer awareness as well as physician reactions to the advertisement. A second campaign launched the following year. These experiments revealed that consumers had been informed while two-thirds of physicians viewed the advertisements favorably. Company executives reported to a concerned congressional subcommittee that they did not intend to continue advertising.[26] History has proven otherwise.

The first crack in the bulwark against DTC advertising had been made by Merck using a relatively small chisel.[27] The next assault against direct-to-consumer advertising was, by comparison, a grenade. The organization responsible for this explosion was Boots, an English chain pharmacy, which had historically served as a pharmaceutical retailer, rather than manufacturer. In an attempt to diversify, Boots had taken the rather unusual step of developing its own medicines. In 1964, the company introduced into its stores a powerful new painkilling medicine known as ibuprofen, which did brisk sales. A decade later, the company sought to enter the American market and first tested the waters by granting a nonexclusive license to ibuprofen to Kalamazoo-based Upjohn, which branded the product as Motrin. By the early 1980s, the patents had expired on ibuprofen, which meant Boots would no longer receive royalties from Upjohn's sales in the United States. Consequently, Boots decided to go around its former partner and introduce some of its own medicine into the US market and, in doing so, created a pain for regulators.

To overcome the sizable lead that Motrin had over its own ibuprofen product, Rufen, Boots initiated a direct-to-consumer advertising campaign. This decision was the brainchild of a young marketing professional fresh out of college who was not swayed by the conventional wisdom of the time that DTC ads were anathema. In 1983, two years after the Merck print campaign to support Pneumovax, a twenty-five-year-old Liz Moench developed a television advertisement featuring a chalkboard talk from Boots's CEO, John Bryer.[28] The advertising campaign by Boots, like that of Merck, was for a limited time and market, targeting the Tampa, Florida, print and television market.[29] By today's standards, the advertisement seems quite tame, merely pointing out that Rufen was less expensive than Motrin and that Boots, not Upjohn, was the company that developed the product (though not mentioning Upjohn by name).

The idea of placing the advertisement was passed under the discerning noses of officials at the FDA and received no negative response. In May 1983, Boots began their limited but combined print and television advertisement campaign. However, the company would soon find that the action did indeed provoke a vigorous response in the form of a politely worded cease-and-desist letter from the FDA. The regulator did not compel Boots to stop, but instead sought a voluntary moratorium on direct-to-consumer advertising. Although compliance would be voluntary, the FDA did demand that any future advertisement should eliminate any content that would suggest how and for what the medicine is used, which of course would step on the toes of the American Medical Association and other physician advocacy groups. (According to the nonprofit reviewer, Open Secrets, hospitals and doctors together have an even more powerful Washington lobby than the pharmaceutical industry based on lobbying dollars spent.[30]) The FDA suggested that Boots's pioneering advertisement would be allowed to continue if it merely focused upon the differences in cost between Rufen and Motrin.

Although it was the target of the Rufen campaign, Upjohn responded with its own ads, not for Motrin (which was still the market leader and hardly damaged by Rufen encroachment) but rather for a new and what would prove to be a surprising medicine Upjohn had developed years before.

Hair Today, Gone Tomorrow

In 1979, Upjohn gained an FDA approval for a new hypertension drug known as Loniten (generic name minoxidil). Although the drug was the umpteenth drug approved for the treatment of high blood pressure, its distinguishing feature was a rather beneficial side effect. From its earliest testing in clinical trials, patients who were balding and also taking Loniten noted a regrowth of hair.[31] Though not yet approved as a treatment for baldness, word of this property spread and Upjohn sought to encourage the momentum (adhering strictly to its effects on blood pressure) by advertising the drug in print and over the airwaves, causing fur to fly in many quarters. Soon the company was recording robust sales, not necessarily for hypertension as tablets were being crushed and mixed with water and alcohol to create a topical treatment for baldness that was administered with an eyedropper.[32]

By the time that Upjohn had been granted FDA licensure in 1988 for its topical minoxidil product to prevent baldness, the ceiling on direct-to-consumer advertising had been utterly shattered. In 1984, a who's who of pharmaceutical giants had testified under oath before Congress in staunch opposition to pharmaceutical direct-to-consumer advertising (including Upjohn), but these commitments proved to be a bald-faced lie. In a true sense of the word, Upjohn would be dismantled as a consequence of the advertising boom, for as we have already seen, increased advertisement-based revenues allowed the company to be acquired by Pfizer in 2002.

No fewer than two dozen additional DTC advertising campaigns would be launched between 1985 and 1990. The FDA would attempt to rein in some of the companies with one example being a rejection of the original name for the hair regrowth formulation of minoxidil as Regaine (not so subtly suggesting that consumers would utterly restore their natural hairline). Ultimately, the name would be tweaked to a more acceptable Rogaine, though it retains the name Regaine in the United Kingdom.[33]

Likewise, the FDA erected barriers for a later campaign for another so-so hypertension medicine with an entirely different side effect. An early television advertisement for this Pfizer product featured happy couples passing a lingerie store, which led the male to smile and sprout devilish skull protrusions. However, the FDA was hard-pressed to allow these advertisements to continue as they deemed the commercials implied men would become "horny." The irony is nearly comical given that the product in question was Viagra, and its rather well-known side effect was a physiological one, not psychological.[34]

The denouement of the DTC ban occurred in 1994 with the rise of the new speaker of the house, Newt Gingrich. The Georgia republican labeled the FDA and its leader, David Kessler, as the "number one job killer" in the nation, citing their heavy hand in regulating pharmaceutical advertising.[35] Kessler had been an opponent of unregulated advertising, left in 1997, and the agency soon lowered or removed many of the hurdles (and safeguards) frequently cited by Gingrich loyalists.[36] One rather troubling action taken in response to congressional pressure was that television advertisements did not have to convey a comprehensive list of potential side effects, just a small number that were considered "major risks."

In the days and weeks after Kessler's departure, industry spending on direct-to-consumer advertising exploded. Whereas spending on television advertisements had yet to exceed a billion dollars per year in 1996, this number would be closer to six billion ten years later (figure 3).[37] Likewise, the number of advertisements would rise from 79,000 in 1997 to 4.6 million in 2016 (figure 4). The rate of increase in DTC advertising spending has slowed in part because of new technologies that cost less than traditional ad buys in print and television. In particular, internet-based advertisements can provide greater efficiency in identifying and messaging to particular markets. Nonetheless, a quick flipping of channels reveals no shortage of television advertisements. Indeed, a 2011 study suggests the average American sees no fewer than nine separate pharmaceutical advertisements each day, which equates to sixteen hours per year.[38] And this number merely reflects advertisements conveyed over the airways on television, not including online exposure, radio, or print.

Direct to Consumer Advertising

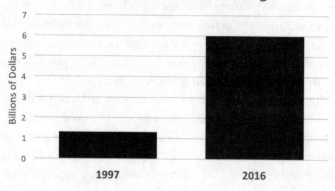

Advertisement Frequency

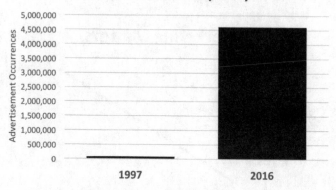

Figures 3 and 4. Rise of DTC Advertising/Comparative Bar Graphs
Figure 3. Pharmaceutical spending grew more than four-fold in the twenty years between 1997 and 2016 (adapted from Schwartz, LM, Woloshin, S. Medical Marketing in the United States, 1997-2016. JAMA. 2019;321(1):80–96. doi:10.1001/ jama.2018.19320). Figure 4. The frequency of direct-to-consumer advertisements grew dramatically from 1997 to 2016 (adapted from Schwartz, LM, Woloshin, S. Medical Marketing in the United States, 1997-2016. JAMA. 2019;321(1):80–96. doi:10.1001/jama.2018.19320).

Although six billion dollars in annual spending on television ads might sound like a large number, it pales in comparison with the total number of dollars spent on overall marketing costs. Because of the opacity that we have and will continue to encounter throughout our story, the exact amount of monies used to promote pharmaceuticals are virtually impossible to divine. In fact, anyone who has ever tried to read the financial statements of a biopharmaceutical company realizes that such costs are collected under categories such as "cost of sale" and "selling, general and administrative costs," making it difficult if not impossible to discern the various actual costs specifically for sales and marketing. Researchers at Dartmouth University suggest that the level of overall spending for pharmaceutical marketing had blossomed from $17.7 billion dollars in 1997 (the year after Kessler left the FDA) to nearly $30 billion in 2016.[39] The bulk part of the spending consisted of 663,000 television advertisements broadcast across the United States and this same report indicated that in the same time period, regulatory oversight had declined precipitously.

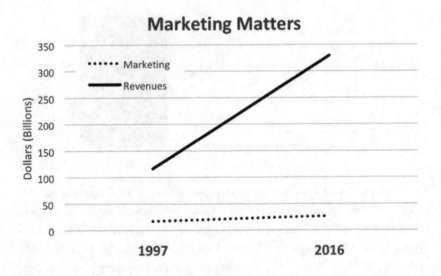

Figure 5. Graph of Cost vs. Revenue Spends

These results compare marketing costs versus revenues, revealing a dramatic return on direct-to-consumer advertising (adapted from Schwartz, LM, Woloshin, S. Medical Marketing in the United States, 1997-2016. JAMA. 2019;321(1):80–96. doi:10.1001/jama.2018.19320).

Beyond television and internet, incentives for physicians to speak about a particular medicine, free samples, and other marketing expenses totaled more than twenty billion dollars a year in 2016.[40] From the standpoint of most pharmaceutical companies, this strategy seems to have worked as intended. Over the same time period that advertising costs increased from $17 billion to nearly $27 billion, annual drug sales rose from $116.4 billion to $329 billion (figure 5). Not too shabby of an investment.

We will end this chapter as it began, with a discussion of the relative costs of research and development versus sales and marketing. A November 2014 report from the British Broadcasting Corporation (BBC) charged the pharmaceutical industry with profiteering, citing that the industry as a whole has a profit margin of 19 percent, on par with the banking industry, more than three-fold higher than automobile manufacturers, and twice that of oil and gas producers.[41] This article further went on to cite information gathered by GlobalData, an analytics firm, which indicated that nine out of ten of the largest pharmaceutical companies spent more on sales and marketing than on research and development.[42]

Although the American public might understand the need for research and development spending, they are potentially less convinced by the benefits of sales and marketing expenditures. Indeed, the BBC report was picked up and expanded by other news outlets, including investigations reported during 2015 in the *Washington Post* and Vox.[43][44] What these stories highlighted was the fact that the rising costs of medicines would be a political hot potato and likely to be a focus for politicians' wrath for years to come.

Unsurprisingly, the reaction to the BBC report was vociferous. An industry advocacy group, the Pharmaceutical Research and Manufacturers Association (PhRMA) stridently declared the numbers reported by Global-Data and the BBC to be "overstated," contending R&D levels generally exceed S&M and citing statistics about legal expenses and other costs that artificially elevate sales and marketing expenditures. Ironically, in making these arguments, the industry was pointing out that pharmaceutical companies' own quarterly and annual financial reports consolidate such a myriad of expenses into a few line items, making it impossible to clearly identify specific costs for their sales and marketing activities as compared to their expenditures on research and development.

A lack of objective data prevents one from concluding which cost is higher and the truth is that there is no magical inflection point that would change the situation were one number or the other prove to be higher. For argument's sake, let's assume that the two expenditures are equal. Recalling our lengthy discussion of Eroom's Law, which you may recall reflects the rising costs of research and development, one can safely infer that sales and marketing expenditures have been rising at a rate at least as high as the rather dramatically declining efficiencies of research and development, which is to say they have both been going up.

As it is clear that someone has to pay for the rising costs of both R&D and S&M, it is likewise reasonable to presume that both sets of costs contribute to the rising price of medicines. Consistent with the theme of this book, the growth of the pharmaceutical enterprise includes an advertising industry that is increasingly reliant upon the billions of dollars in revenues that propel it. Were Eroom's Law not sufficiently problematic to contribute to the rising costs of medicines, it seems likely that such inefficiencies (in terms of pricing at least) can be doubled by equally large expenditures on sales and marketing.

The Burden on Uncle Sam

As we have seen already, most of the costs for new medicines are borne by the United States. This fact has been responsible for considerable gnashing of teeth by politicians, payers (e.g., insurance and federal healthcare providers), and, of course, the individual American consumer of prescription drugs. In terms of the costs of direct-to-consumer advertising, the disparity seems rather appropriate as the United States is one of only two countries in the world that allows direct-to-consumer advertising (the other being New Zealand). Thus, it would seem that one way to decrease costs to American consumers would be the abolishing of this practice, a subject to which we will soon return.

Indeed, government regulation over medicines has been a hot potato for many politicians and bureaucrats. This is a uniquely American problem as most other countries, including Canada and the members states of the EU, do not allow DTC advertisement. The tides in support of this practice have ebbed and flowed, have influenced policy, and have been influenced by political events. In this chapter alone, we witnessed the impact of legislative actions such as the Kefauver-Harris Amendment and of legislative whims, such as the harsh branding of the FDA by Newt Gingrich and their subsequent loosening. Thus, it is important to discuss a few recent events that have dramatically changed the biopharmaceutical landscape and to learn how some of the unintended side effects of certain policies have had a disproportionate impact on pricing.

It is to the subject of the congressional intervention that we now turn, as arguably many key legislative and bureaucratic imperatives meant to promote public health have instead upped the costs of new medicines.

CHAPTER NINE

I'm From the Government, and Am Here to Help . . .

A s we have already seen, the Food and Drug Administration (FDA) has an outsized responsibility to expedite new medical innovation and at the same time ensure the safety, efficacy, manufacturing, and advertising of new medicines. This same agency has identical responsibilities for regulating a myriad of products that altogether, as revealed earlier, represent a quarter of American consumer spending. As a consequence, the agency, which is only modestly staffed (a euphemism for inadequately populated), was recently subjected to intense attempted politicization, which caused further strain to an agency that is thoroughly inundated with crises at any given time.

The heroic people serving in this immense federal bureaucracy have a thankless job. Francis Oldham Kelsey was but one example of an extraordinary civil servant who saved countless lives, and she is joined by many other unknown scientists and physicians who do likewise on a daily basis. Yet, the FDA seems always to be at the whipping post, accused of either slowing progress (think Newt Gingrich) or being feckless in allowing unsafe products to be marketed to the American consumer (think Vioxx). Dr. Kinch frequently gives seminars detailing the history of the FDA and its role in regulating medicines. In conveying a truly sincere respect for the organization, he nonetheless conveys the comparably heartfelt belief that he will know he has something to atone for in the next life if he finds himself serving as an employee of the FDA.

The FDA provides a science-based, nonpartisan service to ensure the health and safety of an entire nation. Yet, this agency is an arm of the federal government. As such, politics invariably creeps into the organization, often in unexpected ways. For Dr. Kinch, an October 2017 visit to meet with FDA leadership in White Oak, Maryland, began with a representative case of the impacts of politics, albeit a relatively benign example. In past visits to the FDA, the televisions in waiting areas would be tuned to any of the major news networks, with each television around the spacious lobbies showing a different channel. In contrast, all of the televisions on that Halloween morning during the Trump administration were tuned to Fox News. On the elevator ride up to the meeting room, Dr. Kinch noted the change and, with an eye roll, was informed that the new mandate was that all televisions in lobbies and public spaces were to convey the highly biased views of the commander in chief. This little incident exemplifies the challenges faced by an already overburdened staff that must conform to the whims of the reigning administration while still tackling multiple Herculean tasks all at once, the effects of which will far outlast any political trend.

Politics aside, the mandate of the FDA is in constant flux, impacted by predictably unpredictable calamities, man-made and otherwise. Arguably, the most famous example occurred in the early 1980s with the discovery of HIV/AIDS. As we discussed earlier in this book, the FDA became the focal point of criticism that claimed it was holding up the development of new medicines meant to control the raging epidemic. The headlines were filled with angry protests by organizations such as the AIDS Coalition to Unleash Power (ACT UP), which famously held a sit-in protest at the FDA headquarters (then located in Rockville, Maryland) on October 11, 1988. Yelling, "Hey, hey, FDA, how many people have you killed today," the crowd blocked the entrances to the building, forcing employees to go home.

Beyond the tragicomical irony of shutting down the agency as a means to demonstrate concern about inaction, this protest came a full year-and-a-half after the remarkable approval of the first effective drug targeting HIV. Although there can be no question that the Reagan administration was exceedingly tardy in recognizing and reacting to what would be the worst epidemic in the United States since the 1918 Spanish flu,[1] once mobilized, the scientific community in general and the FDA in particular demonstrated extraordinary nimbleness and flexibility. Following the isolation and identification of the HIV virus by a French team led by Luc Montagnier, a worldwide campaign was initiated to identify potential therapeutics. Through a combination of rigorous science and sheer luck, a failed compound originally intended for the treatment of cancer proved quite effective in blocking HIV/AIDS. In a time when the clinical testing of a new medicine alone routinely took more than a decade, the time elapsed from the laboratory-based demonstration of efficacy to FDA approval of zidovudine (AZT) was a mere twenty-five months.[2] Admittedly, it would have been even better to have begun earlier, but twenty-five months is a remarkably short time to undertake all of the discovery, development, manufacturing, and safety and clinical testing. It soon became apparent that the canny ability of the virus to mutate and thereby develop resistance to AZT propelled the need for additional medicines.

In this context, recommendations from ACT UP and other activists were heeded, and ultimately Congress passed the 1988 Health Omnibus Programs Extension (HOPE) Act. Among the provisions in this legislation was the creation of the AIDS Clinical Trials Information System (ACTIS), which provided the HIV/AIDS community with information allowing volunteers to participate in clinical trials of experimental medicines. This system proved so effective that it was expanded to include other diseases and, in the age of the internet, is best known by its website designation: ClinicalTrials.gov.

The efficiencies developed and deployed by the FDA during the HIV/AIDS crisis, both to improve clinical trial availability and to test existing drugs for potential new uses, were broadly applied to other medicines. However, as the nation approached the new millennium, the flexibility demonstrated by the FDA would succumb to a seemingly never-ending wave of tragedies that would haunt the agency for years to come. A total of twenty-four FDA-approved medicines would be withdrawn from the market from the period spanning 1997 through 2004. Among the highest profile of these were a variety of popular diet pills (e.g., Fen-Phen, Dexatrim), allergy medicines (e.g., Seldane, Hismanal), and painkillers (e.g., Vioxx, Bextra). Even one of the most popular classes of medicines, the cholesterol-lowering statins, suffered a setback when Baycol was withdrawn shortly after its release following reports of skeletal muscle destruction and kidney failure.

For a time, advertisers seemed the primary beneficiaries of these disasters as the frequency of pharmaceutical advertisements was exceeded only by commercials for attorneys seeking clients for the inevitable class-action lawsuits. On a more serious note, the outcry against the FDA increased by many decibels, with accusations that the high-profile "bad drugs" resulted from a scenario where the regulator was too cozy with the pharmaceutical industry.

These perceived outrages had been largely prompted by a series of legislative events that admittedly seemed to convey a general sense of insider dealing, not because of any reality, but instead because both the regulators and the regulated had been distracted by success and did not take the care to explain the commonsensical actions that unintentionally conveyed an insider play.

Waving Away PDUFA

When we last left off with the extraordinary scientist Louis Lasagna, he was working to provide more transparency in the activities of the FDA and the pharmaceutical industry. In August 1990, Lasagna chaired a presidential advisory panel on drug regulation and testified that "thousands of lives were lost each year because of delays in approval and marketing of AIDS and cancer drugs."[3] The panel also urged the FDA to approve drugs that not only extended the quantity of life, but even those that merely increased their quality of life. In the wake of the HIV/AIDS crisis, the agency had been roundly criticized for allowing a backlog of unreviewed new drug applications to pile up, which itself was the result of underfunding of the regulatory agency. Even the most vocal critics admitted that the FDA was trying as hard as it could, but it simply was understaffed and overwhelmed.

This fact was nothing new but its implications were merely magnified by the HIV/AIDS health crisis.

Rather than merely complaining about the FDA, which seems to be a perennial Washington sport, the panel made recommendations for future improvements. In particular, the Lasagna panel recommended that pharmaceutical companies could be given the ability to pay the agency to hire additional staff "for outside review of new drug applications by qualified experts, who have no conflict of interest." The legislation received the wonky Washington title of the Prescription Drug User Fee Act (PDUFA; pronounced "puhdoofah" for short). The idea here is not to bring people into the FDA who might be biased, but instead to create a fund that could hire more FDA staff to clear its backlog of reviews. Once above water, these additional staff could then assure that future reviews would be conducted in a timelier manner. The FDA would be happy because it could be more appropriately staffed to meet its crucial mission while the pharmaceutical industry would embrace a more rapid turnaround for reviews of new medicines. The proposal seemed rational enough in supporting an underfunded organization.

Invoking the concept that no good deed goes unpunished, the PDUFA law was misunderstood and pilloried from the outset. For example, on the day after the proposal was released, the *New York Times* published a comment from Public Citizen, Inc (a consumer advocacy group founded by Ralph Nader), which stated this approach would "undermine the authority and independence of the FDA." The vocal response largely reflected the assumption that the experts would be hired by the companies to review applications submitted by the same company, a regime that sounded quite sinister indeed. This supposition, however, was grossly inaccurate. Instead, the idea was that the FDA would hire independent staff and dedicate these to a more expedited review of the backlog of applications sitting on the desks of the agency. The application would not be reviewed with greater leniency, but simply would not sit unread on an overworked bureaucrat's desk. Indeed, one might argue that potential safety or efficacy issues might be uncovered, and disaster prevented by some future Frances Oldham Kelsey hired with the additional funding. Nonetheless, the image of an all-too-cozy relationship, generally invoking visions of dark rooms filled with cigar smoke, held sway in the minds of many concerned citizens.

Despite these misperceptions and buoyed by an upswell of patient advocacy from groups like ACT UP, Congress moved forward with PDUFA, which was signed into law by President George H. W. Bush on October 29, 1992 (five days before the election that same president would lose five days later).

Building upon the recommendations from Lasagna's presidential panel, the PDUFA law allowed the FDA to charge a fee, paid by applicant companies, that would not replace congressional appropriations for the agency, but instead would function simply to expand the number of staff available to review new drug applications. When the law went into effect in early 1993, the average fee was set at about $100,000. In response to concerns that the legislation would only benefit fat cat companies that could afford such costs (which in reality constitute a mere fraction of the costs needed to develop a new drug), Congress exempted small businesses and/or those organizations submitting applications to address "rare or unmet public health needs" (a subject to which we will soon return). The FDA in return would be closely monitored to be sure that they were indeed being more responsive to timelines and, of course, to prevent any perception of abuse arising from fees paid by industry sponsors. Moreover, Congress required that PDUFA be reviewed every five years and be subject to a new up or down vote by Congress, which could modify the legislation to improve its intended performance.

Work conducted at Yale by Dr. Kinch revealed a rather dramatic intended outcome of PDUFA. Whereas the number of new medicines approved by the FDA within a given calendar year had only exceeded thirty-one before (in 1991), no fewer than thirty would be approved in the period between 1995 and 2003, largely reflecting the clearance of a backlog of unevaluated applications. Consistent with this finding, fifty-four new medicines were introduced in 1996 alone, double the average rate of approvals in the period from 1950 through 1992.

While the FDA and the pharmaceutical industry were basking in the glow of the outcomes being generated by PDUFA, a bolus of drugs that would later have to be withdrawn due to severe toxicities (including death) were destined to soon capture the headlines. Never mind that most of the drugs taken off the shelves in the period from 1997 through 2004 had been approved before PDUFA was signed into law, the knives were out with the FDA playing the role of the proverbial turkey.[4]

The FDA responded to the withering criticism by tightening the regulatory oversight of both approved and experimental medicines. As we have already seen, the FDA required vigorous testing to identify potential risks from a particular form of cardiac toxicity that contributed to the deadly consequences of Vioxx and Bextra (among other medicines). Pharmaceutical companies thus were faced with the need for additional testing, both in preclinical animal and cell-based models, as well as during human clinical trials. Such changes were again understandable and mostly defensible at the time. However, the breadth of the new rules were ultimately applied even to medicines that would have virtually no cardiac risk (such as monoclonal antibodies) and soon be dubbed yet another "box checking exercise" that contributed to the rising costs of drug development in general and Eroom's Law in particular.[5]

This increased scrutiny of FDA caused it to rather dramatically increase the costs of drug development in a few unexpected ways, yet more examples of unintended, but in this case, quite necessary, consequences.

First, Do No Harm

The term pharmacovigilance is not used much outside the confines of the FDA and the pharmaceutical industry. This mouthful of a word refers to activities meant to ensure the safety of the medicines we take. The first known example of the practice was documented on January 29, 1848, when an otherwise healthy fifteen-year-old girl from Winlaton, England, Hannah Greener, died following a routine procedure to treat an ingrown toenail.[6] A subsequent investigation revealed that Greener had been administered a particularly powerful dose of chloroform as an anesthetic. Chloroform had only come into general use a year before and, while hailed as a needed anesthetic, most of the practitioners using the volatile gas were inexperienced and unaware of the fatal side effects arising from overexposure. As a consequence, the prestigious medical journal *The Lancet* established a group of unbiased physicians, who compiled a list of adverse effects following anesthesia with chloroform. This action would provide a model for future systems meant to track the safety record of a medicine after its approval. As recently as the mid-1990s, a spate of deaths associated with a drug intended to treat individuals infected with hepatitis B virus went undetected. This drug, fialuridine, caused liver failure but the damage had been presumed by individual pathologists to be the result of the hepatitis B infection, rather than the medicine intended to treat it.[7] Only due to stepped up pharmacovigilance was it possible to demonstrate that the medicine meant to address the disease instead worsened patient outcomes.

The situation improved in 2006 when the FDA published guidelines with the wonky title, "Requirements on Content and Format of Labeling for Human Prescription Drug and Biological Products," but which is better known as the Physician Labeling Rule.[8] These principles mandated the creation of a "label" for each prescription medicine (also known as a package insert as this is included when a prescription is dispensed) to provide physicians with a summary of prescribing information (names, doses, and uses for medicines) but more importantly, provides an overview of adverse reactions. Potential reactions deemed particularly serious and even life-threatening were prominently enclosed within a special shaded box toward the top of the profile, and these so-called "black box warnings," as they are colloquially known, would alert physicians as to dangerous problems, perhaps compelling them to think twice before prescribing. Likewise, this information was to be provided to pharmacists and patients (often found as the tightly wound wad of paper accompanying the drug), to allow them more control over their care.

The FDA has also established divisions of pharmacovigilance tasked with detecting, analyzing, and conveying information to health professionals and the general public about potential risks arising from the use of medicines. Teams of "safety evaluators," which generally consist of trained clinical pharmacists, analyze information reported to the FDA about safety and pay special attention to severe adverse events (defined as dangers that could cause death, hospitalization, persistent disability, or birth defects). The regulators also place special attention upon particularly vulnerable populations, such as pregnant women, the elderly, and the very young, to name but a few.

In 1969, the FDA had put into effect a voluntary system whereby drug companies could report adverse effects of products they were marketing. Although more than two million voluntary reports were logged into the system between 1969 and 2003, researchers estimated this represented a mere one percent of all severe adverse events.[9] [10] By 1993, this process had been digitized into a web-based system, known as MedWatch, which allows physicians and consumers to review potential risks and to report adverse events. Any information gained from these systems can be compared with the outcomes of clinical trials conducted in the lead-up to the approval of a medicine. But more recently, a major source of information used by the safety regulators arose from a very different source and this vital system nonetheless has contributed to the costs of medicine as we will now see.

An additional means to evaluate drug safety arrived in the form of legislative mandates driven by the spate of high-profile drug withdrawals in the late 1990s and early 2000s. In what has become known as the Food and Drug Administration Amendments Act (FDAAA), a series of eleven actions, referred to as Titles, were signed into law by President George W. Bush on September 27, 2007.[11] Among the titles was the renewal of PDUFA, with an interesting twist that conferred powers upon the FDA to "assess and collect fees for advisory review of proposed direct-to-consumer television advertisement of prescription drug products," thereby reflecting the prominent role of such advertisements in modern society.

We will for now focus our attention upon Title IX,[12] which would dramatically expand the amount of information gathered on drug safety and, in doing so, unintentionally contribute to the rising costs of new medicines. This portion of the legislation mandated a strict policing of "post-marketing surveillance trials," also known as Phase IV clinical trials. These trials are designed to conduct a more extensive evaluation of drug safety, such as the effects of chronic exposure, or to evaluate risks to special patient populations (e.g., the very young or old or those with potential complicating factors). Such trials had long existed but were generally carried out by physicians and could be invoked by the FDA as a condition for their approving a particular drug.

As an example of the maddening frustration of statistics, a relatively small clinical trial often does not provide enough information to distinguish low frequency adverse event "signals" from the generalized "noise" of human maladies. Although it may seem counterintuitive, a side effect that occurs reliably with a frequency of one in a hundred (which is considered an intolerably high frequency for almost any medicine) would require a trial size of no fewer than three hundred individuals to ensure there is a 95 percent chance of detecting even a single adverse event.[13]

This disconcerting mathematical truth is compounded by a trend toward ever smaller clinical trials. As we will see in the next chapter, smaller sized clinical trials meant for low incidence diseases have become quite the fashion and have unintentionally created concerns about unwanted safety problems. (Note that rare diseases—or those that only effect a small number of people—are not a new phenomenon. What is new is that prior to the mid-2000s the prevailing opinion among investors and large pharmaceutical companies was that you couldn't make money developing drugs for small populations until they decided they could make up for low volume in sales with exceedingly high prices, but we will return to this part of the story later.) Altogether, when you factor in the undermining reality of statistics, the fact that "bad drugs" such as Vioxx invariably slip through the cracks becomes understandable. As the finger pointing from that particular episode began, it was revealed that FDA-mandated Phase IV clinical trials were too often ignored and not adequately enforced, not merely for Vioxx but across the board.[14]

To avoid these nightmares, the 2007 FDAAA legislation increased the authority of the FDA to demand post-marketing safety trials. This new authority dramatically increased the number of commitments by biopharmaceutical companies to conduct Phase IV investigation and indeed, Dr. Kinch's work at Washington University reveals that the rise in the number of Phase IV clinical trials has been tremendous in recent years. Whereas 1999 witnessed 385 Phase III trials and 95 Phase IV trials (roughly a 4:1 ratio), the overall number of trials increased in the following twenty years such that there were 1,634 Phase III and 1,229 Phase IV trials in 2019 (nearly a 1:1 ratio). These outcomes are consistent with the aforementioned comment from a pharmaceutical executive that their company was spending at least as much money on Phase IV as Phase III studies.

Although there can be no question that Phase IV commitments have ensured continued adherence to Eroom's Law, the situation might become far worse. Specifically, a 2015 study published in the prestigious *British Medical Journal* analyzed Phase IV clinical trials and concluded that the sizes of these trials were often insufficient to identify less common adverse events.[15] Indeed, the pharmaceutical industry has repeatedly pushed back against what they view as onerous restrictions associated with Phase IV requirements.

Doctors and Lobbies

With a mind to the old adage of "be careful what you wish for," the granting of an FDA approval to a pharmaceutical company to allow them to begin marketing a new medicine generally marks the beginning of a new set of headaches. Invoking another adage, a coveted approval can be the proverbial straw that breaks a company's back. On the bright side, the granting of a first product approval is certainly a reason to celebrate the much-anticipated generation of revenue, especially for an upstart biopharmaceutical company that has been hemorrhaging cash, perhaps for a decade or more. As is often the case, a sophisticated forward-looking organization will have expended far more money than just research and development costs, as they build and prepare a sales and marketing team to help launch the new product (and book the print, television, and internet ads).

The reality is that the FDA increasingly requires that newly approved products undergo additional testing in the form of Phase IV trial commitments. The outcome is that while the champagne may flow in boardrooms with the receipt of the FDA approval, crucial decisions have to be made as to how to simultaneously meet the demands by the regulator to deliver more data and from Wall Street to deliver not only revenues but earnings. The inevitable outcome is that a company seeking to assuage FDA concerns over safety in the form of Phase IV clinical trials must cannibalize their own sales. Historically, companies have been loath to be their own biggest competitor (diverting a significant portion of paying customers toward clinical trials that the company must underwrite, creating a sort of financial double-whammy). The situation is compounded when one realizes that, for the entire time the new product has been developed, the patent clock has been ticking to a point when generic competition will inevitably subsume the pioneering product.

For these reasons and others, the pharmaceutical industry has developed one of the more powerful lobbies on Capitol Hill.

According to the nonpartisan and nonprofit Center for Responsive Politics, political action committees and members of the Pharmaceutical Research and Manufacturers of America ranked number four out of a total of 4,293 organizations in terms of 2018 lobbying, contributing nearly twenty-eight million dollars to politicians. As such, drug makers rank at the very top in terms of lobbying efforts by a single industry.[16]

Although lobbying tends to leave a bad taste in the mouth, not all efforts are insidious, even as it pertains to the pharmaceutical industry. Few rational-minded individuals would argue against the outcomes of a concerted lobbying effort in the 1990s, which allowed pharmacists to administer immunizations. Prior to these efforts, only physicians were permitted to give vaccines. Given the frequency that individuals visit their local Walgreens or CVS as compared to their physician, this seemed like a practical way to protect millions more Americans against annual killers such as influenza or tetanus. Certainly, the pharmaceutical industry supported such legislation as it would increase the sales of their vaccine products. However, it would be a bit harsh to presume that these efforts to promote pharmaceutical sales were not in the public's interest.[17] Nonetheless, it would be equally naïve to presume that a substantial portion of the $27.5 million spent on lobbying efforts by the pharmaceutical industry was not devoted to help stem the increasing outrage that has been building over drug pricing in recent years.

In a future chapter, we will see how these lobbying efforts have been utilized and indeed have become necessary to overcome the self-inflicted reputational damage to and by the pharmaceutical industry. For now, though, we will focus upon an example of how lobbying and well-intended legislation action caused what is arguably the most intensive strategic change in the business of the biopharmaceutical industry in its multicentury existence, and, in the process, contributed to the surge in drug pricing.

CHAPTER TEN

Odd Couplings

n this chapter, we will focus upon orphans. We are not referring to parentless children, such as the red-dressed star of the *Annie* comic strips and musical. Rather, the subject refers to a designation for a series of diseases that occur at low incidence in the United States. These diseases have historically been underserved if not entirely ignored by a pharmaceutical industry and investment community that presumed there was insufficient profit potential arising from disease that affected only a handful of people.

Those of a certain age may recall the 1992 movie *Lorenzo's Oil* starring Susan Sarandon and Nick Nolte, whose child is diagnosed with a rare genetic metabolic disorder (in this case, adrenoleukodystrophy, a disease that impairs how our bodies process foods). The malady causes progressive neurological failure, which invariably would fate their child to end up in a vegetative state and premature death. Based on a true story, the child, Lorenzo Odone, had the misfortune of inheriting a bad gene but the good luck of having affluent and loving parents with sufficient time and resources to discover a treatment for the disease (the eponymous oil that allows the child to survive).

A central theme of *Lorenzo's Oil* is the repeated frustration experienced as the parents fail to generate interest from the pharmaceutical companies to research and develop a treatment for their son. The film critic Roger Ebert gave the film four stars and stated, "It was impossible not to get swept up in it."[1] Indeed, the audience groaned as the parents repeatedly hit one brick wall after another, generally portrayed in the form of uncaring suit-clad businesspeople accurately stating that, even if a remedy could be found, it would still lose money given the extreme rarity of the disease. Ultimately, the protagonists succeed in developing their own remedy and the film ends with signs of hope, not merely for Lorenzo but for the future of those diagnosed with adrenoleukodystrophy, conveying a montage of faces of children helped by Lorenzo's oil.

Fortunately for society, by the time that *Lorenzo's Oil* premiered on December 30, 1992, a means to address the central problem of orphan diseases had been well under way. On January 4, 1983, almost a decade to the day before the premiere of the film, Ronald Reagan signed the Orphan Drug Act of 1983 into law. Like the president signing the bill, the key piece of legislation had its roots in film and television. On March 4, 1981, the NBC network aired its Wednesday night staple, *Quincy, M.E.* The show starred Jack Klugman (most famous for his starring role in *Twelve Angry Men* and the television adaptation of *The Odd Couple*) as a coroner who gave this "dead" profession new life by revealing the more exciting side of forensics (with no lack of detectives, guns and criminals and years before shows like *Crime Scene Investigations*). This particular episode of *Quincy, M.E.* had been written with help from Jack Klugman's brother.

Maurice Klugman was a Hollywood writer and producer who also happened to have been diagnosed with a rare form of cancer in the late 1970s. Awakened by his diagnosis to the dearth of research devoted to low-incidence diseases, Maurice was demoralized when he read an article in the *Los Angeles Times* about a May 1980 subcommittee meeting. A gathering of experts had been called to testify before the House Energy and Commerce Subcommittee on health and the environment, chaired by California representative Henry Arnold Waxman. The testimony of these luminaries was centered around the issue of diseases of sufficiently low incidence that fell far below the radar of pharmaceutical companies. The subject was considered of such limited interest that only the *Los Angeles Times* sent a reporter to cover the hearing. Indeed, this paper did so only in the interest of local coverage since a Tourette's syndrome patient from Los Angeles had been among those asked to testify.[2]

Although the *LA Times* had buried the story deep in the paper the following morning, this would nonetheless initiate a monumental change in the pharmaceutical industry beginning with a single reader: Maurice Klugman. Simultaneously inspired and outraged by the summary of the testimony he read that morning, Maurice began pitching an idea for a future episode of *Quincy, M.E.*

In the fourteenth episode of the sixth season, the TV coroner investigated the death of a child suffering from Tourette's syndrome who had died in a terrible fall. The plot centered around a request from a researcher, played by actor Michael Constantine, who asked for permission to study the deceased child's brain in an attempt to help find a cure for Tourette's syndrome. The rest of the episode detailed how a lack of profitability caused the pharmaceutical industry to ignore low-incidence diseases like Tourette's syndrome. The injustice compelled the show's title character to crusade for public support in front of Congress to compensate for the lack of compassion by the private sector.

In the course of developing the episode, Jack Klugman joined his brother in becoming ever more outraged by the lack of care or compassion available to patients suffering from rare diseases. In what was an extraordinarily rare circumstance at the time (though commonplace today), Klugman agreed to take up an offer to testify himself before Waxman's congressional subcommittee. Whereas earlier meetings had gone virtually unnoticed, the *New York Times* ran a story by Karen De Witt on page A16, accompanied by a photograph of what was clearly an angry Jack Klugman speaking into a microphone with a clenched first.[3]

Seated next to Klugman was Adam Seligman, a nineteen-year-old man with Tourette's syndrome, who conveyed shocking stories about how the only medicine for his indication was available overseas and "had been confiscated at Customs." The impassioned testimony in favor of incentivizing pharmaceutical companies to develop new medicines for rare diseases came just six days after the first national broadcast of the *Quincy, M.E.* episode on Tourette's. Among his comments, Klugman's appeals included, "'In this whole scenario, there are no villains, no bad guys, but there are no heroes either. What's the dividing line? How many cries before they get heard? We are not talking about orphan drugs; we're talking about orphan people."

The subject of orphan diseases and orphan people had finally broken through and captured public interest.

Nor would this be the last episode of *Quincy, M.E.* to address this issue. In its final season, in an episode titled, "Give Me Your Weak," the cantankerous medical examiner was back at it. Recalling the earlier episode, Michael Constantine returned as he and Quincy advocated for so-called orphan diseases by testifying in front of Congress. Sadly, Maurice would not be around to realize the outcomes of his seminal contributions, as he had succumbed to his rare cancer in May 1981 (two months after the earlier episode had aired).

The return of *Quincy, M.E.* to the subject of orphan indications was an example of art reflecting life. Not to mention an opportunity for a high-profile payback.

In developing the storyline for "Give Me Your Weak," Klugman had the writers include an excerpt from a real-life encounter he conveyed in an interview with United Press International in 1981. In this interview Klugman discussed a heated conversation with an unnamed representative of the pharmaceutical industry. Klugman stated, "I asked why drug companies couldn't find a cure. They told me there are only 100,000 victims of the disease so it wouldn't be profitable to invest $7 million to $50 million in research. . . . I blew my stack. What are they doing, waiting for a popular disease? Something in the top 40? . . . Congress was considering a bill to underwrite drug research on Tourette's disease, but it died in committee. The bill comes up again soon after our show airs. I hope to hell the congressmen see it."

Members of Congress did see it and the Orphan Drug Act sailed through the House of Representatives. This bill granted tax incentives, extended patent protection, and provided subsidies for both private and public sector research on orphan diseases, which it defined as indications afflicting fewer than 200,000 Americans. However, the bill became stuck in the Senate when a prominent Republican, Orrin Hatch of Utah, refused to support the tax credits, a primary incentive for pharmaceutical companies to study orphan diseases.

Klugman struck back with gusto. In "Give Me Your Weak," the character actor Simon Oakland, who had a tendency to play the roles of unsympathetic heels, adopted a persona and position remarkably and surely coincidentally similar to that taken by Senator Hatch. The episode concludes with a large crowd of protestors, who had gathered outside the fictional senator's office window, demanding passage of the Orphan Drug Act. In real life, these hundreds of protesters were all the victims or families of patients with rare diseases, which added to the impact of the television program.[4] This early intrusion of Hollywood into politics, so commonplace today, achieved its goal, and Hatch suddenly had a change of heart with regards to the legislation, embracing the Orphan Drug Act. Quoting the journalist Ezra Klein in a December 2012 interview, "Jack Klugman pretty much rolled Orrin Hatch; not an easy thing to do."[5]

President Ronald Reagan signed the Orphan Drug Act into law on January 4, 1983. The primary provisions that went into effect that day were an extended period of exclusivity, 50 percent tax credits for enabling development, and waiving of PDUFA. Given the importance of this legislation, let's translate each of these different incentives into English.

As you may recall, a period of exclusivity granted by patents is the historical means by which companies had ensured that they could carve out a market for themselves before losing it to generic competitors. As the amount of time and dollars needed to develop new medicines has increased (recalling Eroom's Law), lawmakers in the 1980s began to seek ways to incentivize companies to continue developing new medicines.

One way to do so was to grant a seven-year period of exclusivity, in which other products using the same medicine could not compete with a new drug approved for an orphan indication. This lengthened period of exclusivity was independent of whether the drug was subject to patent coverage. Consequently, this provision of the Orphan Drug Act could allow companies to find new roles for old medicines that would not otherwise be eligible for patenting.[6]

The second provision of the Orphan Drug Act was about tax credits. This in effect offered an opportunity for a company to create a new medicine for an orphan indication at half the cost, as they would receive a tax credit (i.e., deduction) for 50 percent of all expenditures incurred during the product's research and development. Given the rising costs of drug development, the generosity of this tax credit can convey an extraordinary opportunity, perhaps overly so.

The third provision had to do with waiving of PDUFA fees, obviating the charges mandated by the PDUFA legislation. Recalling an earlier chapter, these fees are charged to expedite the review of new drug applications and can easily amount to hundreds of thousands of dollars. However, these numbers fade in comparison with the major impact of the Orphan Drug Act.

The success of the Orphan Drug Act since its inception is readily apparent. In the entire history of the pharmaceutical industry leading up to 1983, a mere thirty-eight drugs had been devoted to the treatment of rare diseases.[7] In the year 2018 alone, thirty-four new medicines were introduced for this same cohort of orphan diseases.[8]

One might wonder in astonishment how it is that this fairly modest reform led to such a robust response and perhaps even reasonably question whether this subset of human maladies might be capturing an overly large fraction of the world's medical expertise and expenditures.

The aforementioned embrace of orphans did not happen overnight. A few brave companies adhered to the spirit of the law and began developing medicines uniquely suited to rare diseases. One example is the founding of a company in Cambridge, Massachusetts, known as Genzyme. As the name suggests, the company sought to develop cures for rare genetic deficiencies of enzymes. Although the story of the founding of Genzyme has been detailed in Michael Kinch's previous book (*A Prescription for Change*), it suffices to repeat that the company utilized the emerging science of recombinant genetics, which expanded rapidly in the latter years of the 20th century, to develop enzymes and other unique ways to address genetic diseases of metabolism, similar to the malady effecting the titular character in *Lorenzo's Oil*. These new protein-based treatments were made possible by complex genetic recombination techniques that tended to be far more complex than the comparatively simple chemicals that had been the mainstay of the conventional pharmaceutical industry. As we will detail in the next chapter, these drugs were far more expensive to manufacture and even more so for consumers to buy.

For now, we will focus our story on how orphan drugs changed the mindsets of consumers, physicians, and insurance providers. By definition, orphan diseases encompass a relatively rare set of maladies. Although admittedly arbitrary, as we stated earlier, Waxman's legislation defined an orphan disease as afflictions affecting fewer than 200,000 Americans within a given year. This is a poorly conceived notion as the population of the United States has narrowed considerably in recent years, which has expanded the number of medicines qualifying for orphan status. In contrast, the EU bases their definition of orphan as a percentage of the population with the disease. Although the American definition is enough people to fill two Rose Bowl stadiums, this number is sufficiently infrequent that it had induced the creation of only a handful of medicines up to 1983. Instead, the pharmaceutical industry had focused upon high frequency diseases such as hypertension (affecting 75 million Americans) or high cholesterol (affecting 102 million).[9][10]

Given the lack of market volume, it was understandable that biopharmaceutical companies would have to charge more for drugs addressing orphan diseases. Whereas conventional hypertension drugs might cost hundreds of dollars per year, an orphan drug would require a much higher price tag just to break even, assuming of course that the costs to develop the drugs would be the same. As we have learned, clinical trials to gain FDA approval generally reflect a percentage of the number of people who suffer from the disease. Although significant price premiums were always factored into the price of orphan drugs to recoup costs, it is only in the last decade or so that prices for such products have grown exponentially so they can achieve blockbuster status.

Take for instance the introduction of the first monoclonal antibody to treat an infectious disease, Synagis, which prevents respiratory syncytial virus in premature infants. Approved by the FDA as an orphan drug in 1998, it was by far the most expensive product marketed to pediatricians at the time, costing then between $600 and $3,000 per patient per RSV season. (The product is dosed on a per-weight basis and the number of doses required depended on when during the typical RSV season the child was born.) Compare that to more recent years, when the prices charged for treatments of rare diseases have routinely exceeded $100,000 and we are rapidly approaching a point where these might cost millions of dollars per year. In fact, in May 2019 the FDA approved the first drug that would exceed the $1 million per patient mark—again for the pediatric market, dwarfing the price of Synagis just two decades earlier. Developed by Novartis, Zolgensma is priced at $2.125 million and is a one-time gene therapy drug for a rare disease called spinal muscular atrophy in infants and toddlers under the age of two. About 1 in 11,000 babies are born with spinal muscular atrophy, or less than 400 babies per year.[11]

Clearly, the provisions of the Orphan Drug Act had the desired effect Congress intended—it incentivized the creation of new medicines for under-served populations. But one outcome they may not have counted on was that the prices of these new orphan drugs are increasingly higher than remedies for more common diseases. As rare diseases became ever more attractive to developers, the loved ones of those afflicted with uncommon diseases may be inspired by the mere hope that the economic incentives may continue to result in new treatments to ease the suffering of the afflicted. However, for that hope to live on, the afflicted must be able to afford the stratospheric pricing.

From the standpoint of an insurance actuary responsible for making decisions whether to pay these costs, they can often justify high prices. Such thinking focuses upon an assumption that such diseases are infrequent—or that the new therapy will offset other costs to treat the conditions. Thus, while certain one-off patients might be expensive, the extreme rarity of these cases means the overall system will not be dramatically affected. Moreover, these same actuaries face what we might call the "*60 Minutes* dilemma," where an insurance company representative must defend a decision not to cover a drug for an orphan disease. This risk might entail a high-profile interview opposite an aspiring television investigative journalist. The resultant and exceedingly negative publicity worsens further still when the statistic-quoting "corporate suit" competes in a split screen against images of a disease-wracked patient and the crying friends and family of an individual denied treatment.

Given this dynamic, a combination of legislated incentives to develop drugs for rare diseases, and the ability to charge enormous prices motivated a larger set of companies beyond Genzyme to enter the orphan drug market. The increased participation would ultimately compel many organizations to find ways to "game" the system. For examples of this, look no further than a diagnosis that spurs abject dread into many: the scourge of cancer.

A Stable Market

As a young academic cancer researcher in the early 1990s, Dr. Kinch was fortunate enough to participate in a collaboration with an established pharmaceutical company. The work was largely academic and intended to discover the underlying basis of metastasis, the ability some tumor cells gain that allows them to break away from a tumor and colonize distant sites in the body. Metastatic cells are thus generally a primary cause of the greatest pain, suffering, and death from cancer. As the work progressed, Dr. Kinch and the team identified a potential opportunity to intervene against this process. In discussions with commercial collaborators, it was asked whether this discovery might be something that the company might want to more fully embrace and develop as a product.

The response was shocking when informed that, "Cancer is generally not a disease that our company emphasizes. Think about it: Patients are on cancer medicines for a short period of time, after which they either expire or go into remission. Either way, the market is gone. We prefer pills you have to take daily for the rest of your life because that is a stable market."

Expanding upon this idea, cancer, unlike the rare genetic diseases as portrayed in *Lorenzo's Oil*, adds a further complication because the duration of treatment is so limited. For a company to earn back the monies invested into research and development, they would have to charge an exceedingly large amount of money. At the time (recalling this was the 1990s), such high costs were largely not conceivable by anyone, including doctors, patients, payors, or even the pharmaceutical companies themselves as Dr. Kinch's experience exemplifies.

All this and more changed with the increasingly widespread adoption of the Orphan Drug Act. Cancer in particular proved a means to manipulate a loophole created by the legislation. We will focus upon how a sudden paradigm shift in business strategy took place, allowing cancer to emerge from its long history of being a pariah to the darling of the pharmaceutical industry.

The results of studies that Dr. Kinch and his team conducted at Yale and later at Washington University revealed that drugs targeting cancer represented fewer than 4 percent of new medicines introduced in the 1940s to barely 10 percent of all new medicines approved in the 1990s. This all changed in the early years of the new millennium as the number of cancer-focused drugs began to grow. In a typical year over the past two decades, oncology medicines now routinely capture more than a third of all drugs approved in the United States (figure 6). Some of this rise reflects the extraordinary fundamental understanding of cancer that has accumulated in recent years. However, at least a portion of the recent popularity reflects both a cause and effect of changing views of drug pricing in general and the Orphan Drug Act in particular.

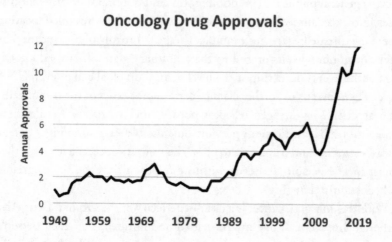

Figure 6. Growth of Cancer Drugs Graph
The number of drugs targeting cancer has grown six-fold from the late 1980s, paralleling the rising prices associated with these vital medicines (results reproduced from data provided by CRIB).

The word "cancer" is ambiguous, suggesting a disease with relatively distinct features, comparable to let us say, something like a heart attack. Patients suffering from cardiovascular diseases share certain commonalities (e.g., high cholesterol with or without hypertension). In contrast, cancer varies far more wildly among individuals. There are indeed some properties that often (not always) distinguish cancer cells, such as a propensity to grow more rapidly or survive when they should die. However, the disease within a single individual often evolves at a breathtaking rate as the end stages of the disease are characterized by extraordinarily high rates of DNA mutation and evolution. This extreme variability might mean that cells that have metastasized to one organ might react quite differently to treatment than cells at another site in the body (despite the fact both emerged from the same parent cell not many months or years before).

Our increased understanding of cancer biology has taught us that each person's cancer has to be regarded as a unique disease, each with its own "temperament" and proclivity to change. Nonetheless, physicians, scientists, and the general public still predominantly tend to lump very different diseases into exceedingly broad categories based upon the presumed location where the disease began. For example, we speak broadly of breast cancer as a type of tumor with its origins in the mammary gland. Increased knowledge of the events occurring at the level of an individual cell or even DNA molecules allows us to further classify certain properties of the tumor cells, such as HER2 or estrogen receptor positive breast cancers. While these generalities and classifications provide some usefulness in lumping different diseases together and being able to grasp their significance, the reality is that cancer in one person (and even within one person) is exquisitely variable and constantly changing.

With this in mind, cancer is a clear beneficiary of the Orphan Drug Act. Although impractical, one might defend an argument that each person's cancer is unique and that a market size of one could readily classify every tumor as being an ultra-ultra-orphan disease. Such an argument is impractical as it is essential to group like-patients into groups so as to have enough subjects to evaluate experimental therapies.

Although the argument for cancer to be considered an orphan disease is quite reasonable and defensible, this has been a point of abuse. Building upon the notion of lumping cancer together into groups, it was appreciated that treatments meant to address one particular tumor type are likely to be relevant to another. In an unconscious attempt to circumvent Eroom's Law, a process arose allowing a drug approved for one type of cancer to be recognized and reimbursed by insurance companies for other cancer applications.

Most Americans are surprised to learn that, within reason, a physician can prescribe any FDA-approved medicine for any indication.[12] Once a drug has been given the nod for marketing in the United States, the FDA largely steps aside in terms of how it is dispensed. For example, if a physician sought to prescribe a cholesterol-lowering statin drug because you broke your toe, they could do so, even if the FDA-approved labeling guidance did not include that indication. Likewise, remarkably few drugs have actually gained FDA approval for pediatric use and instead companies rely upon off-label uses for special populations, such as children.

Despite the fact that physicians are able to prescribe a medicine, the payer (usually an insurance or government organization) is not compelled to pay for this medicine. The payer might inform the pharmacist to go back to the prescribing physician with an alternative set of medicines.

The consequence of this system is that doctors, pharmacists, and insurance companies seem to perform a poorly coordinated minuet. For example, many have experienced the frustrations or delays in obtaining a prescription written for a branded pioneer medicine over a less expensive generic equivalent. Depending upon how much the doctor (not patient) decides to dig in their heels, the standoff will generally end with a compromise. Alternatively, a particularly desperate or wealthy patient might be compelled to pay for the off-label prescription purely out-of-pocket.

A very different situation can arise with cancer medicines. Given that the first generation of oncology drugs were broadly developed to kill all fast-growing cells (which includes many different types of cancer cells), a cancer medicine approved for, say, breast cancer, might have comparable activity against prostate cancer (and many do). Were each sponsor to test all of their medicines against each type of cancer (not to mention the subcategories that vary with regards to HER2 or estrogen receptor), the costs to do so would be prohibitive and likely stymie the development of cancer therapies.

Instead, payers have established or subscribed to catalogs that compile the medicines used to treat different maladies. Rather than requiring an FDA approval to justify paying for a particular chemotherapeutic regime, these consortia of payers relied upon a series of so-called compendia, which serve as recommending bodies for the use of medicines. The compendia, in turn, rely upon peer-reviewed publications of scientific studies to decide which medicines should qualify as reasonable interventions for particular cancers. Thus, a product developed for one cancer might be broadened for use in other diseases if the caretakers of a compendium have reviewed the published literature and determined there is sufficient clinical utility to justify the use of the medicine. Indeed, the resulting strategy of "compendia expansion" has immeasurably expedited the widespread adoption of new cancer drugs.

Leaving aside the fact there are multiple compendia, some of which are inconsistent with one another in their recommendations, the compendia expansion approach has proved largely efficient for advising what medicines should be prescribed and reimbursed. Indeed, this approach was well-intended and is widely regarded, perhaps overly so as we will now see.

Consistent with a theme that rings throughout this book, the unintended consequences of two well-intended improvements in drug development (compendia expansion and the Orphan Drug Act) is that the combination of these two positives has created a negative: increased costs. You may recall that a company receiving a new drug approval from the FDA for an orphan disease might understandably justify a higher price given the small market. If the company later expands the use of the medicine to other cancers, via compendia expansion, they can inexpensively enlarge the number of patients. Thus, the same expensive medicine can quite quickly expand into a large market.

There is nothing inherently insidious about this approach. After all, if one population might benefit from a drug intended to treat another, then it would certainly be inappropriate to do otherwise. However, the situation becomes far murkier when one considers that the default approach to gain the first approval for a cancer drug more often than not utilizes the Orphan Drug Act. The advantages of this approach include not merely the tax credits, increased market exclusivity, and funding provisions but the ability to charge a higher cost for the resultant medicine. This approach has proven so successful that Dr. Kinch's work revealed the vast majority of new cancer drugs are approved using such an approach. In 2018, for example, fourteen of the seventeen new cancer drugs approved by the FDA took advantage of the incentives of the Orphan Drug Act. As we have already seen, these incentives have catapulted drugs meant to target cancer to the top of the league charts in terms of FDA approvals. Cancer medicines now dominate the biopharmaceutical industry.

For Dr. Kinch, as one who led oncology research in academia and the private sector and was motivated to do so by having lost multiple family members to the dreaded disease, the dramatic attention and outcomes arising from new oncology drugs have been heartwarming. In particular, a new generation of immune-based oncology drugs, known broadly as checkpoint inhibitors, have revolutionized cancer care. These miracle drugs have provided miraculous cures for cancer patients, with diagnoses, which would previously have proven to be incurable death sentences. A high-profile example was the extraordinary recovery of President Jimmy Carter, who was suffering from metastatic melanoma and was told in the summer of 2015 that he had but a few days to live. Rather than simply saying his goodbyes to the nation (which he did and the country warmly reciprocated), Carter elected to participate in the clinical trials for one of the new immune-modulating drugs. As the nation became distracted by other news, we largely forgot about Carter, only to be shocked by an announcement in November of that same year that not only was Carter still alive and resuming his vigorous activity in support of Habitat for Humanity, but that the former president was cancer-free. The reversal of fortunes was extraordinary.

Nonetheless, these drugs are not cheap. The same class of drugs used to treat President Carter cost something in the range of $150,000 a year.[13] For the lucky fewer (somewhere between 20 and 40 percent of patients treated with these medicines), the results are stupendous, with loose talk now referring to "cures" for cancer, a concept once thought impossible. In an effort to expand these cures even further, combinations of these pricey medicines are being explored, and preliminary information suggests that a mixture of two drugs (Opdivo and Yervoy) will cost a quarter million dollars per year. Yet, even these costs pale in comparison with other promising therapies, such as genetic manipulation of a patient's immune cells, which will cost more than the combination of these two already-pricey drugs.

Given the high-profile nature of these drugs and seemingly miraculous outcomes, such as Jimmy Carter's, insurance companies were loath to question the ever-rising costs of such extraordinary advances. One might even consider that accelerating price tags desensitized many payers, both institutional and individual, to the benefits arising from a life free of dreaded diseases such as cancer. Perhaps recalling the distasteful debate over alleged "death panels" that were invoked during the debate over the Affordable Care Act, there seemed to have been a hesitancy to speak up too loudly in opposition to the costs of these new miracle drugs. Consequently, the slope of the price increases has continued.

The attention upon high-profile clinical successes and the price tolerance heightened the allure of oncology, both for new and established companies. As is often the case, venture capital poured copious money into companies seeking to market ever more complex, useful, and expensive new drugs. Many payoffs were indeed realized with sky-high initial public offerings (IPOs) for biotechnology companies, particularly those focused upon cancer, recalling the heady days of the 1990s. Likewise, even established companies joined in the frenzy, the extreme example being Bristol Myers Squibb. Buoyed by the scientific, medical, and commercial success of Opdivo and Yervoy, the venerable pharmaceutical giant announced it would scrap its portfolio of drugs meant for other diseases and focus entirely upon oncology (emphasizing its lead in developing checkpoint inhibitors).

Before leaving the subject, it is important to review lessons learned since the passage of the Orphan Drug Act. On one hand, it is evident that the combination of incentives and the ability to price the market according to its relative size created an environment that allowed both large and small biopharmaceuticals to thrive and create medicines for populations of patients that had been long neglected. On the other hand, it is not entirely clear whether the current state of affairs is what Henry Waxman had in mind in crafting the pivotal legislation.

An appalling abuse of the Orphan Drug Act occurred in the early days of the COVID-19 crisis. Sensing an opportunity to salvage a medicine that had failed to be useful for hepatitis C disease or the Ebola virus, Gilead Science began evaluating the potential use of remdesivir in the early days of 2020 for COVID-19. The company knew from experience that the incentives would evaporate once the disease had been officially diagnosed in many Americans. Gilead fought hard against the clock, not merely to assess its usefulness against COVID-19 but even more urgently to be sure that their application for orphan status would be granted before the number of infected Americans reached 200,000. Through intense lobbying, this goal was achieved on Monday, March 23, just as the nation and indeed the world reached arguably its most vulnerable and terrified point during the crisis. Corporate executives might have sighed in relief because a botched rollout of COVID-19 diagnostics meant that the magical 200,000 threshold would not be achieved until April Fools' Day, a week after the FDA had granted them orphan status. However, by that time, the question was moot because the outcry was deafening. Bernie Sanders immediately labeled the action as a "corporate giveaway," while Tahir Amin, a leader of a patient advocacy group, nicely summed up the situation with his quote, "Here's an opportunity for Gilead to come out smelling like roses and instead they've just created a stink."[14][15] Under such pressure, Gilead voluntarily gave up orphan status the next day, a nearly unprecedented move of contrition.

Despite the clear need for reform, it is unclear whether the money and emotions behind the Orphan Drug Act would support a moderation of the key legislature. For Dr. Kinch, a mere mention of revising the Orphan Drug Act triggered an extraordinary reaction. In a 2014 manuscript that reviewed trends in the development of new medicines, he and his team reported the steady rise in approvals for drugs targeting orphan drugs, which had climbed from negligible in the 1990s to more than 40 percent in the 2010s (it now stands at greater than 50 percent). The team pointed out that "given the finite amount of resources available for drug development, an emphasis upon orphan disease necessarily means that fewer resources can be dedicated to diseases that confront society at a higher incidence." The statement seemed innocuous and sufficiently self-evident that they included it in a scientific paper submitted for peer review. The response from one of the six reviewers (theoretically, rational peers from the scientific and medical communities) labeled the authors as "Nazis," accusing them of intending to "allow the small children to die." This utterly emotional response to an objective statement of fact (i.e., the availability of finite resources necessitates a responsibility to husband them appropriately) underlies the fact that the subject of orphan diseases and the Orphan Drug Act is one that holds hostage both the heart and the pocketbook.

Nonetheless, there is periodic talk, including from Henry Waxman himself, that the legislation has spun out of control.[16] A powerful lesson learned is that incentives, when properly delineated, can change behaviors. Given other lessons learned (e.g., about pricing), such knowledge can help motivate future opportunities and we will return to this subject nearer the end of this book.

As impactful as the 1983 Orphan Drug Act would become, one can argue that Henry Waxman and Orrin Hatch's most potent legacy on healthcare, and ironically, in driving up the prices of medicine, would follow a year later: the development of generic medicines.

CHAPTER ELEVEN

Generic, But Not Uninteresting

We have already learned that a distinguishing feature of the pharmaceutical industry is an ever-accelerating treadmill in which escalating research, development, sales, and marketing expenses are invested into a product that will inevitably succumb to competition from generic drugs. While most of our attention has been focused upon the innovator organizations responsible for introducing new medicines into the marketplace, it is time to turn our attention to their inevitable competitors in the generic pharmaceutical industry.

As we began studying the business of generic medicines, it became clear that this part of the pharmaceutical enterprise is every bit as complex as the branded pharmaceutical branch. And just as opaque.

Although manufacturers of generic medicines are widely presumed to provide a remedy to the skyrocketing prices of drugs, we will see that the situation is not always so clear cut. High-profile incidents and lesser-known information suggest that generics companies may be driving up the costs of medicines at least as much, and perhaps even more, than innovator companies. Rather than taking a side for or against any particular company or strategy, we will simply revert to our approach of laying out the information and allowing the reader to decide the relative merits of this interesting set of companies that also strive to deliver medicines to consumers.

In our interview with Bernard Munos, who is himself a vocal critic of the branded pharmaceutical industry, he pointed to data revealing that innovator organizations like Pfizer and Merck generally are no longer the source of the vast majority of medicines that consumers buy.[1] Indeed, objective findings reveal that 90 percent of prescriptions are filled with generic products.[2] Yet ironically, one can now see that the rise of an industry brought into existence with the goal of reducing the costs of new medicines has done exactly the opposite—yet another example of unintended consequences.

To understand the current state of generic pharmaceuticals, it is important to provide a bit of history and witness an extraordinary about-face regarding acceptance of generic drugs by medical professionals and consumers.

Although we have already seen that companies developing branded pharmaceuticals have been around for centuries, the realistic beginning of the modern biopharmaceutical industry began in the 1940s. A combination of scientific breakthroughs and the practical needs of a world at war created an extraordinary demand for revolutionary new medicines. Arguably, the greatest breakthroughs arose from the need to treat battlefield injuries, leading to medicines for bacterial infections, including penicillin and streptomycin. Likewise, increased understanding of deadly poisonous mustard gases facilitated the discovery of new cancer therapies as a direct consequence of events occurring in the Second World War.[3]

As the patents for these crucial medicines began to expire in later years, the branded pharmaceutical industry initiated a campaign to strangle generic competition. The pharmaceutical industry and its lobbying organization, the American Pharmaceutical Association (APhA; a precursor to today's PhRMA), initiated a two-front war against generic medicines.

The first arm was directed at physicians, arguing that their deeply held right to determine what medicines were best for their patients was at risk. The argument unfolded as follows: A prescription they write should be followed to the letter by a druggist. The APhA besmirched "unethical pharmacists," who "place no restraint on the ethical practice of pharmacy."[4]

The underlying argument was that manufacturers of generic medicines were inexperienced and, in an effort to cut costs, reduced quality as well. Thus, physicians were urged not to accept generic substitutes.

Complicating the situation, the industry had a track record of assigning tongue-tying names to generic drugs. Looking at drugs approved in 2015, the list includes generic names such as idarucizumab and isvavuconazonium sulfate, or if you prefer, the branded trade names of Praxbind and Cresemba, respectively. This naming strategy is indeed an old trick, as Bayer had argued in 1899 that the generic name for its branded product, Aspirin, should be 2-acetoxybenzoic acid.[5]

Now place yourself as a physician, always pressed for time with a full waiting room, deciding whether to write out a prescription (being sure the spelling is correct given the potential for disaster) for either "isavuconazonium sulfate" or "Cresemba." The choice is obvious.

Complementing this line of attack, branded pharmaceutical developers joined the leadership of the American Medical Association (AMA) to pen a series of articles that urged physicians to avoid generics. These pieces argued "a pharmacist rarely knows all the facts that a physician knows about a patient and is usually unaware of why the physician has specified one product for another."[6] Using an approach that physicians would ultimately lose control over their patients, the AMA largely stuck by its branded pharmaceutical brethren in fighting against generic interlopers.

The defensive positioning of the branded industry was further strengthened by a parallel campaign to lobby legislators. Beyond pressure on federal lawmakers (a subject to which we will momentarily return), the branded industry placed a stranglehold on generic competition in the individual states. Starting in the 1950s, the branded industry launched a campaign to enact "anti-substitution laws" (meaning laws created to prevent the substitution of a branded drug by its generic equivalent). By 1970, all fifty states had complied. Only the District of Columbia had held out and this was roundly criticized by the AMA and APhA.[7]

Although antisubstitution laws did not formally preclude generic competition, they required a patient to sign a form taking responsibility for any harm that might come from the substitution of a generic medicine for its branded counterpart. Needless to say, the resulting intimidation of the lay public largely suffocated the generics industry.

Despite these obstacles, the generics industry had established enough of a toehold to begin organizing on their own. In 1946, as the first generic medicines began to enter the marketplace, generic industry participants formed the Parenteral Drug Association (PDA), which advocated that their medicines were safe and effective in all ways, including cost-effectiveness. This organization was joined nearly a decade later by the National Association of Pharmaceutical Manufacturers (NAPM), another nonprofit lobbying group, which crowed about the health and economic benefits of generic medicines.[8]

While the generics industry mobilized, the American consumer became increasingly concerned with the prices of new medicines. By the late 1970s, a combination of the economic malaise of stagflation and the ever-escalating costs of drugs compelled the United States Senate Select Committee on Small Business, led by Wisconsin democrat, Gaylord Nelson, to take on the question of generic medicines. Of particular concern was that the branded pharmaceutical industry had created an illegal monopoly by blocking out generic drug manufacturers.

In November 1997, testimony from William Apple, leader of the NAPM, declared antisubstitution laws had been enacted in prior decades to protect the public from "unscrupulous firms that wanted to manufacture cheap imitations."[9] Yet, Apple continued, there was no longer a need for these protective measures. This same committee also heard testimony from an Illinois state legislator who had sponsored a bill to block antisubstitution laws in his state. The Illinois lawmaker revealed a lobbying abuse that arose when his committee was informed that generic medicines would "force inferior quality drugs on the poor." That claim was made by an Black man claiming to be a member of a lobbying group, Operation PUSH, led by the prominent activist, Jesse Jackson. However, further probing revealed the man testifying to be an executive working for a manufacturer of branded medicines.

Compelled by such testimony and increasing concerns held by both federal and state governments, in 1978 the FDA head Donald Kennedy commissioned the creation of a publication of all medicines deemed by the FDA to be safe and effective, including both branded drugs and generic equivalents. The resulting product would take the form of a book and would be entered into the Federal Register. This book, which was first released on Halloween 1980, was appropriately donned in a pumpkin-shaded cover and would forever be known as "the Orange Book." This book essentially conveyed those medicines that could be readily accepted by both physicians and pharmacists as being "therapeutically equivalent" and interchangeable. For the first time since its maturation, the branded pharmaceutical industry had suffered a substantial defeat at the hands of their generic competitors.

The riposte by the generics industry had only just begun.

ANDA One, ANDA Two, ANDA 56-Fold Increase

The next battle between branded and generic drug manufacturers would amount to a draw as evidenced by the clunky naming of a piece of legislation signed by President Ronald Reagan in 1984. The Drug Price Competition and Patent Term Restoration Act was a bipartisan and dual-chamber compromise championed by two former rivals we have already met, Representative Henry Waxman and Senator Orrin Hatch. Known widely as the Hatch-Waxman Act, the new law enabled generic competition by establishing something to be known as an "ANDA."

To provide a bit of perspective, a new drug application (NDA) for a medicine submitted for approval to the FDA can be a monstrous document, consisting of millions of pages of data pertaining to the safety, efficacy, and manufacturing capabilities of a branded pharmaceutical company seeking to market a new drug. Indeed, one industry executive estimated that, if printed and neatly stacked, one NDA would be as tall as the Empire State Building.[10]

The generics industry argued there was no reason to duplicate all the evidence for safety and efficacy given that approved medicines already had established a long track record. Instead, the lobbyists successfully argued that the required information should be limited to demonstrating that a generic medicine would be "bioequivalent" to the pioneering, branded drug. After considerable wrangling, the definition of "bioequivalent" was deemed to include evidence that the product could be manufactured at no worse a quality than the pioneering drug and studies demonstrating that, once administered, the generic medicine is found at essentially the same concentrations as the pioneering drug.[11] Consequently, the "abbreviated"

NDA application (known colloquially as an ANDA) might be thousands or even hundreds of pages long, considerably more compact than an NDA. As an additional incentive for would-be generic manufacturers, the legislation sweetened the deal further by offering organizations filing the first ANDA a period of 180 days of exclusivity (nearly six months), after which time other ANDA awardees could compete.

The same piece of legislation also provided incentives for the branded pharmaceutical industry. Specifically, the law granted an extended term of patent exclusivity to encompass the time that a drug is tested in clinical studies. This seemed a reasonable compromise that could hold off generic competition in the face of ever escalating times (and financial costs) needed to gain an approval for a new FDA-approved drug. However, time would show that the net effect was a huge boon for the generics industry.

Although Hatch-Waxman was a clear setback for the branded pharmaceutical industry, they still had a trick or two up their sleeves. One of the less reputable of these schemes is the so-called "pay for delay." As you may recall, the FDA will grant 180 days of market exclusivity for organizations filing the first ANDA once a branded drug comes off patent. In an attempt to minimize losses, many branded pharmaceutical companies entered into deals with the ANDA holder in which the two organizations would split the profits if the ANDA holder would agree to delay the introduction of their product (and thus delay the lowering of prices for the consumer by nearly six months). Although clearly inconsistent with its intent, this pay-for-delay scheme is technically legal. In the long run, such agreements may nonetheless prove a bad deal for both branded and generic pharmaceutical industry partners. Pay-for-delay agreements gained visibility in early 2020 as they were highlighted by certain candidates in the Democratic primary for president, including senators Amy Klobuchar, Bernie Sanders, and Elizabeth Warren.[12][13][14]

Looking back, while the generics industry certainly existed and was restricted to a small piece of the market up to the time of enactment of the Hatch-Waxman Act, the industry would explode in the years following. Indeed, the backlog of ANDA applications would grow so rapidly that a remedy, in the form of the Generic Drug User Fee Act (GDUFA), was enacted in 2012. This is a simple extension of the PDUFA measures meant to accelerate the regulatory review of branded pharmaceuticals by charging companies a fee, whose proceeds could be used to hire more FDA staff. Similarly, the GDUFA legislation allowed the FDA to charge a fee to review ANDA applications for generic equivalents.

The explosion of generic products utterly redefined the overall pharmaceutical enterprise. Sales of legacy medicines that had been the source of reliable revenues soon collapsed due to pricing pressures from generics competition. Conventional wisdom among industry professionals now presumes that roughly 80 percent of the revenues from a branded pharmaceutical product will be lost in the first year after the entry of a generic competitor, with revenues almost entirely gone within five years. As a result, the pioneering manufacturers of branded pharmaceutical companies often tend to quit the production and marketing of these medicines altogether, abandoning the market to be taken over by generic upstarts.

When Housecleaning Creates a Mess

As periodically seems to dominate the headlines, the story of generic medicines and prices is not always a positive one. For a prominent example of the dangers of bureaucracy, we turn to a story with origins from more than a half-century ago. Levothyroxine (brand name Synthroid) is a synthetic form of a hormone whose natural form is deficient in some patients suffering from an underactive thyroid gland. The symptoms of hypothyroidism can include chronic fatigue, constipation, weight gain, and, if left untreated, heart damage, coma, and death.

Fortunately, levothyroxine was introduced by German-based Knoll Pharmaceuticals in 1955 and provided a cheap and efficient means for treating hypothyroidism for decades. The drug was so ubiquitous, safe, and effective that levothyroxine was exempted from the list of medicines that had to gain a new license following the passage of the historic Kefauver-Harris legislation (following the thalidomide disaster).

This all changed in the mid-1990s, when the FDA was reviewing the list of medicines used in the United States. Despite its continued widespread use and understanding of its safety and efficacy, leadership at the FDA decided that some information on file with the agency about a subset of medicines previously approved by the agency needed to be updated.

This was accomplished by the simple filing of a notice in the Federal Register with the innocuous designator 62 FR 43535.[15] This 1997 proclamation mandated that Knoll, which had sold levothyroxine for forty-two years, must go back and perform new trials to confirm efficacy and safety or, as an alternative, file what is known as a "citizen's petition" to explain why a full data package was not necessary. The FDA justified this action by claiming a lack of information about the drug's bioavailability (where the drug is in the body after taking it). According to Bernard Munos, this was purely an unnecessary "housekeeping" decision by the FDA but its unintended consequences are still felt today.

The implications of this tidiness were immediate. The many patients, some of whom had been taking Synthroid for four decades, were left wondering whether their medicine was still effective and, if they were forced to abandon the Knoll drug, would there be safe alternatives.[16] Although the FDA tried to assure these anxious patients that their mandate was "not a public health emergency," the damage had not only been done but would soon expand quite dramatically. The situation worsened when the FDA declined the requested "citizen's petition" and demanded the full set of trials to assess bioavailability and to provide information about the stability of the drug.

The FDA warned in 2001 that it would pull Synthroid off the shelves unless its demand for updated safety and efficacy data were met. Complicating the situation further, Knoll had been purchased by Abbott Laboratories just months before and the new owner was scrambling to file the necessary paperwork amid the transition.

The consequence was that Synthroid and other forms of levothyroxine would eventually reenter the market essentially unchanged but for one key feature—the prices would be much higher. This justification for this higher price was predicated upon the need for the questionable clinical trials. In the course of researching this book, the example of levothyroxine was cited multiple times as an example of how unnecessary bureaucracy has increased prices.

Bottom Dwellers

Although the Hatch-Waxman legislation met the goal of enabling the generics pharmaceutical industry, it may have worked a bit too well and, consistent with the theme of unintended consequences, a law intended to decrease the price of medicines resulted in some of the most audacious and visible increases in drug costs and altered availability.

The headlines in recent years have screamed with stories about price gouging for drugs such as the EpiPen, Thiola, and Daraprim. In each case, the drugs subject to the price abuse were generic.

The EpiPen is a surprisingly old product featuring an even older drug: epinephrine. The first attempts at marketing of the active ingredient was in 1896, a year after epinephrine (also known as adrenaline) had been first isolated. While first introduced as a means to increase blood pressure (i.e., in heart failure patients), the drug is far better known for its ability to counter the effects of anaphylactic shock following a bee sting or other acute allergies that might otherwise be lethal. A key for expanding this medical advance into a commercial product resulted from an innovator by the name of Sheldon Kaplan working at a defense contractor, Survival Technology, Inc.[17]

The Bethesda, Maryland, company had responded to a Pentagon request for devices that could be used by soldiers in the battlefield following an attack with nerve gas. Kaplan led a project to deliver an auto-injector (a pen filled with counteragent) that could be thrust into the thigh to deliver atropine (a medicine to fight nerve gas). The beauty of the product is the lack of training needed for its deployment (i.e., stick needle in leg, that's it). Atropine-filled pens from Survival Technology were distributed to US coalition troops in the 1990–1991 Gulf War, aping the actions the Iranian military had taken given Saddam Hussein's proclivity toward using chemical weapons against the Islamic Republic.[18] As allied coalition forces gathered to retake Kuwait in early 1991, it was widely presumed Hussein might again resort to chemical weapons.

The developers at Survival Technology similarly reasoned that the same device could be used to deliver epinephrine and would later license EpiPen technology to Merck KGaA.[19] The EpiPen was not alone in the marketplace, facing stiff competition from similar products: Adrenaclick from Impax Laboratories, Twinject from Lineage Therapeutics, and Auvi-Q marketed by Sanofi. In total, work from Dr. Kinch's team at Washington University reveals no fewer than twenty-four FDA-approved manufacturers of epinephrine. However, one by one, the competitors for the EpiPen left the market, largely the result of ever-lowering prices, known in the industry as "the race to the bottom." The Adrenaclick and Twinject were both eventually discontinued, and Sanofi pulled its product due to calibration errors, which tended to deliver the wrong amount of drug.[20]

In the meantime, Merck KGaA sold the rights to the EpiPen to a manufacturer by the name of Mylan in 2007.[21] Mylan is a manufacturer of generic medicines that suddenly found itself alone in the market and took full advantage of the fact. Whereas Mylan purchased the EpiPen at a time when the average sales price was $57, it raised the price again and again, ultimately gaining infamy when the price exceeded $500. Worse still, the company embarked upon a campaign to package two pens per pack, just in case the first pen might fail, thereby doubling the price further. Again, the company saw no reason not to charge these exorbitant rates because they lacked competition that might dissuade them, so they continued their ever more expensive march toward a concept referred to as "what the market would/could bear."

A nearly identical situation arose with a serial offender. Our old nemesis Martin Shkreli ("the PharmaBro") burst on the scene in 2015, capturing the headlines for weeks when it was revealed that he had arbitrarily overnight inflated the price of an old drug (pyrimethamine, trade name Daraprim) by fifty-six fold (from $13.50 to $750). The reality is that by this time, Shkreli had long proven himself a repeat offender in pulling off such price gouging schemes. Having started his business career by short-selling stock futures while he smeared his targets with regulators and the public alike, Shkreli founded a pharmaceutical company named Retrophin. In February 2014, Retrophin acquired a struggling pharmaceutical company and increased the price of its medicine (chenodiol, trade name Chenodal) five-fold. Three months later, Retrophin acquired the rights to a drug that had been marketed since 1988. Tiotropin (trade name Thiola) had been approved using the Orphan Drug Act and was used to treat a rare form of metabolic disease in which patients have a propensity to develop excruciatingly painful kidney stones. In May 2014, Shkreli purchased the rights to Thiola from Mission Pharmacal, which had sold the product at $1.50 per pill, quickly ramping the price to $30, which was particularly painful as the average patient required a dozen pills per day. Although Retrophin continues to charge these high prices, by the end of September 2014, Shkreli was out of a job, having been fired for inappropriate activity on Twitter.[22][23]

Shkreli continued the practice of increasing drug prices at the helm of Turing Pharmaceuticals, which is where he increased the price of Daraprim by fifty-six fold. Despite high-profile attacks from Bernie Sanders and many other critics, the excessive pricing controversy would not be his undoing. Instead, he was jailed for securities fraud that arose during his time at Retrophin. Shkreli was convicted and sentenced to a seven-year stint in prison.

Retrophin, Mylan, and Turing were not alone. As egregious as these high-profile price rises would prove to be, at least the medicines they marketed were still available. Something else even darker arose from the blossoming of the generic pharmaceuticals industry.

The generics industry is characterized by a race to the bottom. What is meant by this is that competition among generics manufacturers drives prices down, which is exactly the intention of the Hatch-Waxman legislation, not to mention the fundamentals of market competition in capitalism. However, as profit margins shrink in both the branded and generics arms of the pharmaceutical industry, many manufacturers simply give up. (Remember most companies in both sectors are publicly traded and driven by their investors to deliver continual quarter-over-quarter and year-over-year increases in revenues and earnings.) A bad outcome arises when only one company is left. A far worse situation arises when there are none.

Save the Children

If you remember nothing else from this chapter, please try to recall two numbers: eighty-five and eighty-three. Eighty-five percent of children diagnosed with leukemia are cured of their disease—forever.[24] That is the good news—great news in fact. By the way, this news is not particularly new: these numbers have been achieved since the 1950s. Childhood leukemia was a death sentence before the time of the Vietnam War. Now, these diseases are cured more often than not. The successes have been so profound that we have largely forgotten about this set of diseases that used to inspire so much dread. This feeling, as with the successes experienced with many vaccines, has led us to drop our guard and now exposes us to unspeakable tragedies.

Now the downside. Eighty-three percent of pediatric oncologists report they are unable to administer their preferred cancer drug due to unavailability.[25] That's right. More than four out of five children suffering from cancer cannot get access to the drugs that will save their lives. In some cases, treatment must be delayed. This is a particularly risky option as one hallmark of pediatric leukemia is the rapid onset from symptoms to death. A persistent shortage of these drugs frequently enters the news cycle and there seems to be no let up.

The latest drug to enter the list of hard-to-find medicines is vincristine, a drug that has been on the market since 1963. A workhorse of cancer management, the prices of vincristine have been so low that many manufacturers have simply bowed out. The vincristine crisis began in 2019 when Teva, a powerhouse in generic medicines, opted out of producing it, leaving a massive hole.[26] This decision created quite the irony as Pfizer, a company known for branded drugs, now remains the only manufacturer of vincristine, a medicine that has been off-patent for decades.

Vincristine is an example of the downside of lowering drug costs too much. Although such examples are rare, they are becoming more frequent as large generic drug makers rationalize their portfolios. The increasingly dire situation with these childhood leukemia drugs reflects the limitations of a free market system, especially in an industry so beholden to the pressures of Wall Street, where the manufacturers of vital goods can leave at will. New thinking will be needed to create alternative approaches or incentives that will both assure available supplies of key medicines (e.g., private or not-for-profit companies whose missions are to deliver off-patent drugs at low margins but still ensure their availability for the purpose of public health).

The Upside of Generic Medicines

Thankfully, the race to the bottom does not always end with only one or even zero companies left in the space. For the most part, generics have met their intended goal of lowering drug costs. According to a 2019 study from the American Association of Retired Persons (AARP), the average cost of generic therapies declined by more than half when comparing 2013 to 2017 (from $751 to $365 per year). In that same time period, the average cost for branded medicines increased from $4,308 to $6,798. This clear divergence in costs is partly attributable to the impact of aforementioned trends (e.g., Eroom's Law) but also reflects the divergent business approaches adopted by companies associated with the branded and generic pharmaceutical industries.

Branded pharmaceutical companies, which have consistently been the pioneers of new medicines, have struggled since the passage of Hatch-Waxman to respond to the rising dominance of the generics pharmaceutical industry. However, new technologies have provided innovator organizations some protection against generic competition through the creation of new types of medicines that are both popular and useful. These new medicines are proving themselves to be far more efficacious, safe, and costly than any previous medicines. Yet these same drugs are particularly complex and challenging to manufacture. Consequently, these new drugs—the latest step in an evolutionary journey of the pharmaceutical enterprise—are among the most expensive products (pound-for-pound) ever created by mankind.

CHAPTER TWELVE

The Costs of Complexity

n the beginning, there were plants . . . and they were good. No, this is not a biblical allusion but a surprisingly accurate representation of the first few dozen millennia of drug discovery. Our earliest medicines were generally whole or ground-up plant products or the chemicals readily extracted from them. Natural remedies for illness and disease are evident in every culture around the globe going back through recorded history. As such, it was only natural that the pharmaceutical industry would look to such sources in the modern era, but corralling nature has proven difficult, which is where we will take our story in this chapter.

It may come as a surprise to many contemporary readers to learn that many spices used in cooking today were in fact cultivated not for their flavors, but as medicines. This very long list includes the use of paprika as a nutritional supplement, oregano for digestive maladies, and cayenne peppers for aches and pains. In fact, the vast majority of spices were cultivated and introduced into widespread use to improve nutrition, digestion, or pain.

A stroll down the aisle of any nutrition store will reveal many supposed remedies, some of which are grounded in fact. The lore behind most holistic remedies is the consequence of stories passed down through generations. While some are supported by objective science (e.g., paprika is packed with beneficial vitamins and minerals), others not so much, and, more likely than not, the perceived benefits result more from the placebo effect than anything in the supposed remedy.[1]

Loose ideas and minimal regulation create an opportunity rife with the potential for abuse. For example, while there is growing interest by the scientific community to objectively realize the medical potential benefits of medical marijuana, questionable and likely overblown claims are driving the rapidly expanding fad and legal availability of products such as cannabidiol (better known as CBD).

The inevitable scams arising from fad products such as CBD raise an interesting question of why the FDA does not more tightly restrict the nutrition market. The answer lies with some familiar characters. When we last left Orrin Hatch, he had recovered from the riposte delivered by Jack Klugman, supported the Orphan Drug Act, and cosponsored the legislation that remodeled the generics drug industry. A decade later, Hatch sponsored the Dietary Supplement Health and Education Act of 1994, which was signed into law by President Bill Clinton.

This legislation resulted from a combination of industry lobbying and celebrity pressure. In this case, the celebrity was the film star Mel Gibson, who worked with the nutritional supplement industry to create and distribute televised pressure pieces meant to support an easing of restrictions on dietary supplements. The most famous of these advertising campaigns featured Gibson's home being raided by over-eager FBI agents, who cuffed the actor for the crime of harboring a bottle filled with vitamin C capsules.[2] The consequence of this pressure campaign was the passage and enactment of the aforementioned law, which allowed manufacturers to introduce dietary supplements without the need for an FDA approval and the loosening of other safeguards for products derived from plants and herbs.

Moving Beyond Supplements

In general, plant-based interventions, including vitamins and spices, are relatively safe and inexpensive. At the same time, these same products can be quite crude, and the desired chemical components might be present in the plant but at a sufficiently low concentration to mediate the intended reaction. Taking a step back in time, this fact was recognized first by various apothecaries and later by early pharmaceutical pioneers who sought to isolate, purify, and concentrate the desired chemicals. As we have already seen, these isolation techniques brought forth a myriad of pure medicines, including aspirin and morphine. Our work suggests that the vast majority of medicines introduced into Western society before 1950 had their origins within plants, microscopic forms of life (e.g., yeast producing penicillin), or animals. For the most part, these medicines were affordable and readily manufactured, providing the mainstay for the pharmaceutical industry through the end of the Second World War.

Given the success of these early products, it is a bit ironic that so-called "natural products" (i.e., products derived from nature) fell out of fashion due primarily to cost. A telling example can be found with the cancer drug known as paclitaxel.[3] The potent chemotherapeutic compound was origi-nally discovered by NIH scientists in the bark of certain yew trees growing in the Pacific Northwest.

While the chemical was potent, it was present at low levels, and a back of the envelope calculation determined that the quantities required for human use would doom all the yews in the United States to be cut down and that would only satiate a fraction of the need for the drug. In desperation, the NIH incentivized the private sector to address the question of supply and demand by soliciting a collaborative agreement with a low royalty rate and access to materials and information gained by federal scientists about Taxol.[4] Despite a suite of incentives, few private sector organizations were sufficiently compelled to attempt to increase production. It only took one.

Bristol Myers Squibb received the contract in 1989 and within a decade, the company had not only gained an FDA approval, but had managed to rack up at least a billion dollars in annual revenues (the first cancer drug to reach this coveted mark, earning paclitaxel "blockbuster" status).[5] But there were problems.

Paclitaxel was expensive to purify, a recurring problem with natural prod-ucts. Nature has a rather annoying tendency to make highly complicated molecules that are not easily generated in the laboratory, much less scaled up for a manufacturing plant. As such, the potential inability to generate enough material to be viable as a commercial product can limit enthusiasm for natural products. Occasionally, human intervention can improve production efficiency. Indeed, paclitaxel's production today occurs through a "semisynthetic" process in which raw material produced in cells from yew trees are chemically prepared in a way that dramatically increases the yields from the manufacturing process.[6] Nonetheless, manufacturing costs remain comparatively high and one week's worth of paclitaxel (even for generic forms of the drug) routinely exceeds $13,000.[7]

To avoid the high costs of complex natural products, the pharmaceutical industry has been emphasizing what are known as synthetic drugs. Not to be confused with an entire class of illicit hallucinatory and narcotic medicines, our usage of the term refers to remedies that are manufactured using entirely chemical processes (rather than natural products or semisynthetic modifications of natural materials). These laboratory-derived drugs tend to be smaller and more straightforward than natural products. To use a technical term, a clunky natural product molecule tends to be complex, made up of many different and often exotic chemical structures that frustrate efforts to increase the ease and efficiency of manufacturing.

While the portion of a natural product responsible for the desired therapeutic activity might be located on one part of the molecule, the rest could stabilize the structure of the molecule; for example, preventing it from degrading too quickly in the body. However, this necessary but "extraneous" structure might itself, by pure chance, find itself able to interact with other molecules in the body, which in some cases can be problematic, but occasionally quite helpful. Specifically, such interactions can alter how the molecule interfaces with the body.

Another cancer chemotherapeutic agent known as doxorubicin (trade name Adriamycin) is an example of this phenomenon. This natural product is described in oncology textbooks as conveying the ability to kill cancer cells by inserting itself into tumor DNA and blocking its function, thereby freezing a tumor cell in its tracks. Upon closer inspection, at least nine different mechanisms that allow doxorubicin to kill cancer cells have been described and its range of activity reflects a complex structure allowing the drug to do many different things at once.[8] This diverse activity might appear to be an asset, since killing a tumor cell in multiple ways would seem a distinct advantage (think of the innumerable horror films in which a failure to finish off the antagonists facilitates the return of the murderer). However, in a world dominated by a nervous regulator always on the lookout for potential side effects, the idea of a clunky molecule that acts in multiple ways proportionally increases the risk for unwanted toxicities.

Beyond safety, synthetic medicines are also attractive largely because such products can be manufactured in bulk, sometimes for pennies a dose. Moreover, unique manufacturing methodologies might themselves qualify for patent protection. As we will see in the next chapter, patents are a primary means by which pioneering branded pharmaceuticals can hold off unwanted competition from generic manufacturers. Beyond the drug itself, a more efficient means of producing a drug might be patented at a later date and thereby allow the pioneering organization to retain a competitive edge. In particular, such companies seek the ability to produce at lower costs and thereby remain financially competitive with companies producing generic materials.

With the exception of a few products derived from animal and plant sources, most of the new medicines introduced from the 1950s through the 1970s were synthetic medicines. However, the world would start to change in 1982 with the dramatic introduction of an innovative new product with old roots.

Sugar Fix

The subject of high drug prices driving down the use of much-needed medicines seems to be rampant in the media in recent years, and no drug better exemplifies the issue than insulin.

Nineteen twenty-two was an annus mirabilis in medicine, arguably the most dramatic single year in biomedical research until 2020. The most dramatic findings of that year were the outcomes of four rather dowdy scientists working in relative isolation amid the glitter and bustle of the "Roaring 20s." In that remarkable year, three Canadians (Frederick Banting, Herbert Best, and James B. Collip) researching in the Toronto laboratory of a Scottish scientist (James J. Rickard Macleod) discovered and performed some of the most hasty and dramatic clinical investigations ever recorded. The impact of their discovery would bring dying children back from death's door and ultimately save millions worldwide. The largely forgotten details behind this story highlight and foreshadow contemporary issues that threaten the lives of many today.

Just eleven days into this remarkable year of 1922, a fourteen-year-old boy lay unmoving, nearly comatose, in the pediatric ward of Toronto General Hospital. Leonard Thompson had been diagnosed three years before with type-1 diabetes,[9] an autoimmune disease usually diagnosed during childhood. For unknown reasons, the body's defenses in these children have inexplicably decided to destroy the insulin-producing cells of the pancreas and do so with gusto. Those diagnosed with type-1 diabetes are unable to process sugars and for most of history were fated to a death spiral that included diabetic ketoacidosis. Craving sugar but unable to process it, the body will instead metabolize fats, creating a buildup of toxic byproducts (known as ketones) that accumulate and ultimately poison the blood and organs, causing the organs to shut down and patients to enter an inevitable and irreversible coma, dying soon thereafter.

Leonard was an outlier. He had survived three years because his parents were quick to embrace a starvation diet that minimized calorie consumption and thereby delayed the dreaded buildup of ketones. Like all the "lucky" children treated in this manner, Leonard lived only because he was slowly being starved to death with the "Allen Starvation Diet," the brainchild of a Morristown, New Jersey, physician.[10] As 1921 came to an end, the inevitable seemed to be catching up, as a thin and sickly Leonard was entering the end stage of his disease. The child had been diagnosed with ketoacidosis and was hospitalized in the diabetic ward amid other children dying of the disease.[11] Despite being packed with patients, these pediatric diabetic wards were among the quietest suites in most hospitals, as the majority of patients were either too sick to cry or were lying comatose as their parents and physicians waited for the lethal chemicals in their bodies to accumulate and end their silent suffering.

Leonard Thompson was given a chance at survival, actually two chances. Building upon results hastily but successfully conducted by Banting and his team using dogs in the laboratory, Thompson was injected with a preparation of insulin from the pancreas of a fetal calf.[12] Unfortunately, the batch of drug had been sloppily prepared and was full of contaminants. These impurities triggered a painful abscess.

Nonetheless, enough insulin had been delivered, just barely so, to allow the child to live days longer, albeit suffering from the abscess. The Canadian team worked night and day to improve the purification of insulin from the calf pancreas, and did so just in time. Two weeks later, they returned to the quiet hospital ward and, amazingly, convinced Leonard's parents to let them try again. This time, however, the results were remarkable. Within hours, Leonard began to show clear signs of improvement. The treatments continued and Leonard began to eat more, gain weight, and ultimately, the boy would survive another thirteen years, perishing from another killer, pneumonia, in 1935.

Encouraged by the extraordinary results with Leonard Thompson, the Canadian team treated another dozen patients, one at a time, learning from each experience about how to prepare and deploy their vital medicine.[13] A mere few weeks after their first human experiment, Banting's team conducted their most audacious experiment.

The doctors entered the hushed ward, which was filled with more than four dozen comatose patients silenced by diabetic ketoacidosis.[14] The team progressed from bedside to bedside, injecting each child with a bolus of insulin before moving on. By the time the last patients were being injected at the far end of the long ward, the doctors began to hear cries emerging from where they had begun. These were not the cries of agony characteristic of grieving parents, but rather of unexpected joy. Adding to the cacophony were occasional higher pitched yells from awakened children. Indeed, the insulin treatment proved so effective that the mausoleum-like nature of the ward soon rang with energy and noise, beautiful noise, of ecstatic families. Based on such dramatic successes and buoyed by scientific talks given first at Yale University and other prestigious New England and Canadian schools, word began to spread about the new miracle drug known as insulin.

From the beginning, money and power would play a role in who would get access to this new insulin miracle. An example of this limped into the Toronto clinic of Frederick Banting on August 15, 1922. Elizabeth Hughes was an underfed fifteen-year-old girl, five feet tall and weighing a mere forty-five pounds. Her malnourishment did not reflect a lack of means but rather her participation as another exemplar of the Allen Starvation Diet.[15] As his Manhattan practice grew, Dr. Frederick Allen opened the Physiatric

Institute for Diabetes and Metabolic Disorders in April 1921.[16] This would prove to be poor timing given what was to come.

Elizabeth (Lizzie) was admitted to the Allen Institute as one of its first patients. Like other patients admitted to the Institute, Lizzie was immediately put on a crash diet and rapidly shed pounds off her already slight frame. The precocious teenager was the youngest of three daughters of Charles Evans Hughes, an American political titan. Although his stature has largely been forgotten, Hughes was among the most powerful American politicians of his day (or any other day for that matter). Lizzie was born in 1907, swaddled in the governor's mansion weeks after her father took the helm of the state of New York. Charles would later be appointed to the United States Supreme Court in 1910. He left that position six years later to run for president and captured the Republican nomination. Hughes lost a surprisingly close contest to Woodrow Wilson at a time when America was melding in solidarity behind a soon-to-be wartime president.

Hughes was favored to repeat as the Republican presidential nominee in 1920 (which was nearly guaranteed to be a Republican victory given Wilson's poor health and the debilitating stroke he suffered in late 1919). Despite these extraordinary tailwinds, Hughes declined the invitation to represent the Republicans in 1920. The politician's family was reeling after his eldest daughter, Helen, had succumbed to pneumonia in 1920. As we know, his youngest, Elizabeth, had been given the virtual death sentence of juvenile diabetes a few months before that.[17] Instead, Hughes would later settle on becoming the forty-fourth secretary of state under Warren G. Harding before returning to the Supreme Court to serve as the eleventh chief justice of the United States.

Given these bona fides, the entry of the frail Lizzie Hughes into the Bloor Street office of Frederick Banting is of particular significance to our story, both in expected and rather surprising ways. Lizzie had experienced only limited success by following the Allen Starvation Diet, but her family had heard news from up north about Banting's pioneering work. The list of families seeking the new insulin cure had swamped the ability of the Toronto clinic to meet demand.

Despite his notoriety, Banting was not a terribly sympathetic personage, acting largely as an unappreciative jerk both before and after his monumental discovery. Complaining to Best, who was on vacation in Maine,

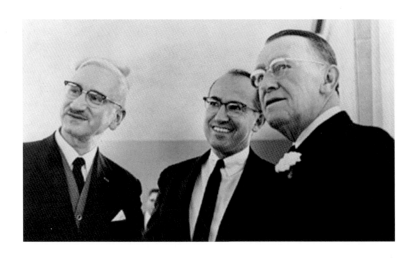

ABOVE: Albert Sabin and Jonas Salk meeting with Basil O'Connor at the March of Dimes in 1961. *Courtesy of March of Dimes.* BELOW: Trump signing the executive orders for Gilead's remdesivir (with Gilead CEO).

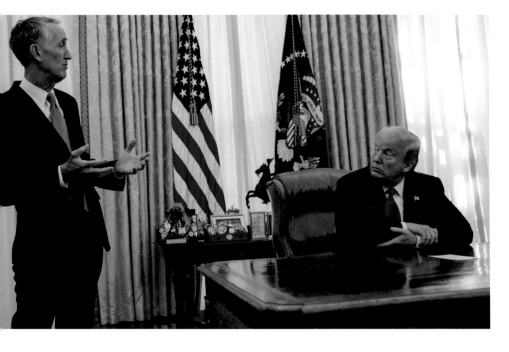

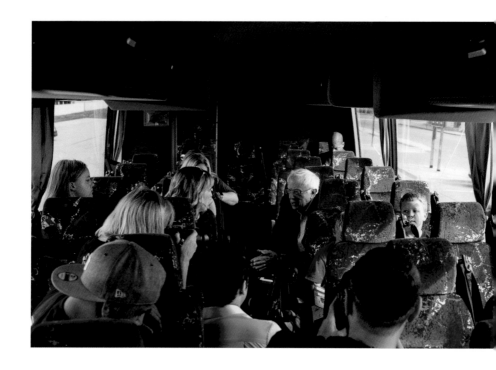

ABOVE: Bernie Sanders, medical tour to Canada in 2019. *Credit: Brittany Greeson for* The New York Times. BELOW: Martin Shkreli. *Credit: C-Span.*

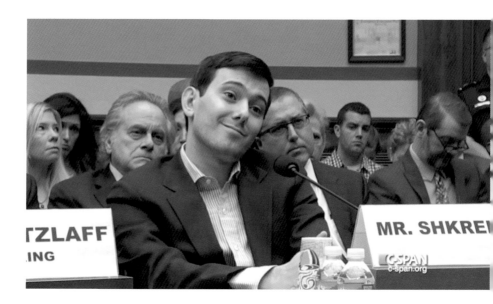

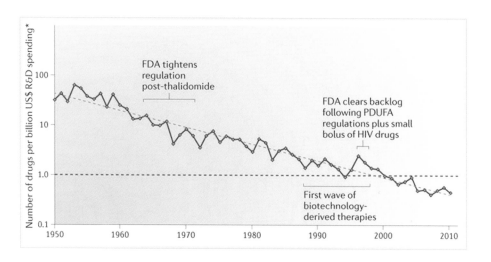

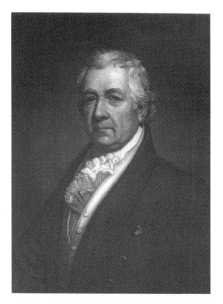

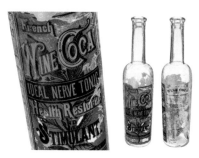

TOP: Eroom's Law. *Credit:* Nature *Magazine.*
CENTER: Samuel Latham Mitchill.
BOTTOM: French Wine cola.

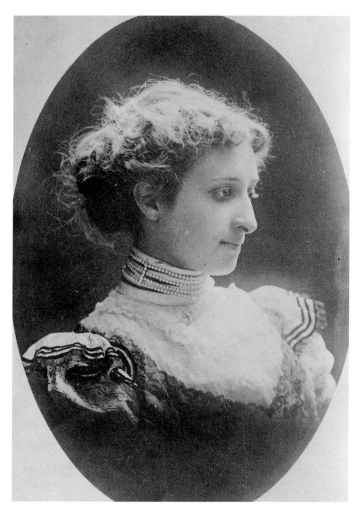

ABOVE: Cora Dow. *Courtesy of Library of Congress, Bain News Service.*
BELOW: One of Cora Dow's famous fountains.

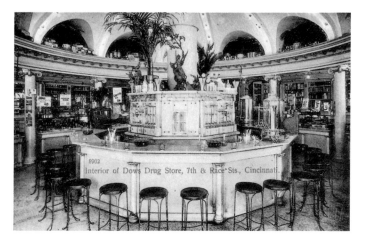

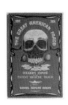

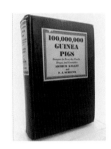

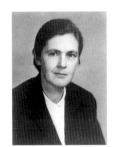

ABOVE LEFT: Upton Sinclair's *The Jungle* on the cover of *Collier's* magazine that included a headline or article from Samuel Hopkins Adams. ABOVE CENTER: *100,000,000 Guinea Pigs.* ABOVE RIGHT: Frances Oldham Kelsey. BELOW LEFT: Louis Lasagna. BELOW RIGHT: John Lechleiter, the Eli Lilly CEO responsible for Year YZ.

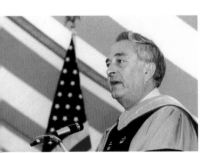

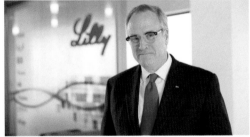

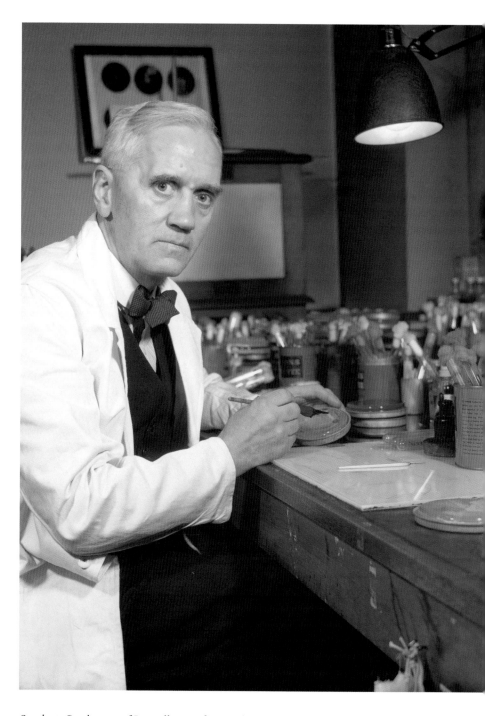

Synthetic Production of Penicillin: Professor Alexander Fleming, who first discovered the mold *Penicillium notatum,* here in his laboratory at St. Mary's, Paddington, London (photo taken in 1943).

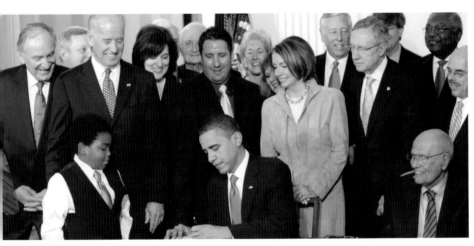

President Obama signing the Affordable Care Act. *Credit: The Washington Post Company.*

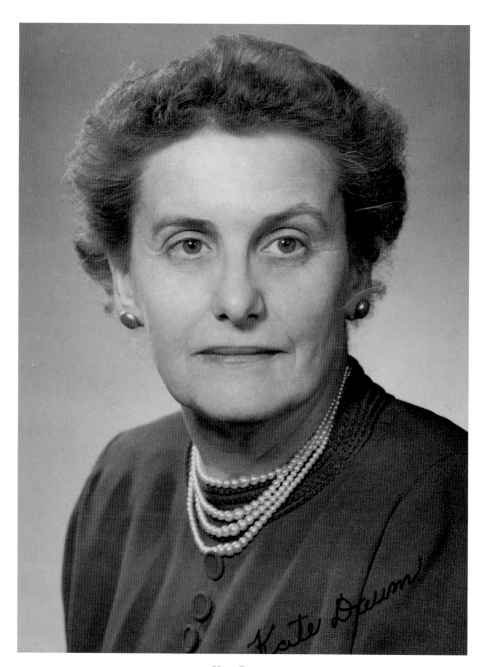

Kate Daum

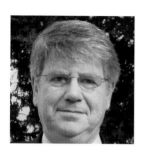 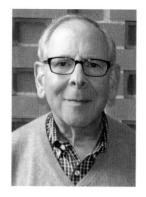 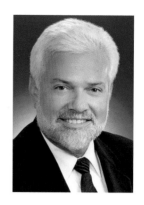

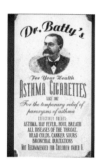 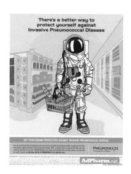 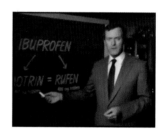

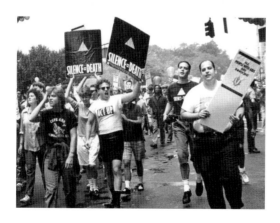

TOP LEFT: Bernard Munos. TOP CENTER: Charles Muscoplat. TOP RIGHT: Andrew Dahlem. MIDDLE LEFT: A completely Batty idea: Cigarettes for Asthma. MIDDLE CENTER: A 1981 Pneumovax Direct-to-Consumer advertisement. CENTER RIGHT: The first TV advertisement: May 19, 1983 Boots CEO touting Rufen. BOTTOM: ACT UP Protest. New York City, 1988.

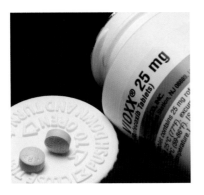

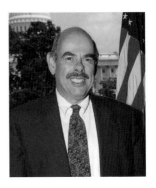

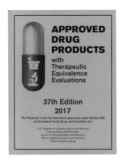

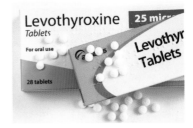

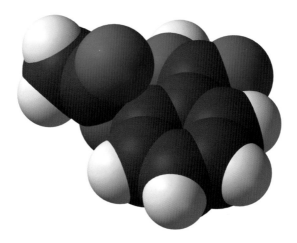

TOP LEFT: Vioxx. TOP RIGHT: Henry Waxman—the driving force behind the reform of medicines in the 1980s. CENTER LEFT: The Orange Book—The cover of the FDA listing of approved drug products was colored to commemorate the day of its release, Halloween, and thereafter has remained known as "the Orange Book." CENTER RIGHT: An example of unintended consequences arose with a bureaucratic directive to update information for levothyroxine, resulting in a dramatic increase in price. BOTTOM: The molecular structure of aspirin.

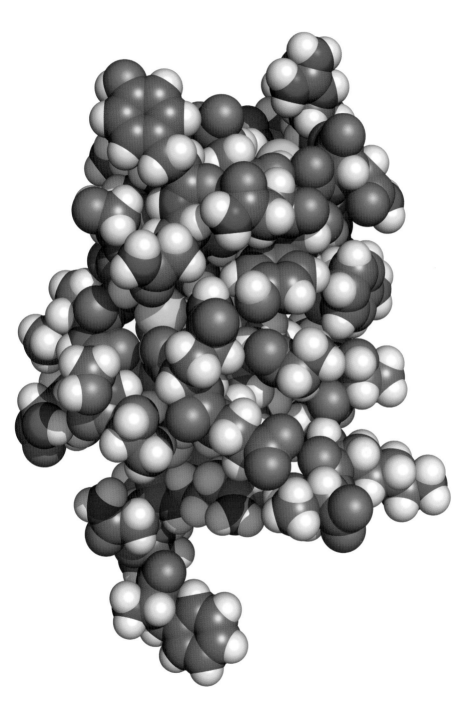

The molecular structure of insulin.

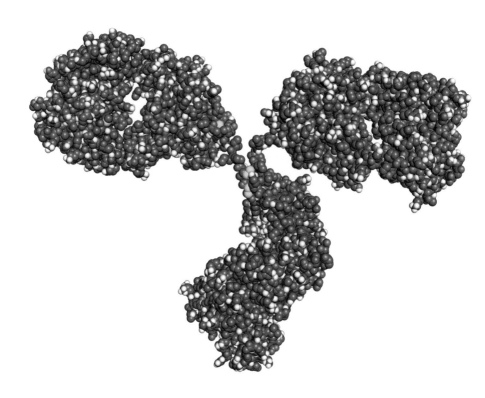

Monoclonal antibody structure.

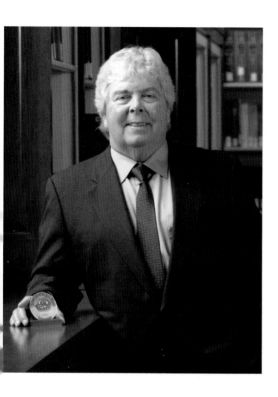

Herbert Boyer (ABOVE) and Stanley Cohen (BELOW)—Biotechnology pioneers.

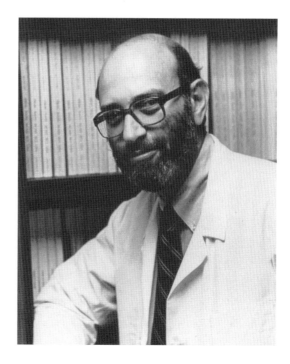

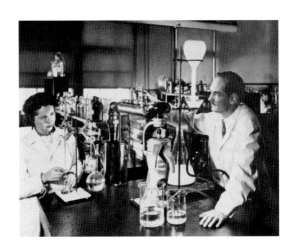

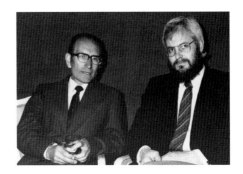

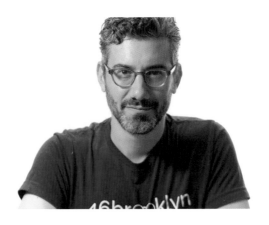

TOP: George Hitchings and Gertrude Elion.
CENTER: Georges Köhler and César Milstein.
BOTTOM: Eric Pachman—Founder of 46brooklyn.

The AMNOG procedure

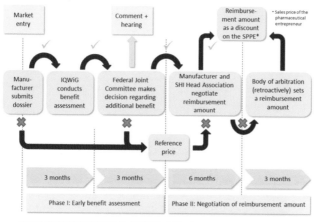

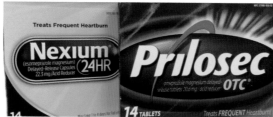

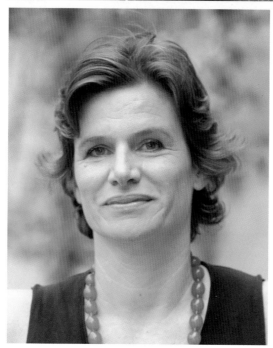

TOP: The AMNOG process overview.

CENTER: Nexium/Prilosec.

BOTTOM: Mariana Mazzucato

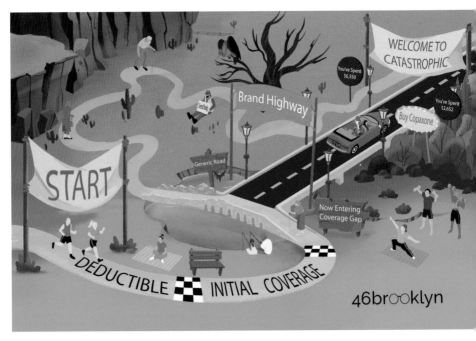

The Race to Catastrophic (from 46brooklyn).

Banting whinged, "You are a lucky one to be out of the heat that prevails here at present, and even worse than the heat as a disturbance is that diabetics swarm around from all over and think that we can conjure the extract from the ground."[18] This was, at a minimum, a callous remark about families simply desperate to save the lives of their children.

One letter did ultimately attract Banting's attention. A mother was inquiring as to the discovery of insulin, describing her daughter as, "pitifully depleted and reduced."[19] Although insulin was still in short supply and the lines for the vital substance were long, this particular mother was notable for being the wife of the rich and powerful Charles Evans Hughes. The depleted Lizzie was elevated to the top of the list.

Not only was the decision impacted undoubtedly by the patient's finances, but her stature meant that the American press would closely track Lizzie's progress.

And progress she did. The emaciated girl responded well to insulin, quickly gaining a taste for and the ability to metabolize an ever-increasing array of foods that would have been lethal before she began receiving insulin treatments.[20] Lizzie would grow in height but more importantly, her emaciated frame began adding weight at a rate of more than two pounds a week. By Thanksgiving, Lizzie had returned home and weighed 105 pounds, more than twice what she weighed during her August admission to Banting's clinic. Indeed, a 1930 photograph of Elizabeth, a year after she graduated Barnard College, reveals a healthy woman with plump cheeks. It is estimated Lizzie received 4,200 insulin injections over nearly six decades and lived to the ripe age of seventy-three, expiring from a fatal heart attack in 1981.

Lizzie's story would go on to personify the opportunities insulin offered. Unintentionally, her story would also highlight the economic disparities associated with access to expensive breakthrough medicines—and in today's world that seems to be equally true for drugs that have been around for decades, such as insulin.

According to a study published in January 2019 in *The Journal of the American Medical Association*, researchers at the Yale Diabetes Center revealed that more than a quarter of all diabetic patients had underused their insulin within the past year.[21] That is one of four people who suffer a life-threatening disease and at a time when the cure for their disease was about to celebrate its one hundredth birthday. Worse still, many of these patients did not inform their physicians of this decision and follow-up studies revealed that these same patients, unsurprisingly, had lost control over their blood sugar levels, doomed to suffer complications from a deadly but manageable disease.

Editorializing on this outcome, Elisabeth Rosenthal of *Kaiser Health News* recounted the all-too-familiar stories of the impact of insulin rationing and underuse.[22] She related the story of Alec Smith-Hold, a young restaurant manager, who was found dead of diabetic ketoacidosis in his apartment, three days before payday and with an empty vial of insulin located near the body. For the remainder of our story, we will continue to utilize insulin as an example of the pricing problem and, for now, we will return to the story that was all the rage in 1921.

Lilly-White Progress

Throughout 1921, George Henry Alexander Clowes was closely watching the progress being made in Toronto from afar. The precise definition of "afar" in this case is 528 miles, the distance from downtown Indianapolis to Toronto's General Hospital. Having been in the audience for the fateful speech at Yale University, George Clowes was destined to undertake a journey from Indianapolis to Toronto multiple times, both to track the progress of the insulin discovery and to nurture its widespread application. As the groundbreaking work advanced from the laboratory to the clinic and began to show promise, a lack of material severely hampered the drug's development. Clowes offered the services of his employer, Eli Lilly & Company, whose claim to fame centered largely upon innovative manufacturing technologies.[23] The international partnership ultimately culminated in a refinement of the techniques used to isolate and purify insulin from the pancreas of slaughtered cows (and later pigs).

As this was a comparatively early example of academic cooperation with the private sector (something seen as scandalous to contemporary academics), the Lilly offer was attractive, as escalating demand for insulin experienced its own form of a sugar rush. Herbert Best would move from his academic position to Connaught Laboratories, a Toronto-based firm tasked with producing insulin for the Canadian market. As a result of

Clowes's advocacy, Eli Lilly would be granted a nonexclusive license to market the product in the United States by mid-1922. A nonexclusive license is a contractual arrangement whereby a patent estate owned by one organization (in this case, the University of Toronto) can be licensed to multiple partners (one of which was Eli Lilly). By contrast, an exclusive license would grant the use of the patents to only a single licensee, thereby quashing competition. The University of Toronto elected to make insulin available to many manufacturers, but, in practice, the experience gained by Eli Lilly scientists in the early months of scaling up the production of insulin would provide sufficient know-how to fuel waves of intellectual property and trade secrets that would allow the company to outcompete all others for years to come.

In the months after Eli Lilly began to produce and distribute insulin, the price of the life-giving product plummeted as the product began to become widely available. Similarly, a Scandinavian professor, August Krough, visited Toronto in late 1922, leaving with an agreement to create Nordisk, an organization (originally a nonprofit institution that later transformed into a for-profit company) to market insulin in Europe. Notably, Eli Lilly and Nordisk (known as Novo-Nordisk after a merger) remain today among the largest insulin manufacturers in the world.[24] The reason for this dominance is a word and concept that we have encountered already but is worth discussing further: patents.

Patents 101

The concept of a patent is not fully understood by many.[25] At its core, a patent is a simple trade. The trade involves information for exclusivity. Let's take this apart a bit. The advancement of virtually any technical field relies upon an accumulation of information about a new technology or improvements made to increase its efficiency and usefulness. If only one person or group entirely controls information flow (i.e., keeps a secret), then the wider society is likely to be held hostage. At the same time, that company is therefore at risk were someone to steal an idea and set themself up as a competitor. As important, the wider field of knowledge will not advance if the ideas behind a new invention remain opaque.

An enlightened idea was to enact a trade whereby the publication of information for all to see (in the form of a patent) would be traded for a period of exclusivity in which the originator of the idea can obtain governmental assistance (e.g., legal enforcement) to prevent competitors from stealing their ideas. Thus, a patent is a simple trade: knowledge for a finite period of exclusivity (usually twenty years).

While patents are designed to promote technological advancement in the long term, they also incentivize entrepreneurial inventors to innovate for shorter-term financial gain. In the case of the University of Toronto, access to patents provided licensing revenues to spur companies to manufacture and sell insulin. The inventors (the university) would receive royalties (usually payments based upon a percentage of commercial sales) from companies and could, in turn, invest these royalties into their academic and public good priorities. The companies in turn are granted a legal means to exclusively market their products until the patent expires and other companies predominate (e.g., generic manufacturers). An exclusive license means that only a single partner is given rights to practice the invention, which contrasts with a nonexclusive license, where more than one company is able to commercialize a particular invention. In our example, Eli Lilly could tell the world about their new technologies for manufacturing insulin while assuring that so long as their patents remained active, they would not have to fear that their ideas might be stolen by a competitor. In interviews with current and former Eli Lilly executives, they have consistently conveyed that Eli Lilly had a long tradition of passing along a portion of the cost-savings in manufacturing to the patient in the form of lower prices that were made possible by new manufacturing technologies.[26]

As a whole, the patent process tends to work rather well. The public benefits in the short term from the fact that entrepreneurs have incentives to create new or improved means of doing things (like treating diabetes). Over the longer term, the situation gets even better because the expiration of a patent term can promote competition to make generic medicines available at even lower prices. Moreover, one must keep in mind that the fundamental trade that characterizes a patent means that the invention had been disclosed years before, allowing competitors to potentially make (and likely patent) newer improvements to that invention.

Although fundamentally sound, the situation can get somewhat out of control for new and emerging fields. Having established this framework, we will continue to follow the story of insulin and how a miracle drug helped create generations of new breakthroughs—and headaches.

For most of the past century, insulin was manufactured using material collected from the pancreases of slaughtered cows and pigs. The processes for harvesting and purifying the material improved over the decades and were protected by patents and an occasional trade secret (information deemed so sensitive or difficult to protect via patents that it is not considered worth disclosing publicly). Despite these incremental improvements, insulin still came with its own set of risks. Significantly, cows and pigs are not humans, and from the viewpoint of our humble immune systems, there can be very real and dangerous differences between species.

The immune system has evolved over millions of years to distinguish friend from foe, identifying and eliminating potential lethal bacteria or viruses. This friend/foe decision-making is quite precise, distinguishing even seemingly trivial differences. As it turns out, animal-derived insulin varies ever so slightly from its human counterpart. Proteins are made from fundamental structural units known as amino acids, and the structures can be thought of as beads on a string. Using this analogy, human insulin is composed of two strings, one with a strand of twenty-one amino acids and the other with thirty. Cow-derived (bovine) insulin differs from its human counterpart by only three of the fifty-one total amino acids and pig-derived (porcine) insulin varies by only a single difference. Although this may seem a trivial difference, it can be sufficient to mobilize the immune system to reject animal insulin as foreign, with catastrophic consequences. Although Lizzie Hughes would receive 4,200 doses of bovine and porcine insulin without rejecting it, there was no guarantee that the next one she received would not be a "black swan," recognized and rejected by the immune system. In that case, she would have been fated to reject all animal-based insulin products and could once again run a risk of succumbing to diabetic ketoacidosis. Sadly, many people over the years did indeed experience this fate. Yet, help would be on the way in the form of new technologies.

Transformation

In 1973, two California scientists started a revolution. In a manuscript published in the *Proceedings of the National Academy of Sciences*,[27] Herbert Boyer of the University of California San Francisco and Stanley Cohen of Stanford University reported the successful cloning and expression of a gene from *Xenopus laevis* into *Escherichia coli*. Translating this into English, the scientific duo was able to isolate a particular piece of DNA from an aquatic frog and place this into a common bacterium isolated from the human gut, which was then compelled to manufacture a frog protein.

While this might seem a bit of humdrum esoterica, it was a monumental discovery. The study generated considerable excitement and angst among many scientists and nonscientists alike, ultimately compelling contemporary futurists to warn of an impending apocalypse. Indeed, such ideas inspired a young Michael Crichton, already known for the techno-thriller, *The Andromeda Strain*, to pen another science-gone-mad novel you may have heard of: *Jurassic Park*.

Although the world did not end as imagined by Crichton, a new one did indeed begin. The technological ability to produce proteins from one species in another gave rise to a true revolution in medicine, one that continues to gain momentum decades later. The first product conveyed in this revolution was a rather well-worn one: insulin.

Rather than isolating insulin from cows or pigs, scientists at a small bio-technology start-up founded by none other than Herb Boyer by the name of Genentech utilized this "recombinant DNA technology" to manufacture bona fide human insulin.[28] Unlike animal-derived products, this insulin was indistinguishable from self-produced insulin and therefore would not be rejected by an overeager immune system.

In addition, the ability to produce insulin in a controlled laboratory or manufacturing ecosystem removed many of the variabilities often encountered when insulin had to be harvested from cadaveric animals. The resulting recombinant insulin (named Humulin) gained FDA approval in October 1982. This human material was safer and more reliable than any insulin prepared since the 1920s. Although the product had been developed and the bulk of research and development done by Genentech, the company ultimately awarded an FDA approval was Eli Lilly & Co.

The Indianapolis-based company not only recognized an opportunity for an improved product, but the threat that might be posed by an upstart company armed with advanced technology. Lilly therefore licensed the technology, patents, and production capabilities from Genentech, allowing the California-based company to enjoy a steady stream of licensing revenues while Eli Lilly deployed its sales force to promote the new product.

The benefits conveyed by human insulin came with a hefty price tag. Humulin was marketed at a price twice that of animal-derived insulin. This cost increase in part reflected the relative nascence of the technology, which had required years to optimize the efficiency of manufacturing. Yet, the premium also reflected the improved safety of the drug. Officials at Eli Lilly and Genentech assured the questioning public that this recombinant product would obviate periodic disruptions in insulin availability caused, for example, by sudden changes in the availability of cows or pigs.[29]

The licensing deal with Eli Lilly was part of a larger strategic plan enacted by the Genentech. As its name conveyed, the South San Francisco company was determined to become the dominant player in recombinant DNA technologies. Over a remarkably short period, the scientists at Genentech delivered one innovation after another, staking out a dominant position in biotechnology akin to the later rise of Google or Amazon in the internet era.

In particular, Genentech continued to address more and more complex problems and product types, culminating in an entirely new and extraordinarily powerful class of protein therapeutics.

Actively attempting to avoid the double entendre that size means everything, the mass of a molecule is generally a measure of its complexity. We will first introduce the concept of a "mole." This concept is neither the furry and annoying creature that destroys gardens nor the beauty mark associated with famous actresses such as Marilyn Monroe. Rather, a mole in the lingo of a scientist is a highly specified number of things. Specifically, a mole is exactly $6.022E23$ things. In other words, a mole is the number 6,022 with an additional twenty zeros after it. This is a very large number. For the lightest of elements, a mole of hydrogen atoms weighs one gram.[30] For aspirin, which is composed of many more atoms, the weight of a mole (also known as an atomic weight, or more accurately, molecular mass) is 180 grams.

With these numbers in mind, the so-called molar mass of insulin is 5,808 grams per mole (grams per mole is hereafter shortened to the descriptor

"Dalton"), thirty-two times larger than aspirin. You may recall from our discussion of natural products that larger molecules tend to be far more complex and challenging to manufacture. Recall that paclitaxel broke the hearts of many a chemist and nearly broke the bank (not to mention the potential clear-cutting of many forests) and it is humbling to realize this challenging product came in at a paltry 854 Daltons, a fraction of insulin's heft.

A key to understanding the power of recombinant DNA technology is that bacteria, rather than the chemists, are responsible for manufacturing the molecule. As a result, complex biological creatures (and yes, a bacterium is a pretty darned complex being) have the ability to produce highly elaborate molecules and this fact helps us understand the true power of the biotechnology revolution begun by Cohen and Boyer.

With this in mind, Genentech scientists pioneered how to produce larger and more complex products. For example, Genentech nabbed an FDA approval in 1993 for dornase alpha, a 3,700 Dalton enzyme for the treatment of cystic fibrosis (taking advantage of the Orphan Drug Act in doing so) and in 1987 for alteplase, a whopping 70,000 Dalton drug that dissipates certain clots involved with heart attacks. Even bigger things were soon to follow.

Although the company hoped to rule the biotech world as dominantly as, say, Microsoft or Google would dominate the digital arena, Genentech was not alone in this race, being joined by other innovative technology firms with names inspired by genetic technologies, such as Amgen, Biogen, and Celgene. Nonetheless, Genentech would position itself as an industry leader based not solely on its products, but its ideas.

Thickets and Stacks

In its science-based approach, what Genentech did particularly well was not only to teach the world about the fundamentals of biotechnology, but to develop the business case using a sophisticated and aggressive approach for developing intellectual property. The company was an early leader in realizing that every bit of information pertaining to the science, clinical application, delivery, or manufacturing might be leveraged into patents. The company would quickly expand this knowledge to include an increasing array of opportunities, both to identify molecules that change during disease, as well as to develop new medicines meant to correct these defects. As the knowledge base expanded in terms of size and complexity, the company would engage flocks of patent attorneys to submit new patent applications for review by an ever more harried set of Federal examiners at the United States Patent and Trade Office (USPTO).

The result was an accumulation of knowledge that would create far more value than had the company focused solely upon developing the next new drug. The result of this savvy approach would lead to the interchangeable concepts of "stacks" and "thickets."

The fundamentals behind these ideas are quite straightforward. A single patent might be regarded as a potential hindrance to competitors, rather like a speed bump. As any driver who has encountered such a barrier knows, a speed bump can be avoided merely by driving around it. Following on this example, Genentech created more and more speed bumps, placing them both wide and deeply enough to frustrate competitors seeking an easy way around them.

Once enough of these individual barriers have been erected, this is often referred to as a "thicket" of intellectual property. To imagine this, think of a forest thicket but rather than benign leaves, this thicket is filled with sharp, thorny objects. For example, if one is developing a new medicine, the core intellectual property might be the chemical definition of the drug (i.e., its chemical formula and structure), which is known in the patent lingo as its "composition." Composition can also include the physical formulation of the drug, adding another layer to the thicket of patents meant to protect an invention. Beyond composition, other features of the thicket might protect the product by identifying the types of diseases to be targeted, characteristics of the patients suffering from the disease, how the drug is manufactured and delivered, or the doses used. This is just a small sampling of the various "methods of use" that comprise a patent thicket.

The requirements for a patent boil down to whether a claimed invention is "useful" and novel, collectively known as "nonobvious." The first word seems obvious enough but nonobvious needs a bit of useful clarification. A nonobvious invention is one that would not be obvious to a person who is an expert (a person deemed to be "skilled in the art")[31] in a particular field. Therein lies the rub. If you or anyone else is aware of a fact, either because you read about it in a journal article or heard news of it from a seminar or even in a lunchtime conversation with a friend, then the fact is considered "obvious" by a patent examiner and that claim will be rejected in a patent application. The result of this requirement for nonobviousness means that the disclosure of a finding must remain a water-tight secret (known only to others within the organization or protected by legally binding confidentiality agreements) until a patent has been submitted.[32] Pinkie promises do not qualify nor does telling a spouse or other relative. Many patent applications have been tossed out due to such indiscretions. Loose lips sink not only ships.

Returning to our example of creating a thicket of obstructions to block competitors, the information protected by patents can extend from a core identification of a new molecule, its usefulness in terms of who is treated and at what doses, but can extend considerably further. The scientists and attorneys at Genentech were masters of such strategies as they extended the patentability to include methods of manufacturing a particular molecule and new technological features involved in the manufacturing or delivery of the molecule (e.g., patenting the delivery of a drug orally, in the muscle, intravenously, or via other sites). Even seemingly esoteric information, such as the pairing of your new medicine with some other new or old medicine, was deemed worthy of patenting.

Utilizing the analogy of an onion in reverse, the consequence of the strategy was the creation (rather than the peeling back) of more and more layers to an onion. To understand the importance of this approach, consider that a patent term is limited (generally to twenty years) and the research and development of a drug frequently requires a decade or more, all while the patent clock is ticking. When deployed strategically, each new layer of onion could be added sequentially to hold off potential competition. Consequently, the patent of the core composition of matter (i.e., the identity of the drug) might expire after twenty years, yet the ability to produce the drug might provide a few extra years, while patents protecting the dosing regimen or identity of patient populations who benefit most from the drug extend it a few more years. Ideally, from the standpoint of the company, such a strategy would continue ad infinitum, but realistically, one can only push such an approach as far as the USPTO examiners will allow.

Nonetheless, the strategy of discovering new drugs, how they work, and how best to manufacture and administer them disproportionately benefited the earliest entries into the biotechnology race. As one example we have already seen, patents filed by the home institutions of Herb Boyer and Stanley Cohen would dominate the use of recombinant DNA technology, the fundamental lifeblood of biotechnology, for the first two decades of this booming industry. Likewise, Genentech's early emphasis upon creating ever-improved means of manufacturing new medicines would create a dominant position for the company for years, even decades, to come.

Now we arrive at the related concept of "stacks." The business and legal teams at Genentech and other biotechnology innovators were as savvy as their scientists. Rather than deploying their thickets of patents solely as a means to exclude competition, early pioneers of the industry realized the potential of "renting" their ideas to even their most fierce competitors. This approach had manifold advantages. By allowing others to have access to their intellectual property, the parent company could earn substantial royalties from products developed by others (not merely their own products). Indeed, during Genentech's first decade they generated more revenues from their intellectual property than from products directly marketed by the company. Adding to this advantage was the fact that dominant early players in the industry could refute claims by nervous regulators and legislators that industry pioneers were establishing an exclusionary monopoly and unfairly discouraging competition.

As the low-hanging fruit were harvested to capture the fundamental ideas to create and produce biotechnology products, the growing thickets of patents meant new entrants into the biotechnology field had to enter into royalty-bearing licenses for a growing number of patents. The term "royalty stack" therefore refers to the large amount of monies required to pay for the legal agreements and licenses needed to advance a product. These costs form a stack of paper patents piled on the desk of a corporate attorney and come right off the top line of revenues for the sale of a drug. These "stacking charges" for a new biotechnology product could easily amount to a third of all revenue. Let's take this concept apart a bit with a hypothetical example.

Let's say you are an entrepreneur who has discovered a new biotechnology product to treat or even cure a disease. Even if all your ideas and your product are completely novel and belong to you, the royalty payments required simply to "rent" the patents required to commercialize your product could amount to a third of the revenues of your product, not including costs of research of development, manufacturing, marketing, and other business expenses. That means that for every dollar you might earn, thirty-three cents fly out the door before you even research or develop it, much less manufacture, distribute, and advertise the product.

With this in mind, two trends unsurprisingly dominated the biotechnology industry in its first few decades. First, there was much money to be made in both developing new ideas and patenting them, even if your company never intended to make a tangible product. As a matter of fact, many biotechnology companies were created and thrived simply from renting out their intellectual property. At a fundamental level, one can argue this is a good thing and indeed, the biotechnology industry tended to thrive in places brimming with good ideas (like the university towns along either coast of the United States).

On the other hand, the second trend is that all these payments had the inevitable consequence of increasing the price of new medicine. As an exemplar of this, we need look no further than the revolution—and the price ballooning—brought forth by the discovery and utilization of monoclonal antibodies.

CHAPTER THIRTEEN

Smart Bombs and
Dumb Money

A discussion about the impact monoclonal antibodies have had on health outcomes and the price paid for those outcomes deserves its own chapter. As a young scientist in the mid-1990s, Dr. Kinch recalls with vivid clarity a lecture given at a specialized biotechnology conference by an unlikely presenter for such a gathering—a career politician. Senator Thomas Richard Harkin of Iowa spoke in front of a room of scientists, pointing out in graphic detail the impressive accuracy and effectiveness of the cruise missiles and smart bombs used in the Gulf War. These images were imprinted on the minds of all in the room, especially as the war had concluded only months before. Harkin then dropped his own bomb. After describing advances made in America's war on cancer, infection, and all the other biomedical achievements of the 20th century, he pointed out that in aggregate, the collective funding for biomedical research ever spent had amounted to less than a single year of the Pentagon's research and development budget (not including procurement, paying troops, etc.). This stinging point elicited the intended head-shaking and murmurs. Senator Harkin concluded by asking what if we could develop similar smart bombs for the body, with the ability to target debilitating diseases? Wouldn't that be amazing?

Only we were. And yes, it most certainly would be amazing . . . and life-altering.

The missiles being developed were admittedly a bit smaller than those that rained down upon Baghdad, but are nonetheless just as dramatic in their outcomes.

In May 1975, a rather extraordinary paper was submitted for publication by investigators from the Medical Research Council Laboratory of Molecular Biology in Cambridge, England. The authors were César Milstein, an Argentinian-born biochemist who had already established a passion for studying antibodies, and Georges J. F. Köhler, a German postdoctoral research fellow on temporary loan from the Basel Institute of Immunology. The paper sent for consideration would ultimately enable the creation of yet another new type of specialized medicines, tiny guided missiles that would allow physicians to target disease and treat millions of people and generate countless billions of dollars in revenue.

Antibodies are a highly specialized protein that have evolved over the millennia to help the body defend itself against disease. These proteins are produced by a particular set of immune cells in the body, known as B cells, and are characterized by being both highly conserved and outrageously diverse. The conserved portions of antibodies reflect the fact that evolution relies upon the ability of antibodies to interface with crucial proteins and cells of the immune system to enable the body's defenses to eliminate potential disease-causing proteins, particles, and cells. Prominent among the targets for antibodies are age-old nemeses of human health such as viruses, bacteria, and cancer cells, to name but a few challenges that we all experience, sometimes on a daily basis. Clearly, these different threats are unique from one another. Further, within any single threat, let's say bacteria, there are at least a billion different bacterial species (and this is likely a dramatic underestimate).[1]

How then, you might ask, can antibodies recognize more than a billion potential threats? The answer is that the body has developed a rather extraordinary ability to recognize more than a trillion different potential threats (even after eliminating those antibodies that might cause the immune system to harm the host). The ability to do so is ingenious, involving a limited number of immune cells (T and B cells) that cut and paste different sequences into the guidance systems of immune-based weapons and then mutate at an extraordinarily high rate. It is well beyond our intention to convey the details of this complex system as part of this particular book but it suffices to say that the survival of our species, and all other mammals, is largely due to the evolution of these amazing antibody systems.

Having established that each of us has the capacity to produce trillions of different antibodies, Milstein became obsessed with the question of how he might be able to isolate just a single version of one antibody that targets a protein of interest to study how these vital proteins function (both the antibody and the target).

One might ask why Milstein simply did not immunize an animal and propagate the antibody-producing B cells in the laboratory. Indeed, animal-derived antibodies had been used for almost a century before Milstein's work as evidenced by Robert Koch's antisera for anthrax, tetanus, diphtheria, and other landmark drugs of the late 19th century. Although scientists studying antibodies had used animals for such missions (e.g., by immunizing mice or rabbits), there are two limitations with this approach. First, the antibodies found in the blood of immunized animals are polyclonal, reflecting proteins produced by a large number of different B cells. Although certain technical tricks can minimize the number of different antibodies, even the best of this voodoo results in animals with at least twenty different forms of an antibody. Milstein wanted to perform in depth analyses of one antibody binding to one target and appreciated that the variability among twenty or more antibodies would confound his research.

Milstein also appreciated that the ability to isolate a single B cell clone (in this case, a clone refers to a collection of cells all derived from a single pre-cursor). However, he realized the number of times that a cell can divide and remain viable is finite and limited by a number of features, most notably the lengths of DNA chromosomes, a limitation meant to prevent cancer. Beyond a few dozen rounds of cell division, a roadblock known as the "Hayflick limit" prevents further cell division and survival.[2]

While recognizing this limitation, Milstein was at the same time inspired by cancer cells, many of which can be endlessly grown in the laboratory (a property known as immortality). Milstein recognized that certain B cell tumors are myelomas, a particular form of B cell tumor that retain the ability to produce antibodies. The antibodies emanating from myelomas are identical, reflecting the same target that the B cells recognized before they turned malignant. Yet Milstein did not particularly care to be limited by studying only the molecules being targeted that happened by pure chance with being immortalized by the few myelomas propagated in laboratories around the world. He wanted to make antibodies with the ability to bind targets he would specify.

To meet this need, Milstein and Köhler developed an ingenious methodology to generate "designer" antibodies derived from a single clone of mouse B cells. He did so by merging (in a literal sense) a mortal B cell targeting a molecule of interest with a myeloma cell. The chemical used to create this Frankenstein-like cell (known as a hybridoma—a term that marries the words hybrid and myeloma) was polyethylene glycol, a close molecular cousin of the toxin that poisoned all those children decades before during the Elixir Sulfanilamide disaster.

Avoiding the technical details, it suffices to state that Köhler and Milstein achieved their spectacular vision. They named the creation "monoclonal antibodies" and these tiny missiles conveyed the extraordinary specificity that Milstein had envisioned and conferred them with immortality, which meant that the antibodies could be produced with a high fidelity and indefinitely.

Although developed solely for the purpose of supporting basic research, Milstein recognized the potential that monoclonal antibodies could serve for medical purposes. For example, some antibodies might be used to target certain diseases, which of course is the reason underlying the evolution of the immune system in nature. Appreciating this vision, Tony Vickers, an administrator at the Medical Research Council immediately saw the opportunity.[3] Vickers contacted government officials at the British National Research Development Corporation, which oversaw intellectual property concerns for the MRC. However, this office declined to patent the invention, noting an inability to "identify any immediate applications" for the technology. This would prove to be a costly mistake.

Instead, the first award of a patent for monoclonal antibody technology went to the Wistar Institute in Philadelphia, when they used the techniques developed by Milstein and Köhler to generate antibodies against key molecules on tumor cells. The scientific duo did receive a non-shabby consolation, namely the Nobel Prize, but neither man nor their institution were able to capitalize upon the countless billions of dollars that would eventually be generated by monoclonal antibodies, a fact that apparently frustrated Margaret Thatcher.[4][5]

The prime minister was right to be put out, as monoclonal antibodies would eventually rise to become a major source of innovative new medicines. Yet many hurdles would first have to be overcome before they could be widely deployed. For example, Milstein's work focused exclusively on mouse-derived antibodies and this triggered a crucial limitation that, ironically enough, arises from the immune system itself. The fact that an antibody has been derived in a mouse causes the human immune system to regard a mouse monoclonal antibody as "foreign" and so attacks it. The results, at a minimum, include the fact that the mouse antibody will eventually be targeted by human antibodies that aim at its "mousiness" and cause it to be rapidly cleared from the body. An even greater negative consequence is that the severity of this human reaction to mousiness could include the same anaphylactic reactions that can be elicited by a bee sting (or food allergy), which often resulting in death (or if available, may compel quick action with an overpriced EpiPen).

Nonetheless, the first monoclonal antibody approved for human use was introduced in 1986, just over a decade after Milstein's first demonstration. The problem of "mousiness" was avoided in this case because this drug was designed to eliminate T cells that cause rejection in organ transplant patients. Stated another way, this drug was designed to help eliminate the same cells that are responsible for the immune responses that might otherwise reject the antibody (not to mention the transplanted organ). While this proved to be a clever trick, additional breakthroughs would be needed to allow monoclonal antibodies to be used more broadly.

An equally clever fix to the problem of mousiness was solved using a technique known as protein engineering. This approach was a form of DNA engineering in which most of the mouse parts of the antibody genes were replaced with equivalent human gene sequences. This approach created a "chimeric" molecule that was mostly, though not entirely, human.[6] Although this technique helped delay an immune response, the remaining mouse sequences could render the antibody drug susceptible to being recognized as foreign, though in practice, such a response might take years to arise.

Eventually, a blend of ingenuity and cutting-edge genetic technologies fixed the mousiness problem altogether. The approach known as "humanization" was more laborious (and thus expensive) but swapped out virtually all the mouse portions of a monoclonal antibody and replaced them with human ones. This was a particularly tricky proposition because even a slight change in the shape of an antibody can either render it useless or cause the drug to recognize something in a normal cell and trigger unintended collateral damage. Later technologies were invoked to replace the immune systems of mice with human genes, allowing an otherwise normal-looking mouse to produce a fully human antibody. Later still, the need for mice was bypassed as other techniques were introduced, allowing antibodies to be created by modifying viruses that normally attack bacteria (known as bacteriophage).

These improvements in technology allowed monoclonal antibodies to rapidly evolve from an academic theory to a very real means to target diseases. When combined with a rapidly expanding understanding of disease processes, as well as opportunities for reversing these diseases with the aid of the immune system, these antibody-based guided missiles would lead to the next revolution in medicine, which as we've learned throughout our story, always comes at a price.

The one thing that all the different advancements in antibody technology shared was that each would be protected with a thicket of patents. Thus to deploy the technology, an antibody product would face stacks of patents, each requiring the negotiation of a complicated license and the payment of substantial royalties (usually a large amount of money needed simply to sign a licensing deal, not to mention additional payments at key milestones, followed by a percentage of gross revenues). A standard rule of thumb for antibody drug companies in the first decade of the new millennium was that the royalties needed to pay for these licenses would immediately shave a third of revenues off the top, just as we described for biotechnology innovators of recombinant DNA technology in Chapter Twelve. Let's review that statement. For every dollar charged by a manufacturer for an antibody production, a third of the money, off the top, would be devoted solely to pay for the intellectual property underpinning the technologies needed for the discovery and creation of the drug.

Compounding the situation, antibodies are quite large and complex proteins (150,000 Daltons as compared to aspirin at 180 Daltons; nearly a thousand times larger). Whereas small molecules like aspirin can be synthesized at large scale in vats generally using rather simple (and inexpensive) chemicals, developers must rely upon adaptations of nature to generate monoclonal antibody products. To facilitate this, technology again intervenes, and spectacular discoveries arose starting in the 1980s that allowed companies to create specialized microscopic antibody factories in the form of cells grown first in a laboratory and then scaled up to produce this material en masse in factories. Each of these improvements and modifications, of course, came with their own stacks of royalty payments and contributed to the high costs of monoclonal antibody therapeutics.

Not that all of these improvements were protected using patents. As you may recall, a patent is a simple exchange of a period of exclusivity in exchange for revealing information about technological improvement to the world. A patent is not technically required to sell a product but most pharmaceutical companies are reluctant to advance a product, given the risks of millions and billions of dollars, without a certainty that this product will be free of generic competition, which would only have to invest a fraction of these costs to ensure bioequivalence.

In many cases, companies elected to keep key information about antibody production as a trade secret. As previously discussed, a trade secret is just that: a bit of information that is only known within a company. If one wished to keep the existence of a novel tool or procedure to themselves, they might choose to keep this a trade secret to prevent its competition from learning about it in a patent.

Indeed, both authors worked for an employer who kept certain trade secrets for manufacturing. In those days, we might have been terminated with antibody-based guided missiles on the spot for publicly saying certain three-letter-utterances, such as E-Y-P and F-E-P. EYP stood for enhanced yield production and FEP for further enhanced production. Both techniques referred to ways of manufacturing monoclonal antibody therapeutics with far greater efficiency than conventional techniques of the day. The actual details of the secret recipe were never known to us, and indeed were the purview of only two or three people in the company (much like the Colonel's Secret Recipe at Kentucky Fried Chicken).

Yet, this same example reveals a fundamental problem with trade secrets. One morning, we came to work to learn that a colleague had been charged the night before with insider trading. Beyond the illegality and embarrassment to the company, the executive charged was responsible for developing both the EYP and FEP procedures and was one of its few secret-holders. On one hand, the secret would remain in place for a time, protected by federal guards. Yet, the company necessarily and immediately fired the executive and thereby released them from service as the treasured secret-keeper, an awkward situation to say the least.[7]

Independent of the extraordinary advances in manufacturing technologies and the requisite royalties and secrets, the price to manufacture monoclonal antibodies is and will likely always remain considerably higher than for smaller molecules (traditional chemistry-based drugs). This might not be an issue except that monoclonal antibodies have progressed well beyond a seeming fad, marketed only by a small number of renegade biotechnology companies. Today, monoclonal antibody therapy has arguably become the mainstay in many of even the stodgiest pharmaceutical companies. Why the change?

In a word, money—copious amounts of money.

One reason why monoclonal antibodies have come to dominate the market is because these products are so expensive to produce that the price point can be raised further without raising eyebrows, akin to a decision to add a fancier upgrade to a six-figure sportscar. What is the big deal about an additional few thousand extra dollars when you are paying so much already? Except it wasn't always this way.

MAbs Up Close and Personal

In the last chapter we briefly touched upon a product named Synagis, a monoclonal antibody developed and marketed originally by MedImmune, where both authors of this book would work for a time. However, prior to joining MedImmune, Dr. Kinch and his wife would encounter this breakthrough product in a very personal way.

In 2000, the Kinches' son Grant was born many weeks premature. After spending his first ten days in the neonatal intensive care unit, the baby was released and his relieved parents presumed that was the end of the story. However, the first visit to the pediatrician's office changed this assumption. By this time, it was late autumn, with cold and flu season rapidly approaching. Although a cold for new parents is always a time of concern, certain causes of the cold can be deadly for premature infants. Because the lungs of these smallest of our species are among the last organs to develop, pathogens that infect the lungs can quickly turn deadly. Of particular note is a germ known as respiratory syncytial virus (RSV). This virus causes a minor cold in adults and older children, but can be fatal for neonates, especially premature babies. Not only are the lungs of premature infants underdeveloped and very small, but their immune systems also are less advanced than full-term infants, having missed out on the transfer of healthy components from the mother's immune system, typically transferred during the final weeks of gestation.

The Kinches' pediatrician recommended their son receive a monoclonal antibody drug that had been approved only a year or so before. This medicine, palivizumab (trade name Synagis), happened to be one of the earliest monoclonal antibody drugs approved by the FDA, and as we mentioned earlier, the first monoclonal antibody ever approved for an infectious disease. Dr. Kinch and his wife, who were both academic scientists and at the time studying monoclonal antibodies, were amused at the fact that their son had been prescribed one of the very few drugs of this type.

The Kinches' amusement was short-lived as they learned that the price tag for this drug was just over six hundred dollars a month and repeat doses would be needed each month of the cold and flu season for the next two years. Admittedly, their insurance company picked up much of the cost, but at first, it was reluctant to do so, concerned about the outrageous price tag of the vital medicine. The Kinches were informed that a cost of two thousand dollars per year was excessive but, after a back and forth between the insurance company and their pediatrician, the treatments proceeded.

Fortunately for the Kinches, Synagis would produce the desired outcome as it would for thousands of other children born prematurely. Within the first six months of its first sale, Synagis became one of the most successful biotechnology product launches in history at that time.[8]

We will return to this particular story later in the book but for now, the story seems rather quaint, quite like a modern viewer smiling at the naïveté portrayed in a 1960s settings such as Mayberry, North Carolina. For today, a mere few thousands of dollars for a monoclonal antibody therapy, any monoclonal antibody therapy, would be considered the deal of the century. Now the price tag for such therapies routinely exceeds ten thousand and increasingly touches on hundreds of thousands of dollars per year. Given the opaqueness of an industry dominated by royalty stacks and trade secrets, building an extra hundred dollars or two of profit into an already-expensive product was more feasible than with drugs having a lower price point. Over time, the extra hundreds became thousands, then tens of thousands of dollars.

The sticker shock experienced by the Kinches' insurance company clearly had been desensitized in order to allow such escalations in price. Rest assured that savvy pharmaceutical company executives and canny investors were watching. Big money was to be made with monoclonal antibodies as evidenced by the initial year over year revenue growth of Synagis. Twenty years after the first monoclonal antibodies were introduced, global sales of just the eight top-selling monoclonal antibody products exceeded $64 billion in 2018 alone; while the entirety of monoclonal antibody sales were projected to exceed $110 billion that same year.[9] For the biopharmaceutical industry, this is certainly a market worth defending and, in the case of monoclonal antibodies, a strong defensive posture was virtually guaranteed.

Objective Truth:
A Perverse Dis-incentive

In discussing the high prices of monoclonal antibody and other biologics products, Charles Muscoplat identified a disturbing point that is rarely discussed outside the chatter of industry professionals. Very rarely (and perhaps never) are studies designed to pit one costly monoclonal antibody against another in a head-to-head comparison of cost versus benefit, especially for medicines meant to treat chronic conditions.[10] He continued that this tendency seems to reflect a fundamental fear that "a statistical quirk" might indicate that your product is not superior to your competitor, potentially risking billions of dollars in annual revenues. As an example, Muscoplat revealed that his investigation has failed to identify any head-to-head cost-benefit studies for biologics-based medicines drugs meant to treat asthma, ulcerative colitis, RA, or ankylosing spondylitis, lucrative indications that can annually command tens or hundreds of thousands of dollars.

Indeed, a search for evidence of competitive cost-benefit studies of some of society's most expensive diseases (including chronic autoimmune diseases) verified Muscoplat's assertion (or more accurately, a lack of any evidence that such studies have ever been conducted). This surprising outcome might soon change with a trend, known colloquially as biosimilars, that holds the potential to revolutionize healthcare and its expenses.

Similar to What?

Another attraction of monoclonal antibodies was a reputation that this new class of drugs would not be subject to the inevitable capitulation to generic competition that was destroying conventional small molecule medicines. A combination of patent thickets, trade secrets, and experiences gained in manufacturing of antibody products was thought to be sufficient to prevent interloping generics companies from crowding into the monoclonal antibody market. This idea proved correct for a time as, for example, pioneering biotechnology companies vigorously argued that the concept of "bioequivalence," the measure of how much drug is in the body and for how long, would be insufficient to ensure the safety and efficacy of generic monoclonal antibody and other biologics-based products.[11] In particular, larger and more complex protein therapeutics often are quite finicky, requiring specialized formulations, and are subject to detailed modifications as compared to smaller and more conventional chemical drugs. We will present a few examples of these peculiarities and show how the biopharmaceutical industry has changed radically in recent years.

Largely due to particularly intensive lobbying, the United States government and the FDA were particularly hesitant to enable generic biologics. Europe, on the other hand, became an early adopter, gathering the bruises that often accompany pioneering efforts. Returning to the example of insulin, a series of applications to sell a biosimilar (a term for generic biologics) for a recombinant DNA-derived form of insulin (known as insulin glargine) were submitted in Europe by Marvel Life Sciences in 2007.

Despite the hopes of European leaders that biosimilars might slow the rapid acceleration in insulin drug prices, each of the applications from Marvel was rejected. The European Union regulatory authorities were concerned that the biosimilar forms of insulin had failed to demonstrate sufficient similarity to the original drug.[12] The increased complexity of insulin in general and the reliance upon trade secrets by manufacturers of innovator drugs (including insulin) proved to be a consistent source of frustration for would-be biosimilar entrants. There is an old saying in bio-pharmaceutical manufacturing, "process is product," and this has proven itself with biosimilars.[13] Consequently, in-house secrets (akin to EYP and FEP) would prove a particular hindrance for biosimilar manufacturers to produce a product with the quality of the innovator drug.

Insulin, as we have seen, is only a fraction of the size of an antibody and with far less complexity. Thus, the situation only worsened for monoclonal antibodies and, for a time, it seemed that the strategy to emphasize biologics solely for the reason that they were impervious to competition had proved prescient.

Suddenly, the unexpected intervened and would ignite a wave of interest in biosimilars. Innovator companies decided to take on biosimilar development themselves in an effort to capture sales of popular products away from competitors. Stated another way, innovator companies opted to enter the generic space.

In 2015, the paragon of big pharma, Pfizer, purchased Hospira. The company had spun out of another major pharmaceutical company, Abbott, in 2004, and Hospira's headquarters remained in the Chicagoland area. Hospira's business was primarily known for its focus around hospital products, hence its name.[14] However, Pfizer's rationale for the purchase was to gain access to its biosimilar programs. All the while much of the world thought of Hospira as a manufacturer of rather drab hospital products used for infusions, the company was quietly becoming a biotechnology juggernaut. In particular, Hospira focused upon the development of the tools, techniques, and experience to generate biosimilars. Recognizing an opportunity to tap into a potential burgeoning market, Pfizer swooped in and is now poised to become a dominant manufacturer of generic medicines, albeit generic biologics. Likewise, other innovator organizations such as Biogen, Novartis, and Amgen are repositioning themselves to manufacture and market not only innovative new medicines but generic knock-offs of the flagship products of their biopharmaceutical rivals. Such is the multibillion-dollar lure of biologics in general and monoclonal antibodies in particular.

Nailed It

As monoclonal antibodies changed in reputation from a niche phenomenon to a desired commodity, they became "the next big thing" and largely still are perceived as such. As a result there was a flurry of activity piling into monoclonal antibody products. Everyone, it seemed, wanted in. Stale and stodgy pharmaceutical companies, many with roots founded in the 18th century, suddenly wanted to lead the 21st by embracing new technologies. The result was a dramatic restructuring of the biotechnology industry.

Paraphrasing an age-old truism, when the only tool you have is a hammer, every problem looks like a nail. The problem here being that the hammers are monoclonal antibodies and other high-priced biologics that seem to have a price tag set by Pentagon bureaucrats at tens of thousands of dollars each. Given the potential that an antibody-based drug would be less susceptible to generic competition, many companies were disproportionately attracted to monoclonal antibody-based therapeutics. Given in part to their exorbitant prices, many of the first monoclonal antibody products were directed at life-threatening disease, especially cancer, where a higher cost could be justified. Indeed, monoclonal antibody-based therapeutics enabled the revolution in cancer therapy as portrayed in *The End of the Beginning.* While expensive, some of these medicines hold the potential to utterly cure an otherwise fatal disease, which obviates many arguments quibbling over price, until of course such prices become overwhelming, as we will soon see.

Increasingly though, monoclonal antibody therapeutics are utilized in less life-threatening indications. It seems one cannot turn on a television today without seeing at least one advertisement for a new monoclonal antibody drug for psoriasis. By the 2019, the list of FDA-approved monoclonal antibody drugs for psoriasis had expanded to include adalimumab (trade name Humira), certolizumab (Cimzia), efalizumab (Raptiva), guselkumab (Tremfya), infliximab (Remicade), risankizumab (Skyrizi), secukinumab (Cosentyx), and ustekinumab (Stelara). Despite this competition, the prices of each new drug have increased, not decreased. Newer generations of medicines are also being developed for the same indication. With neither malice nor disrespect for the very real suffering of patients with the most debilitating forms of psoriasis, it is important as a society to ask how many more drugs are needed for that particular disease and whether there is a ceiling for the amounts we (including insurers) are willing to pay for the use of expensive technologies for indications that are not life-threatening.

The long list of antibody drugs targeting psoriasis also reflects a herding tendency that many pharmaceutical industry executives interviewed for this book or in private conversations have defensively asserted was an unfortunate artifact relegated to the past. Despite these sentiments, our data reveal a strong and continued predisposition toward fast-follower (me-too) drugs, with the extreme version of this being the renewed emphasis by "innovator companies" upon biosimilars. Without revisiting that topic yet again, the third decade of the 20th century, a time when modern biomedical science identified new understanding of disease and how to treat it, many pharmaceutical companies remain disproportionately focused upon generating "me-too" drugs. These medicines target psoriasis, immune oncology, and other indications perceived as "popular" by the pharmaceutical sector; safe propositions but unlikely to deliver transformative improvements.

Group Think and Lack Thereof

With the amounts of money being generated, it is unsurprising that the go-go years of biotechnology in the 20th century were awash with speculation. As is often the case, dumb money follows smart and there was (and still is) no absence of dumb money in biotechnology. We have already discussed the impact of industry consolidation, and driving this exuberance is that companies focused upon biologics in general and monoclonal antibodies have been gobbled up at a particularly high rate, despite the fact that many of the acquired companies were indeed turkeys. One example would be the aforementioned company just up the road from MedImmune, which you may recall had the lavish headquarters referred to as the Taj Mahal. It seems the emperor's clothing was indeed limited in that the company failed to produce the presumed lucrative pipeline and its prior double-digit billion-dollar valuation soon evaporated and the company was ultimately put out of its misery.

Like other "hot technologies," there was a rush by many investors to seize upon the perceived riches to be made in biotechnology, especially with monoclonal antibodies. In our respective roles in helping guide early-stage academic and nonprofit entrepreneurs through the maze of activities needed to advance a project toward commercialization, we frequently encounter would-be entrepreneurs with rich relatives, neighbors, or grateful patients with sufficiently deep pockets that they offer to bankroll a project with "millions." In his day job, Dr. Kinch works with would-be academic medical entrepreneurs to help them advance their work. At least twice a year, he will meet with physicians who explain they have already received a verbal commitment from a wealthy patient to bankroll the creation of a company to advance their idea for developing a new medicine.

While this might seem an attractive prospect, experience has taught us that "dumb money," meaning financing from individuals or organizations inexperienced in the drug development process, is generally the best way to assure that a particular venture will fail, often by creating unrealistic expectations about valuations and ignorant of the tedious, expensive, and time-sensitive activities needed to advance an experimental medicine through the thicket of intellectual property and regulatory challenges. Without distracting from the focus of our story, it is important nonetheless to point out that dumb money tends to beget dumb money. A combination of naïveté and excess cash can create speculative ventures that rarely meet expectations.

Given that medicines and diseases are highly relatable, medical research seems to be particularly sensitive to this tendency and perceived "hot technologies" such as monoclonal antibodies particularly so. As a consequence, periods of economic thriving and high stock market valuations have a tendency to create their own bubbles, advancing otherwise half-baked ideas, and, sometimes, even these raw projects find a champion among otherwise-rational companies. Hence, more resources are invested in a project that will inevitably fail. Thus we return once again to the elements responsible for the continuation of Eroom's Law.

Before ending this section, let us take a look at where some less-than-realistic investments have been, and continue to be, made. One example is an oft repeated (and possibly still in progress) development of a monoclonal antibody therapeutic targeting rhinovirus (a frequent cause of the common cold). You might ask why a multithousand-dollar drug would be deployed to combat the cold, but this is a question that clearly many others had not asked before sinking their monies and reputations into such a subject. Another favorite was an approach to develop a monoclonal antibody against cocaine. The idea here was to create a guided missile that would bind molecules of cocaine and thereby remove it from the body before it could stimulate the nervous system, thus ostensibly making cocaine no longer a desirable drug, and thus obsolete. To accomplish this goal, ultrahigh purity cocaine was (legally) procured from the Drug Enforcement Agency. The material was used to develop and test monoclonal antibody drugs and was locked away in an approved safe. Any amounts deployed for research were scrupulously documented. The idea behind the cocaine project faced two obstacles, however. First, a user could overwhelm the antibody by simply snorting even more cocaine. Perhaps more compellingly, monoclonal antibodies are among the few medicines that are even more expensive than high-quality powder cocaine. Nonetheless, key individuals high on such ideas championed this cause for a time, expending resources that might have been invested more intelligently.[15]

Future Shock

In the not-so-distant future, we may look back on the cost and complexity of monoclonal antibody therapeutics as quaintly as we compare a Model-T with a modern Tesla. A new generation of therapeutics has been on the rise and promises to eclipse antibodies in virtually every way, including costs.

Oncology, as we have seen throughout our story, has a tendency to function as a sort-of gateway for expensive medicines and new technology. We saw this in terms of public acceptance of escalating pricing associated with difficult-to-manufacture medicines, such as paclitaxel, and as a prominent indication for even more complex and expensive drugs such as monoclonal antibodies.

These reactions are relatable, as cancer is a disease that inspires dread like almost no other. Recent years have witnessed extraordinary advances in the treatment of cancer, largely due to targeted therapies that exploit unique molecular signatures that render cancer cells susceptible to therapy and thus allow for the reprogramming of the immune system to assist in eliminating cancer. All of these improvements have come at a cost, with most medicines bearing price tags measured in tens or hundreds of thousands of dollars. As these prices became more commonplace, they were increasingly accepted by even non-life-threatening diseases such as rheumatoid arthritis and psoriasis. It is important to reiterate that patients suffering from these diseases embrace these new therapies with open arms, but again, the prices of these remedies have increased the perils of our overall healthcare system.

With the idea that oncology often provides a glimpse into the future of medical technology, what does that future seem to hold? Based upon a review of the scientific literature and medical conferences, one striking trend is the emergence of next-generation therapeutic strategies that are far more complex, and expensive, than even monoclonal antibodies.

One approach that has demonstrated considerable promise is the use of human immune cells engineered to produce modified types of monoclonal antibodies. This technology, known as chimeric antigen receptor T cell therapy (or CAR-T) is a blend of technological advances in understanding genetic manipulation, immune system function and cancer targeting. The idea here is that a modified form of a monoclonal antibody can be used as a homing beacon to identify cancer cells. This antibody is reconfigured so that it can be expressed within patient T cells, where it stimulates those T cells to find and kill tumor cells. This reprogramming of the immune system entails isolating T cells from the blood, manipulating their DNA to "insert" the modified antibody gene, and then growing the cells in the laboratory to a sufficient number of hearty cells, which can then be infused back into the patient, where they will be free to seek out and kill tumor cells. Although this sounds a bit like science fiction, an increasing number of studies have demonstrated the utility of CAR-T technology as a safe and effective means for treating cancer.

All the manipulations required to create and introduce CAR-T cells reflect a new high-water mark for medical therapy. Again, these treatments come at a price, often in the range of at least a half-million dollars per treatment. This hefty price tag does not include the hospitalization and other expenses associated with cancer therapy. Yet, given the dire view of cancer,

Medicare administrator Seema Verma announced in August 2019 that her organization would be willing to pay for these treatments.[16] The stock prices for many companies exploring CAR-T therapies shot up and while certainly generous, the announcement by Medicare raised questions of whether and where the resources needed to cover the costs of such expensive therapies will be found.

A second question pertains to whether and how Medicare and other payers will respond to the application of CAR-T therapy beyond cancer. For example, CAR-T therapies are being developed for the treatment of multiple sclerosis and inflammatory bowel disease, which raises questions about whether there is a limit to where such ultra-expensive therapies will be tolerated.[17]

And CAR-T cell therapies are themselves comparatively cheap when placed alongside certain experimental and FDA-approved gene therapies. For example, a drug approved by the FDA in December 2016 for the treatment of spinal muscular atrophy, a form of muscular dystrophy, was launched with a price tag of $750,000 while a second therapy for the same indication, as we mentioned earlier, launched in 2019 with the eye-watering price of more than two million dollars.[18]

These announcements bring to mind two important points. First, scientific advances in both our understanding of the cause of disease and designing new modalities for treatment have enabled the creation of drugs that are transforming health. Many cancers that had been virtual death sentences, such as metastatic melanoma, can now be cured. The pain and suffering caused by other diseases can be ameliorated or in some cases eliminated altogether by a panoply of new medicines.

Thus, the second and more unfortunate point. Given there is a finite availability of resources available to be devoted to healthcare, the ever-accelerating price of these new medicines will, at some point if not already, reach a point where crucial decisions will need to be made about who does and does not have access to these latest innovations. Public debates invariably seem to result in non-constructive finger-pointing and claims of "rationing," "death panels," and the like. Yet these debates are crucial.

A confounding aspect overhanging the debate about the price and benefits of new medicines revolves around the questions about the credibility and, frankly, greed, of the pharmaceutical enterprise and associated industries (i.e., investors, insurance companies, pharmacy benefits managers, hospitals, physicians, and pharmacies). According to Gallup, the biopharmaceutical industry now ranks among the least-respected institutions in the world and the lowest rated industry in the United States.[19] Thus, we will now turn to the question of how this came to be by citing a few examples.

CHAPTER FOURTEEN

Reputation Decimation

The pharmaceutical and biotechnology industries have revolutionized modern health and indeed society, fostering the innovation behind countless medicines, with vaccines and antibiotics being but two of their orthogonal contributions to society. As a consequence, infectious diseases have largely been eliminated as major sources of death in the modern world, replaced by other diseases. Indeed, even today's biggest killer, heart disease, has been somewhat tamed with agents meant to treat hypertension and cholesterol while treatment of the second largest killer, cancer, is at last demonstrating the potential for curative regiments by harnessing the untapped power of the immune system to combat malignancies.

Despite these remarkable breakthroughs, Andrew Dahlem, a recently retired pharmaceutical industry executive, shared this rather dismal comment about the industry's reputation: "When I started in this industry, we were the most respected in the world. Today, we rank below tobacco."[1] Dahlem's sentiment was reinforced and explained during a 2016 Forbes Healthcare Summit that gathered together several industry executives.[2] In an uncomfortable exchange, the moderator asked about the causations of the decline in pharmaceutical reputation. After the CEOs of Astellas, Eli Lilly, Gilead, and Pfizer pontificated, largely pointing their fingers outward to blame others (a subject to which we will soon return) the boss of Regeneron, Leonard Schleiffer, spoke up, stating unequivocally, "We dispelled some of it (i.e., the reputational decline) last year, because we blamed it on the extremists, the people who come in, dial up a product that's off patent, raising price ten-fold, and they're evil-doers, that's why we're not liked," he continued. "But the real reason we're not liked, in my opinion, is because we as an industry have used price increases to cover up the gaps in innovation. That's just a fact."

This idea of self-induced reputational trauma is consistent with the central thesis of this book, reflecting the impact of Eroom's Law and other features in what seems to many to be the end of the long-standing model of how new pharmaceutical products are developed and distributed. Yet, there is more to the story of how the pharmaceutical industry quickly deteriorated in estimation from first to worst.

In this chapter, we will provide examples of how the pharmaceutical industry rather efficiently destroyed its reputation and did so in an impressively brief period of time. We will also review why it matters.

Although many link the industry today with some of the biggest scandals and challenges facing modern-day America, such as opiate addiction and unaffordable medicines, this was not always the case. Looking back no further than the mid-1950s when Jonas Salk made his announcement that he had developed a vaccine for polio, church bells across the nation peeled with excitement and seemingly every kid wanted to grow up and be a research scientist or doctor.

Wellcome News

If searching for a relative paragon of virtue for the pharmaceutical industry, one can hardly do better than consider the story of Burroughs Wellcome. In the final two decades of the 19th century, the United Kingdom looked with dismay at the fact that the nascent pharmaceutical industry seemed to be burgeoning everywhere except for their small island. Perennial rival France, under Louis Pasteur, was rapidly advancing efforts to discover the sources and remedies for infectious diseases, a human scourge plaguing civilization from its inception. Likewise, the Germans under Robert Koch, propelled by a mature chemicals industry, were vastly ahead of the British. Even the former colonies in the Americas were far surpassing most inept British efforts to develop a pharmaceutical industry. Beyond the fact the British Empire dwarfed most rivals in virtually all other terms of economic and diplomatic might, the shortfall in developing medicines had a strategic significance for a powerful colonial nation that required medicines to sustain its populace and military prepared-ness around the globe. Yet Britain remained largely alone and without domestic sources of medicines.

Two Yankees would soon end this isolation. Silas Mainville Burroughs was born in 1846 in Upstate New York, the son of a prominent US con-gressman. After receiving training as a pharmacist, Silas moved to London in 1878 to work for the British subsidiary of the American firm, Wyeth pharmaceuticals.[3] Two years later, Burroughs had partnered with another American expat, Henry Solomon Wellcome from Almond, Wisconsin, to start a company focused on "ethical" medicines, mostly acquiring medicines being produced in America and distributing these in the United Kingdom. Over the following fifteen years until the death of Burroughs (at the young age of forty-eight, the victim of pneumonia), the company blossomed, pro-ducing their own version of medicines and scientific instruments that had been discovered in America and elsewhere.[4]

From its inception, Burroughs Wellcome built its business around a concept of trust. This was the conclusion of a detailed biography of the organization that showed the company sought to gain the trust of medical professionals and the public by ensuring accessibility to affordable and reliably high-quality products. These principles would carry the company beyond its growth and trendsetting days in the United Kingdom and lead it to even greater prominence worldwide.

With Burroughs's death, Wellcome refocused the company to begin the process of discovering new medicines via internal research and development activities. In 1896, the Wellcome Chemical Research Labo-ratories was founded in Beckenham in Southeast London, followed by the 1902 foundation of the Wellcome Tropical Research Laboratories in colonial Khartoum (the present-day capital of Sudan).[5] In 1904, Henry

Dale, a prominent biologist, was recruited, reluctantly at first, to create an academic-like infrastructure within the company to study potential opportunities to discover new medicines. He was hesitant because few academics would soil their reputations at the time (and for many years to come) by working with the private sector. Nonetheless, this unusual formula worked, allowing Dale to lead efforts that would identify medicines that perturb the function of adrenaline, a key regulator of physiology and disease. Despite the self-soiling of his reputation, Dale's work at Burroughs Wellcome would earn him the highest academic honor: a Nobel Prize. From a business standpoint, these efforts to bridge the divide separating academia and industry supplied Burroughs Wellcome with a wealth of new product opportunities.

The timing of these events in the early 20th century was fortuitous as it coincided with Robert Koch's discovery of antisera (antibodies produced in animals that had been immunized against human pathogens). The transfer of knowledge from Germany by Burroughs Wellcome scientists would greatly benefit the United Kingdom in the coming Great War against Koch's homeland, when antisera from Germany were understandably no longer accessible to the British. By war's end, Burroughs Wellcome was also positioned to commercialize the recent discovery of vitamins in the Cambridge, England, laboratory of Frederick Gowland Hopkins.

An emphasis upon academic-inspired research also led the company to revolutionize drug development and become a prominent player in the birthplace of its founders. As the world entered into its first truly global conflagration, Burroughs Wellcome opened an American research center in Tuckahoe, a suburb of New York City. In the early years of the second world war, Burroughs Wellcome hired a new chemist, George Herbert Hitchings, who had trained at Harvard and Case Western Reserve before joining Burroughs Wellcome. Upon joining the company in 1942, Hitchings was determined to create a world-class research institute on this side of the pond as well.

As brilliant a scientist as Hitchings was, his eye for talent was even more impressive, and two years later Hitchings hired a young, dynamic New Yorker named Gertrude (Trudy) Belle Elion. Elion's extraordinary story was summarized in *Between Hope and Fear*, but for here, it suffices to state that she and Hitchings began a professional partnership unparalleled for the good that would be conveyed to both science and human health.

Starting in Tuckahoe and continuing when the company expanded into a much larger research and development facility in North Carolina's Research Triangle Park, Elion and Hitchings discovered a string of medicines that revolutionized the treatment for a wide array of diseases, including cancer, gout, organ transplantation, malaria, bacterial infections, and herpes. However, it was Elion's final contribution—in 1987—that would both earn her and Hitchings the Nobel Prize. In a true sense of irony, this remarkable achievement would also doom Burroughs Wellcome to ignominy and destruction.

In 1983, Elion officially "retired" from Burroughs Wellcome but continued to work in their research laboratories. In that same year, a French scientist, Luc Montagnier, announced the discovery of a virus responsible for a global pandemic that would become, and remains to this day, one of the greatest threats to public health around the world. With the identification of the human immunodeficiency virus (HIV), the National Institutes of Health (NIH) began a partnership with pharmaceutical companies to test any and all potential experimental and approved drugs for the potential to block the virus. Elion led the efforts at Burroughs Wellcome and, within weeks, the team she led had identified a promising drug candidate originally created in the 1960s in the Detroit laboratory of cancer researcher Jerome Horwitz.

Prompted by an ongoing public health emergency and further reinforced by highly organized patients' rights advocates, Burroughs Wellcome and multiple federal agencies (including the National Institutes of Health as well as the FDA) synergized to expedite the investigation and approval of that medicine. Officially branded with the generic name zidovudine (trade name: Retrovir), the drug would be more widely known as AZT.

AZT provided the first hope for patients diagnosed with AIDS, a dreaded disease that was inevitably fatal. Yet the discovery of AZT was soon to be followed by a raft of additional drugs, many again emanating from Burroughs Wellcome. These discoveries marked a zenith for the scientific reputation for Burroughs Wellcome, but the beginning of a debilitating trend in terms of the public's view of the company in particular and the pharmaceutical industry as a whole.

Oh, the Humanity

In an opinion piece printed in the *New York Times* on August 28, 1989, the editorial board summarized their judgement of Burroughs Wellcome with the title, "AZT's Inhuman Cost."[6] The editorial decried, "At $8,000 a year for users, AZT is said to be the most expensive prescription drug in history." The polemic continued, "The average cost of bringing a new drug to market is $125 million. The maker of AZT, the Burroughs Wellcome Company of North Carolina, refuses to state its costs, but it's hard to believe they reached a fraction of this sum." The *Times* was merely reflecting a wider outrage in the nation for a drug whose price, at $8,000 a year, seemed a discount for Burroughs Wellcome, which initially intended to price the medicine at the round number of $10,000 per year.[7]

The fact that the world's most prosperous nation balked at the high price tag paled in comparison to the outrage sincerely felt around the world. The pricing of AZT would be declared to be extortionate. National leaders, particularly in sub-Saharan Africa, where the disease had struck the hardest and killed the most, threatened to dismantle the patent system and begin manufacturing their own generic versions of the drug. These ripples coalesced into a durable shock that would haunt Burroughs Wellcome and the reputational damage undoubtedly contributed to its merger with smaller and lesser known Glaxo (another UK-based company). Just a few years later, Glaxo Wellcome would undergo another megamerger to create GlaxoSmithKline and in doing so leave behind the tainted name altogether.

Other price cuts would follow but it was a classic case of too little, too late. In 1998, the company announced it would slash the cost of AZT for poor women by 75 percent.[8] Ultimately, the patent would expire in 2005, by which time the drug had been rendered largely worthless due to the rise of AZT-resistant HIV strains.

To our knowledge, the story of AZT was the first time that a perception of excessive drug pricing captured headlines around the world. Perceptions that the pharmaceutical company was taking advantage of the public at a time of a terrible pandemic were accompanied by the reality that much of the preclinical and clinical research needed to discover AZT and then demonstrate its utility had been underwritten by the American taxpayer. (The world would encounter a similar story in 2020 when Gilead priced remdesivir, a potential treatment for COVID-19 that reduced the average hospital stay from fifteen days to eleven, at more than $3,000. Further, they would only make the product available in the United States to avoid the demand for lower pricing sure to come from other governments around the globe.)[9]

As the HIV crisis continued, Burroughs Wellcome had made one misstep after another, incrementally lowering the price of the drug and failing to appreciate the true harm caused by the inaccessibility of the drug to the general public, both in the developing world and even in wealthier western countries. As a consequence, a century's worth of extraordinary goodwill that had been generated toward and by a company founded in 1880 would be lost in the span of a few years.

In subsequent years, the experiences faced by Burroughs Wellcome would be repeated again and again by numerous companies, both as a consequence of escalating costs to develop new medicines and because of increasing opacity in drug pricing strategies. Other high-profile crises, such as prominent drug toxicities (e.g., Merck's Vioxx and other disasters around the time of the new millennium), and unseemly marketing practices (such as those conducted by Insys Therapeutics that contributed to opioid over-prescription) would continue to detract from the industry's contributions.[10] This combination has created the perceptions, and indeed realities, that pharmaceutical companies allow greed to belie their stated commitments to promote the betterment of patients and society.

In Their Defense

The industry believes that they are being unfairly characterized as villains, or at the very least their plight is significantly misunderstood, as they pursue their missions to bring new medicines to market. One only needs to recall nightly TV advertisements during the entirety of the COVID-19 crisis to appreciate the adulation they think they deserve. The COVID-19 ads were placed primarily by the various trade associations for developers and manufacturers (PhRMA and NAM), using (mostly female) employees from member companies to extol the virtues of the industry's ongoing contributions to quickly finding treatments and cures for the devastating virus. The industry undoubtedly hoped the implications from these particular ads would extend to the public's general opinion of their work in other areas as well. From those ads one might not fully appreciate that their frenzied contributions to the global COVID-19 calamity were being generously funded by governments and nonprofit organizations the world over. Yet the companies had retained the pricing rights in most cases. Even this does not distract from the fact these companies had agreed to prioritize this work for the general good and were putting their collective expertise to work.

As we have noted throughout our story, the COVID-19 experience has provided many examples to highlight the broader issues in bringing critical (and not-so-critical) medicines to market and the challenges faced by the pharmaceutical enterprise in pricing them. Historically, most pharmaceutical companies and their trade representatives have cited the rising costs to develop medicines as one of the major causes for rising prices experienced by the consumer. By any objective measure, Eroom's Law has been a seemingly self-perpetuating cause and effect to help explain the ever-accelerating costs to develop a new medicine. As we have seen, steady adherence to Eroom's Law reflects in part the harvesting of low-hanging fruit (i.e., easily addressed diseases and relatively simple and easy to develop medicines), the increasing costs of clinical trials (both to ensure safety and efficacy in light of increasing knowledge of both health and disease), and the cautious regulator approach.

Although the data (as it exists) does support the foundations of Eroom's Law, the underlying data used to develop the concept that the resulting increases in R&D lead to increased prices is utterly opaque, largely due to industry decisions not to disclose these findings.[11] As a consequence of this opacity, industry defenders are unable to refute arguments such as that from a 2016 Harvard study which concluded, "There is no evidence of an association between research and development costs and prices; rather, prescription drugs are priced in the United States primarily on the basis of what the market will bear."[12]

Given the self-inflicted wounds to the reputation of the pharmaceutical industry, the additional damage caused by such conclusions on pricing has understandably led the public and their elected representatives (from both sides of the political spectrum) to call for punitive measures against the pharmaceutical enterprise. No less than President Trump and his GOP administration claimed it would execute several executive orders in the summer of 2020 to rein in drug prices (actions that had not been taken as of when this book went to press).[13] These orders[14] were seen primarily by industry insiders as a political stunt leading up to the 2020 election and dismissed by CEOs across the board on quarterly calls with investors as nothing to worry about while they refused to meet with the president.[15] Taking their collective outrage one step further, the Pharmaceutical Research and Manufacturers of America president and CEO Stephen J. Ubl said in a statement that "this administration has decided to pursue a radical and dangerous policy to set prices based on rates paid in countries that he has labeled as socialist, which will harm patients today and into the future."[16] He called the proposal "a reckless distraction that impedes our ability to respond to the current pandemic."[17] While expected, this reaction by the industry exhibited a lack of self-awareness about its current reputation, as the political stunt was used particularly because it had broad public appeal, across political lines and up and down the income ladder. What the industry was either missing or purposely ignoring was that public sentiment had turned against them, even during an urgent public health crisis where their expertise was desperately needed (i.e., the COVID-19 pandemic).

The pharmaceutical enterprise continues to turn a deaf ear to an increasing crescendo of public sentiment about the prices of drugs. According to a 2016 poll from the Kaiser Family Foundation, roughly eight in ten Americans believe that prices for prescription drugs are unreasonable and support various ideas to lower costs, such as allowing Medicare to negotiate with drug makers and enforcing price caps on high-priced medicines for certain illnesses such as cancer. The survey also points out that two-thirds of Americans favor the creation of an independent group to oversee prices, and nearly nine in ten believe drug makers should be required to disclose information on how prices are set.[18] Likewise, an AARP survey among older Americans produced similar results, causing Nancy LeaMond, AARP's chief advocacy and engagement officer, to state: "The public is making it increasingly clear that profiteering by drug companies at the expense of Americans is unacceptable. People are worried about high drug prices, and many are struggling because they can't afford their medications."[19]

The Rest of the Story

While we would suggest the sentiment of such a conclusion is supported by facts, the magnitude of the charge may be a bit amplified. For example, while it is true that R&D costs have gone up, such increases are not solely due to inefficiencies explained by Eroom's Law. Other reasons persist. The move toward more complex therapeutic types, say the steady progression from small molecules to antibodies and other complex biologics, has also contributed to the rising costs. This claim is certainly not intended as an apologist view because it is not clear that an expensive biologic solution is always the best answer to problems that might be solved by less expensive therapeutic modalities. And yet the pharmaceutical industry is ever-more frequently drawn to these expensive solutions for manifold reasons, all of which are driven by their need to expand their profits.

Another confounding factor arises when one considers the ham-fisted responses of the pharmaceutical industry to Eroom's Law. The changes meant to reverse this steady trend included industry consolidation, which decreased the critical mass of organizations actively involved in drug development and the emphasis upon outside contracting to CROs. Neither response slowed Eroom's Law.

Consistent with another law, that of unintended consequences, these reactions by the pharmaceutical industry as a whole likely guaranteed the continuation of Eroom's Law for at least another generation. For example, industry consolidation and outsourcing facilitated the creation of "middleman" organizations, usually venture-backed startup companies, which in turn were required to generate profitability to keep the doors open and satiate their investors, who were also seeking a hefty return.

While an individual company might mitigate the risk of a high-profile failure of an individual program by acquiring a company that has succeeded, the ecosystem as a whole still suffered the same large number of failures (if not more missteps since smaller and younger companies have less of a track record to draw upon to minimize risk). These added layers of venture-backed companies thus served to create an entirely new layer of complexity and profit seeking (perhaps two layers if you consider the start-up biotechs themselves as one and their venture backers as a second layer). The costs to create and maintain these new industries fueled further inefficiency. While the successful lambs would still be led to the slaughter (i.e., acquisition from an established company), the premium paid for those lambs had to include those other lambs that never made it that far. Stated another way, though individual companies might seek to avoid the risks of product failure during research and development, the industry as a whole could not. In trying to circumvent this problem, the industry compounded the problem.

The same argument can be made for contract research organizations. This entirely new industry was created to do the same activities that pharmaceutical companies had historically performed in-house at cost. While these services looked like a cost-savings to pharmaceutical executives eyeing a quick and efficient solution for their burgeoning research and development costs, these quite savvy individuals failed to consider the fundamental fact that CROs, like themselves, operate with the goal of maximizing profitability. By lowering their initial charges to create attraction and then charging ever more once that client has become dependent upon their services, the CRO model has created a relationship that can become quite lucrative and parasitic; thereby decreasing efficiency further and facilitating further adherence to Eroom's Law.

Exacerbating the situation, these CROs have recently been subjected to waves of mergers and acquisitions. As we have seen with the pharmaceutical industry itself, the costs of consolidation contribute to rising prices and have further perpetuated Eroom's Law. Even more problematic is the fact that these waves of consolidation have largely caused CROs to be exported offshore, leaving comparatively few headquartered in the United States despite the fact that this nation is the primary user of the services.[20]

In researching this book, we were surprised to learn that many of the costs for activities such as mergers, acquisitions, and external contracting are not factored into conventional research and development costs. To be generous, it is certainly safe to say that these costs are not counted in the same way by different companies. Thus, inconsistencies in reporting could suggest that the pace of Eroom's Law is increasing even faster than the already-damning numbers suggest.

As we have seen, issues involving opacity are not limited to research and development. For example, the costs to market and how these activities are accounted for (e.g., booking Phase IV trials as marketing costs) can vary by organization, with implications for how such costs impact pricing.

What Goes Up Doesn't Always Come Down

A problem that continues to plague the pharmaceutical industry arises from temptations to pursue fast-follower drugs. As you may recall, a fast-follower (or me-too) medicine is a minor chemical variation to an existing drug that has already demonstrated it is safe, effective, marketable, and profitable. The attraction to this approach is that the pioneering drug (the first of its type) will have identified and presumably overcome the risks that often derail innovative new medicines. One would presume that a second, third, or later entrant into a crowded field would lower drug prices much in the same way that the price of a Sony PlayStation is kept in check by competing products from Nintendo, Microsoft, Wii, or Ouya.

Something rather odd tends to happen with pharmaceuticals. Let's return to popular statin drugs as an example. The first statin was a drug called lovastatin (trade name Mevacor). As recounted in *A Prescription for Change*, the second, third, fourth, and fifth statins that followed lovastatin charged more, not less, than Mevacor. Paradoxically, these products were progressively embraced by more and more patients, their doctors, and insurers. This trend persisted even after lovastatin had succumbed to generic competition.

This trend was not unique to statins and the lesson learned in many boardrooms was to forego the risks associated with being a pioneer in a new type of medicine and instead let your competitor risk the expensive research, development, and marketing failures. Once a successful market is established, you can then swoop into the market with a lower-risk competitor, which will be viewed as the shiny new object and thus will harvest a bounty that was in fact created by your earlier competitors.

When confronting industry executives with this model, they dismissed such approaches as an artifact of the past. Nonetheless, analyses of a database Dr. Kinch and his team developed to study clinical trials has revealed ongoing tendencies toward this approach in drug development. A prominent example pertains to immune oncology, a burgeoning field in which the immune system is reprogrammed to facilitate the elimination of cancer. In looking at, for example, monoclonal antibodies that target a prominent set of targets (known as PD-1 and the PD-1 receptor), dozens of different drugs are being developed as fast-follower drugs, most of which are unlikely to provide anything more than incremental improvements (if any) over medicines already in use. And yet history has taught us that those minor improvements are likely to yield even greater revenues than the early innovator medicines.

Unless safeguards can be put in place to actively discourage fast-follower medicines, the health system may be weighed down by the considerable resources that continue to be invested into these medicines instead of inspiring and rewarding transformational new medicines. Indeed, financial penalties or fees could be placed upon drug applications to make fast-follower drugs much less attractive. Ideally, such fees could be directed into a fund meant to support research of drugs to address unmet medical needs or to make medicines more affordable to low income individuals, much as the PDUFA fees are redirected to support the FDA in adequate staffing of qualified reviewers and officials.

We will soon convey a particularly lurid story of fast-follower drugs in a future chapter but will close out this part of our story with an anecdote obtained while researching this book. The fundamental question we sought to address was seemingly simple, "How does a pharmaceutical company determine the price of a medicine?" The answers were surprising.

CHAPTER FIFTEEN

How Are Drug Prices Determined?

B oth authors have an extensive history and contacts in the pharmaceutical and biotechnology enterprises. While engaging with
past colleagues and sincerely asking what we presumed would be
a straightforward question, neither of us was ever able to get a conclusive
answer. Indeed, the mere asking of a seemingly innocuous question abruptly
ended multiple phone calls and nearly terminated one friendship, resulting
in an uncomfortable silence for a time. And more than a few former colleagues still working in the industry reminded us that they were "good
people who've dedicated their lives to doing good things for human health"
(which we agree with in most cases), and one friend, who is currently a general counsel at a midsized biotech company in Maryland, who agreed that
prices were outrageous but given the "pressures on publicly traded companies
there wasn't really anything anyone could do about it."

Indeed, the opacity underpinning the decision-making for medicines is
similarly experienced by the vast majority of individuals, including many

in executive management of large pharmaceutical companies. This lack of transparency often comes as a surprise even to savvy financial analysts as evidenced by headlines such as that posted on *Endpoint News* on January 9, 2015. The pharmaceutical industry newsletter led with "Blueprint scores first FDA OK for a precision GIST cancer drug, just ahead of a rival treatment. And the price is a big surprise."[1] The article goes on to describe how the small biotech company was reveling in the approval of its first drug, noting that industry analysts were shocked that the company intended to charge $32,000 per month, nearly twice the cost that even the most aggressive analyses had anticipated.

Nonetheless, we persisted in our effort to determine how the price of a medicine was determined but must warn you that this will be, by far, the shortest chapter in this book. The brevity does not reflect the importance of the question but rather the availability of information to support a reasoned discussion of the subject. We will therefore not sugarcoat what we do and do not know and get straight to it.

For nearly all conventional consumer products, the price charged reflects a confluence of information about the costs of materials, labor, infrastructure, transportation, and, of course, profit, to name but a few of the larger parameters. With medicines, this understandably is a tad more complicated given the extraordinary costs (in both time and dollars) required for a regulatory approval. Compounding the situation, we already know that only a handful of select (and some might argue lucky) products ever reach the market, as most fail either before or during clinical trials. Therefore, the determination of the price to be charged for a new medicine must necessarily compensate for the risks and costs incurred by other, unrelated products that will never enter the market.

As we learned from Bernard Munos, an increased scale of a pharmaceutical company paradoxically leads to greater inefficiency and thus higher costs. In part, this scaling of inefficiency reflects the need to support aging pipeline products as well as currying favor with key opinion leaders and pleasing the demands of aggressive sales forces. As large pharmaceutical companies have become frustrated by their continued adherence to Eroom's Law, many have opted to outsource much, if not all, of their research and development activities to contract research organizations and/or by in-licensing or purchasing upstart biotechnology companies. Both of these options contribute to drug pricing as the organizations providing these services and products have to meet their own payrolls and understandably seek to be rewarded.

Although such pressures may compel established companies to raise the price of new medicines, these stressors are not unique to "big pharma." Legacy companies such as Merck or Pfizer are no more likely to increase the price of a medicine than a recently founded company. Looking further, even the most lean and successful biotechnology company invariably has obtained capital from venture and other types of investors, who in turn have their own expenses and profit motives. Moreover, these venture capitalists themselves invariably hedge their bets by investing in a portfolio of companies, only a fraction of which will prove successful. Therefore, these investors must themselves pay for the failures in their portfolio by maximizing the costs of the relatively few medicines that their companies bring to market.

Another line of thought considers that effective medicines hold the potential to improve the quantity and quality of life. Without sounding over philosophical, this raises the question, "What is a life worth?" Although a loaded question, there is actually an answer, or at least an opinion. In 1968, a team composed of a Johns Hopkins economist, a member of the White House Budget Office, and a professor at Brandeis University published a paper assessing the cost-effectiveness of treating chronic kidney diseases.[2] In a paper that would become a landmark for insurance company actuaries, the investigators introduced the idea of quality-adjusted life year (QALY), which can be roughly translated as the average value a year that a person spends in full health, free of disease. The value of a QALY is admittedly arbitrary and can vary widely (and is guaranteed to be controversial, regardless of the outcomes) but is often cited in today's dollars to range from $50 to $150 thousand per year.[3]

Using parameters such as QALY, the price of drugs that cause dramatic health improvement might be at least guesstimated. As we have already seen, a fraction of otherwise terminal cancer patients are utterly cured of their disease by a new generation of immune oncology drugs. Deploying QALY, one might be able to justify the high costs of these medicines, which are offered routinely with annual prices that exceed a hundred thousand dollars.

Calculating the real benefits of medicines would seem to require intelligence and computing capacity that would far exceed the capacities of even grand masters of five-dimensional chess. We presumed the information needed to calculate a fair price might also reflect the costs of research, development, manufacturing, distribution, advertising, and a myriad other factors, each of which would be weighted to one degree or another to come up with a final number. However, we were shocked to learn that none of this seems to factor into the equation of the pricing of medicines. Indeed, there does not seem to be any equation at all.

The presumably complex answer to the question of how much a new drug costs boils down to a simple economic question: "What will the market bear?"

If one googles the question, "What will the market bear?" they can expect to be greeted with countless opinions extolling or condemning the basic tenets of capitalism. At one extreme are views that defend the practice as a justifiable means to reward the risks associated with delivering a highly desired product. The polar opposite view conveys criticisms suggesting this practice is both the cause and consequence of dysfunction in the modern healthcare (and other economic) systems.

Probing the idea further, it becomes clear that pricing practices may not entail massive poring over spreadsheets and four-dimensional strategy but rather a "spitball" approach to assign an almost random number to a drug. In general, it seems that if a drug is better than an existing competitor, it might be assigned a price above that drug (usually considerably higher). For, a new product that only demonstrates equivalent safety and effectiveness as an existing standard of care might launch with a price just a bit lower. Very often, the price of that drug will quickly rise beyond the price charged of its competitor. Likewise, companies will raise the price of existing drugs seemingly at will but not based on any type of objective formula. For example, a sudden increase (or decrease) in the cost of manufacturing or marketing does not seem to be reflected in the price tag. In fact, the price increase can simply result from the need to show a growth in revenue and earnings to the company's investors from one quarter to another.

Like it or hate it, the pragmatic reality is that pharmaceutical companies are certainly not alone in charging as much as they believe they can get. Yet there are some unique features of the pharmaceutical enterprise that distinguish it from, for example, the costs of other technologies or consumer products. The basic tenets of supply, demand, and competition don't seem to apply to the branded prescription medicines we buy. Look no further than the story of statins, where the fifth statin, which conveyed no significant medical benefit over the first four, commanded both a higher price tag and sold more pills at that inflated cost than any of its predecessors had.

Would we pay more and stand in line for a fifth version of a mobile phone, which had no improved capabilities or features that were better than the previous four? Continuing with the iPhone analogy, would Apple let Samsung (or any other manufacturer) be the first to introduce an improved phone, waiting years to let others blaze the path, only to finally enter the market with a higher priced product (that was no better) and find that consumers embraced it? If the answer to either question is no, then why does this seem to be standard practice for the pharmaceutical industry? And why do we tolerate this dysfunction?

Another distinguishing feature of the pharmaceutical industry is that the products it manufactures can determine the difference between life or death, health or disease. Given this importance, it is essential that we address these inconsistencies. As we progress toward the final chapters of our story, we will suggest some potential remedies to help balance the need and opportunity to allow ever more people to gain access to vital medicines.

The increasing price of drugs reflects the compensation structure for many physicians and hospitals. For example, many oncologists and cancer treatment centers have historically favored drugs that are delivered via long-term infusion. Indeed, the costs of infusion are now a key feature that supports the revenues of many physicians and hospitals. These revenues and profits play a key role in rising prices and are yet another example of the larger enterprise surrounding pharmaceutical products.

At the outset of researching a book on drug pricing, we presumed the proverbial buck stopped at the desk of pharmaceutical companies. Looking further, we were surprised to learn that while the pharmaceutical industry can rightfully be accused of many missteps and of consistently undermining their own credibility (be it through inappropriate pricing or marketing activities), this vital but troubled industry may not be the key component setting prices or even receiving the majority of profits from the expensive products they manufacture.

To understand this jarring finding, we must leave the pharmaceutical industry for a time and turn to a far more mysterious player, including organizations that may be household names but whose impact and power are incompletely understood by almost everyone.

CHAPTER SIXTEEN

And You Thought Pharma Was Opaque

The pharmaceutical enterprise is an ever-expanding behemoth that consists not merely of an expanding number of scientific and medical industries that discover, develop, or manufacture medicines, but it also includes an entirely different set of businesses that control the distribution of medicines that arguably profit even more from the rising price of medicines than the pharmaceutical manufacturers. We have already seen the increasing role of the advertising industry, which was well established long before the first pharmaceutical direct-to-consumer spending. Here we will introduce an industry that was created (without irony) in an attempt to curb drug prices. Yet the exact opposite has happened.

Our story begins with hepatitis C, a disease that has a fascinating backstory from the perspective of both science and drug pricing. Summarizing the science in just a few sentences, hepatitis is a medical term reflecting inflammation and damage to the liver. An acute (though deadly) form of the disease is generally associated with food contamination (known as hepatitis A), while a separate form of chronic hepatitis is an infection caused by hepatitis B virus (HBV). HBV-mediated disease was all but eradicated with the discovery of the responsible virus in 1968 and the deployment of a vaccine roughly a decade later.[1] All the while this quiet but extremely important public health advance was taking shape, another form of chronic infectious hepatitis began to show itself, slowly replacing HBV as the major form of deadly hepatitis in the United States. The cause of this second form of chronic hepatitis was attributed to a new blood-borne pathogen, soon to be dubbed hepatitis C pathogen (HCV).[2] HCV is a fascinating virus but frustrating in the sense that it has resisted all attempts to target it with vaccination.

Buoyed in part by knowledge gained while combating HIV, pharmaceutical scientists were eventually able to develop other medicines that effectively eradicated HCV in infected individuals. Whereas HIV drugs tend to hold off the virus, stalling it in its tracks but not eliminating the infection, HCV drugs can be curative, utterly liberating patients from this otherwise chronic and fatal disease. This first major breakthrough arose with the discovery of sofosbuvir (trade name Sovaldi), which, when combined with another drug (ledipasvir), was demonstrated to be curative when administered as part of a twelve-week course of therapy. Sovaldi was hailed as a major breakthrough and one that justified a high price tag, which was set by its developer, Gilead Sciences, at $84,000.

In mid-December 2014, a St. Louis-based company named Express Scripts announced its intentions to drop Sovaldi from its formulary of medicines.[3] This action was taken in favor of another anti-HCV drug from AbbVie (a spin-off of Abbott Pharmaceuticals) that had been recently approved by the FDA. In making the announcement, the chief medical officer for Express Scripts touted the action to delist one drug over another as "unprecedented." The rationale was that the Gilead drug listed for $84,000 whereas AbbVie priced their medicine at $83,319.

At first glance, this action appears both righteous and yet rather puzzling. The righteousness reflects the fact that it seemed that someone was (finally) taking a stance to support the American public against the rapacious activities of the pharmaceutical industry. A line in the sand had been drawn and a public defender (namely Express Scripts) was looking out for the interest of the average Joe. Looking further, things became a bit murkier.

The confusion centered around the fact that the price difference between the two drugs, while being a few hundred dollars, was miniscule (a difference of less than one percent). Nonetheless, the action taken by Express Scripts on that cold December morning was touted by many, including Dr. Kinch in a prior book, *A Prescription for Change.* Looking back just a few short years, we now see that these initial reactions reflected a naïveté and utter misunderstanding of a business that arguably plays as big a role in driving the high prices of medicines as the drug manufacturers themselves.

In this chapter, we will seek to demystify and shed a bit of disinfecting sunlight on an industry created with the best of intentions, it seems, but yet another example of unintended consequences that allowed it to become a major cause (rather than solution) of escalating drug prices. In researching this part of our story, a relative lack of understanding of, and objective information available about, an industry known as "pharmaceutical benefit managers" (PBMs) has proven to be so opaque that even the most reasonably intelligent medical or business professionals are as confused as we were in trying to grasp a basic understanding of how this industry works. After hearing repeated complaints from credible sources, we decided to learn more about pharmacy benefit managers.

An important consideration in framing this story is the question of who decides what medicine will be taken by a patient. Let's be certain about one thing: The patient today has virtually no say in what drug they will be putting into their bodies (except of course to simply refuse to take a prescribed drug in a potentially self-defeating protest). It is likewise naïve to think that the physician, who was responsible for writing the prescription, will be able to dictate what medicine is finally used. Yes, a physician can certainly influence the decision-making, but the final decision will generally be made by the institution that pays for the medicine.

For many Americans, the payer is a private insurance company. As we will revisit in the next chapter, much of the country relies upon the federal government in one form or another (either as an employer, retiree, or recipient of Medicaid or Medicare) to act as their "insurance company." The business of Medicaid, Medicare, and private insurance is immeasurably complex, with its own version of opacity, and well beyond what we could address in this book. However, it will be necessary to gain at least a rudimentary and generalized understanding of how the system works in terms of the multilayered decision-making associated with prescription medicines.

For now, a few rather commonsensical points must be stated. First, a decision whether to pay for a medicine and, if so, which medicine to approve, is generally made with a degree of good faith from all parties involved. Yet the organizations that make these decisions do so with an eye to their own business prospects and profitability. As the complexity of this decision-making has grown (a subject upon which we will expand), many insurance companies and governmental payers (e.g., Medicare Part D plans) elected to bring in outside help to better inform their decision-making. Over time, these "third party administrators" evolved into the pharmacy benefit management (PBM) system of today.

As a disclaimer, it is important to point out the authors are neither deep experts in understanding the complexities of the insurance industry nor government benefits. However, we did interact with such experts and will attempt to translate and generalize the primary features of an admittedly complex system that, like the pharmaceutical industry, prefers opacity over transparency. Consistent with the approach used throughout this book, we will do so by providing a brief history of how the present system evolved and mutated over time.

From Washington to Washington

Like the pharmaceutical industry, the reimbursement or coverage of new medicines by insurers (be it private sector or governmental) is a relatively new phenomenon. The earliest government-mandated health coverage in the United States arose with the passage of the Social Security Act, which was advocated and signed by President Franklin Delano Roosevelt on April 19, 1935. Title XIX of that historical legislation provided aid to states to support medical assistance though it did not specify support for prescription drugs. An amendment creating Medicare for the elderly and disabled as well as Medicaid for low-income individuals would occur three decades later and be signed into law by President Lyndon Johnson in 1965. Yet neither addressed the question of prescription drugs.

Nonetheless, the first precursor organization to modern PBMs had been up and running for six years. Based on our research, the first example of an organization that provided coverage for prescription medicines, albeit to a limited choice of medicines (to be known hereafter as a "restricted formulary"), arose in the state of Washington with the creation of the Group Health Cooperative of Puget Sound. This member-based organization of pharmacies was established in Seattle in 1947 and was built upon a proposition that savings could be realized by the direct purchase of drugs en masse directly from pharmaceutical companies rather than from intermediate distributors. This organization mandated that the savings earned would be passed along to its members. Were a physician to prescribe a medicine outside of the restricted formulary, special permission would be required before the cooperative would consider underwriting these rare exceptions. As a demonstration of the cost savings realized by the creation of this novel mechanism, a 1966 study revealed the pharmacies that participated in this group paid $0.96 for an average prescription whereas non-member pharmacies spent twice as much. This sounded like a pretty good deal and the model began to spread.

Similar agglomerations of pharmacies sporadically came together in different geographies (e.g., the California Pharmaceutical Association created a nonprofit known as Paid Prescriptions, Inc., in 1964) or were driven by special advocates (e.g., the United Mine Workers established a similar group in 1950 to assist union members suffering the effects of chronic diseases).[4] Such programs soon flourished, gathering momentum by recruiting an ever larger number of pharmacies at a time when the industry was dominated by independent mom-and-pop shops staffed and owned by individual pharmacists.

As revealed in congressional hearings to the Subcommittee on Environmental Problems Affecting Small Business of the House Select Committee on Small Business, some of these same shops soon began to suffer. For example, geographically defined organizations began to set prices that either seemed so low that they would threaten the existence of non-members, or so high or bureaucratic (e.g., requiring copious paperwork) that even founding members became increasingly boxed out of the market and feared losing existing and future customers. In particular, these networks were declared to be guilty of price fixing and collusion. Recognizing the bias of those testifying, nonetheless, a read through the congressional record of the testimony and submitted exhibits from the 1971 hearings seems to align this new model more closely with the mafia than as a staunch public defender.[5]

As evidence of such a concern we will look at testimony provided in mid-June 1971 by David Fleming, a counsel to the California Pharmaceutical Association, who singled out one particular company, which will play a key role for our story.[6] The company, Pharmaceutical Card System (PCS) was pilloried by Fleming. Established months earlier in 1969 in Phoenix, Arizona, PCS had launched by sending letters to pharmacists claiming to have established relationships with a variety of popular insurance companies.[7] For an upfront membership fee of fifty dollars followed by annual payments of eight dollars, PCS would either allow individual pharmacies to opt into a treasure trove of potential customers or be entirely cut out, risking the loss of long-time customers. For those opting in, PCS would manage prescription flow, setting a defined "maximum allowable cost" (MAC), the top price for each medicine that every member pharmacy would be required to honor. In other words, a pharmacist could not charge more than the MAC to their customers, regardless of whether the pharmacy suddenly had an increase in cost (e.g., due to particularly high local increases in rent or wages). In a second mailing a few weeks later, PCS included an implied threat that "third-party prescription programs are here to stay and are growing by leaps and bounds." These communications were submitted into evidence for the 1971 congressional investigation. Testimony by Fleming and other pharmacists continued that, in the face of overwhelming pressure, individual pharmacies were in effect being held hostage, facing either imminent loss of their customers or surrendering most of their profits to PCS and other third-party conglomerates.

Facing dual pressures from expanding pharmacy chains such as CVS and this new breed of conglomerates, which would later be known as pharmacy benefit managers (PBMs), the family-run corner drugstore was accelerating toward extinction. The proverbial last men standing, the chains and PBMs, would then be left to confront one another.

Following the tale of PCS a bit further, the company did fulfill its self-professed destiny and grew by leaps and bounds. In 1972, McKesson, a major pharmaceuticals distributor, purchased PCS and added capabilities to the business model, emphasizing opportunities to deploy robotics to improve the efficiency of dispensing.[8] In 1994, McKesson sold the PCS brand to Eli Lilly for nearly $4.5 billion at a time when the pharmaceutical company was, depending on your perspective, diversifying its business into related businesses (e.g., consumer products, cosmetics) or distracting itself from its long-standing core business.[9] The distractions proved more accurate and Lilly offloaded PCS to a pharmaceutical chain, Rite-Aid, for a third of the cost it had paid for PCS five years before.[10] A year later, Rite-Aid likewise off-loaded PCS to another PBM, AdvancePCS, reflecting a phase of consolidation within the PBM industry.[11] AdvancePCS eventually became a powerful brand. In 2003, just three years after being valued at one billion dollars, AdvancePCS was sold to Caremark for $5.3 billion. In 2007, the pharmacy giant CVS purchased Caremark primarily to gain access to AdvancePCS, paying $26.5 billion for the right to do so.[12] [13]

The ups and downs in the pricing of PBMs such as PCS was occurring amid a consistent period of increasing drug prices. The question, which has become quite a vigorous debate, is a matter of determining how much of the steadily rising costs of medicines was due to PBM growth and evolution at the same time.

To understand the debate, it is important to explain a term we have already encountered a few times in this chapter and one that you have probably heard before: "formulary." A formulary is simply the array of medicines that a particular pharmacy will provide. This is essentially the same as the brands available at a grocery store, but with a rather prominent difference. Whereas not every grocery store carries every brand and flavor, one can simply go to a different store to find it. A formulary, as dictated by a PBM or insurer, limits the availability of medicines for which they will pay. As we have already seen, you can of course obtain any drug for which you have a prescription. However, you will have to pay full price for that medicine out of pocket unless it is included in the formulary of your insurer (or the PBM with which your insurer has contracted).

Armed with this tidbit of knowledge, let's return to the example of Express Scripts' blocking of Sovaldi. This action essentially meant that Express Scripts' 83 million customers (roughly one in four Americans) would no longer be able to access this HCV drug. As a consequence, Gilead Sciences, which marketed Sovaldi, was pressured into lowering the price of the drug.

Lowering a price is not necessarily a bad thing and, indeed, it is quite a good thing, right? Let's be clear, the lower price is generally not realized by the consumer but by the insurance company. One can argue that since insurance rates reflect how much insurance companies have to pay for products, then the savings would undoubtedly be realized (eventually) by consumers. However, concerns about opacity, which will be explored further below, raise questions about the benefit of PBMs and whether the consumer benefits at all.

A simplistic view of PBMs, either as a positive or negative force, is dangerous. Neither case can be made unambiguously, and it is necessary to look more deeply into how these companies operate and make their money. It brings us back to our question from the previous chapter: What is the price of a drug?

Our investigation of this simple question is complicated by the extraordinary opacity of how PBMs work. Multiple people interviewed for this book (including both pharmaceutical and insurance executives) reiterated the extraordinary view that no one knows the price of a particular drug. Further, an even more radical issue is that the complexity of the relationships between drug manufacturer, insurance company, and the PBM has been designed to ensure that no one can ever know the answer to that simple question—including the parties involved.

How can this be? One would think such an answer to be impossible given the extraordinary spotlight that has been placed upon the costs of medicines by Congress and in the media. And yet, we would argue that an unintended consequence of this emphasis has triggered a deepening and broadening array of unknowable facts.

To shed some light upon this paradox, let's define terms that most reasonable people believe they know but may not.

Discounts, Rebates, and Bundling, Oh My!

We are all, whether consciously or not, familiar with the concept of drug discounts. Ubiquitous pharmaceutical advertisements often conclude with a statement such as that which accompanies the television commercial for Nexium: "If you can't afford your medication, AstraZeneca may be able to help." The "help" often comes in the form of a discount. Essentially comparable to coupons for food items often found within the inner bowels of Sunday newspapers, these discounts are provided to patients by pharmaceutical manufacturers. Rather than printed on paper, these discounts often take the form of a piece of plastic indistinguishable from a credit card. Like American Express, however, this form of credit is not accepted everywhere and may expire. For example, Medicaid and Medicare Part D (the prescription arm of elder benefits) consider the use of discounts as a kickback, our first subtle suggestion that this practice is not quite as simple or forthright as a more conventional coupon for mustard or ketchup. Moreover the expiry of these cards can be problematic for patients who have acclimated to or whose health has become dependent upon the medicine (and its discount).

Although discounts can be the source of gastric distress, patients are altogether excluded from the other two forms of pharmaceutical price discounts: rebates and bundling.

A pharmaceutical rebate, unlike its more conventional consumer counterpart, is not issued to the end user (i.e., the patient) but rather to the pharmaceutical benefit manager. These PBMs, as you may recall, are often contracted by insurance companies to help manage the claims and distribution of medicines. The idea is that a PBM can leverage massive buying power to obtain better prices for the products it manages. A payer (e.g., an insurance company or organization such as Medicare) will then bargain with a PBM to establish a "negotiated price" that the end users (the patients) will have to pay for their medicines. It then becomes in the best interest of the PBM to obtain the drugs from the drug manufacturers at the lowest possible cost.

With this in mind, a rebate is a discount offered, generally by pharmaceutical manufacturers, with the goal of including their medicine in the PBM's formulary. Let's take that sentence apart a bit. If a pharmaceutical company wants to market their medicine to the customers represented by a PBM, then their products need to be included in the formulary. To achieve that end, a pharmaceutical company will often provide an incentive, in the form of a rebate to the PBM, to ensure their drug is included in its formulary. Some PBMs may return some of the price savings offered by the rebate to the insurance company or the consumer. Or they can instead pocket the savings. In a statement by the CEO of PhRMA, the trade association for the pharmaceutical industry, "Even though more than a third of the list price is rebated back to payers and the supply chain, health plans do not pass along these discounts to patients with high deductibles and coinsurance."[14]

Keep in mind that the PBM is also making money by collecting an administrative fee from the insurance company for managing the costs and distribution of medicines. The PBM also makes money based upon "the spread," which is simply the difference between the amount charged to the insurance company minus the costs paid to the pharmacy. Consequently, a canny PBM makes money from both ends; from the upstream manufacturers and/or from distributors of the medicines, as well as the downstream insurance companies.

This seemingly simple idea now leads to the subject of "bundling." Let's say you are a manufacturer with a portfolio of products that you want to have included in the formulary of a large PBM (or insurance company if they are not using PBMs). A PBM may negotiate a rate for one drug that is profitable but insist on including this as part of a bundle for a rate for another drug that is not. In this case, the manufacturer may make a profit on one part of the bundle but lose money on something else. Yet, if the company were to limit the bundle only to profitable products, the PBM may walk away and take their clients with them. Indeed, one pharmaceutical executive pointed out to us a situation where they had a bundle of five products with a PBM and lost money on four of the five drugs. Yet the fifth drug made so much money that the pharmaceutical manufacturer determined it was worth losing money on the other four. And when it came time for the manufacturer to update its prices, the fifth drug would necessarily garner the highest price increases.

In such a manner, the conventional concept of pricing based upon supply and demand can become perverted and distorted.

How bad is the situation? No one truly knows.

The reason for this ignorance is not stupidity but the lack of transparency. The negotiated prices between a PBM with both the insurance provider and the manufacturer are strictly confidential and considered a trade secret. This fact precludes anyone (including both parties as well as the public) from knowing the magnitude of "the spread" collected by the PBM nor the amounts of administrative fees and rebates.

Compounding the situation, there is growing evidence that in an effort to maximize spread (i.e., profit) PBMs may end up indirectly inflating the prices of both branded and generic medicines. This is the conclusion of 46brooklyn Research, an Ohio-based nonprofit created to help increase the transparency of drug pricing. The team at 46brooklyn aggregates information about the prices paid by Medicaid and other agencies, based on public records, to assess trends in the pricing of both branded and generic medicines. Rather than focus upon a static price, the nonprofit tracks these therapeutics over their lifetimes and takes a unique approach by estimating the cost for one month of treatment.

This approach has revealed dramatic increases in the costs of both branded and generic medicines. For example, the median price of one month of treatment with a newly approved medicine rose from $150 in 2006 to $1,551 in 2018. Although outrageous, this outcome is not particularly surprising given that the focus of the pharmaceutical industry has disproportionately focused upon oncology and other high-cost, low-incidence indications (driven largely by incentives conveyed by the Orphan Drug Act). Another contributing factor is that the types of medicines approved have trended more toward expensive biologics (e.g., monoclonal antibodies) rather than less expensive products. Nonetheless, these results reveal a staggering increase in price that will come as a surprise to very few.

46brooklyn's findings do not stop with branded medicines. An analysis of medicines that lost patent exclusivity between 2005 and 2019 revealed that more than three-quarters of generic equivalents were priced at a level either comparable to or within 15 percent of the price of the branded equivalent. As more generic competitors entered the market, one might reasonably expect that the greater competition would decrease the price, but this is simply not the case.

With medicines, comparing prices are about as simple and transparent as comparing the prices paid by two passengers sitting next to one another on a commercial airline flight. Thankfully, certain federal payers, such as Medicaid, regularly update the national average drug acquisition cost (NADAC), which is the average price they pay for a medicine. By comparing the NADAC with the list prices charged by a pharmaceutical company (known as the average wholesale price or AWP), one can see dramatic differences, with AWP often being more than ten-fold higher than the NADAC.

The problem is that when PBMs are negotiating with payers (e.g., private insurance), they use the overpriced AWP as the set-point, despite knowing that this price is artificially high. PBMs therefore tend to benefit the most from higher rebates from manufacturers, most of which end up in their pockets (as we've previously indicated, the amount, if any, that is shared with insurance companies is unclear due to the opacity of the relationship). The leadership at 46brooklyn playfully refers to the difference between the AWP and the NADAC as the "Supply Chain Profit Opportunity" (SCPO) or "Sick-Po." Over time, the SCPO has increased across the board but especially for generic medicines, because the NADAC tends to decrease for generic medicines due to increasing competition, whereas there is no competition for branded drugs. For drugs such as childhood leukemia drugs that periodically experience shortages, the AWP (and SCPO) increase particularly dramatically, as do the profits garnered by supply chain providers, namely PBMs.

In recent years, insurance companies (i.e., payers) became increasingly aware that the middlemen (i.e., PBMs) are reaping huge profits from the approaches described above and have begun to acquire these businesses for themselves. The most prominent example of this was the March 2018 announcement that Cigna would acquire Express Scripts for $54 billion. Although impressive, a real demonstration of the power of PBMs had been revealed months before with the December 2017 announcement that CVS Health would acquire Aetna for $69 billion. This allowed both rivals to compete with a third competitor, UnitedHealth, which controls Optum, another pharmacy benefit manager.

A widely held concern about these waves of insurance and PBM mergers is that consolidation will restrict access to medicines. Stated another way, the new insurance/PBM conglomerates may opt away from including less lucrative medicines in their formularies. Such concerns have been related by many practicing physicians, who themselves have been contractually limited to an increasingly narrow base of medicines. Another potential concern is that insurance companies might not let employers separate pharmacy benefits from their coverage. An insurer can then demand a penalty payment for each member each month. This would create, according to Eric Pachman of 46brooklyn, a "worst case scenario" that essentially penalizes employers, who in turn will be forced to pass along higher insurance costs to their employees.

The resulting behemoth drug managers have gained unprecedented leverage and are able to pressure pharmaceutical manufacturers (rarely a source able to garner public pity) and to preclude small competitors. The consequence of such relationships has simply served to increase the overall price of medicines rather than increase their efficiency. The pharmaceutical companies address these pressures by issuing ever more rebates and discounts, which is a form of "funny money" paid to PBMs/insurance companies that doesn't seem so funny to a public that needs these medicines and are the ones who increasingly are paying the price for these inside deals.

In researching this book, we met with Steve Miller, a representative of the pharmacy benefit manager Express Scripts. Defending the industry, Miller pointed to a 2018 article published by Peter Bach of the Memorial Sloan Kettering Cancer Center in New York. Using information on retail sales, Bach's report estimated that pharmacy benefit managers received gross annual profits of $23 billion, which pales in comparison to the $323 billion earned by pharmaceutical manufacturers. The combination of wholesalers and PBMs captured at least a quarter of the profits. Moreover, such estimates are based upon insight into an industry that has fought diligently to retain the secrecy of its business arrangement. Therefore, such estimates must be taken with a very large grain of salt (presumably in combination with an overpriced hypertension medicine to counteract the elevated sodium intake).

Miller made another point in defense of his industry, which was centered upon medicines where PBMs play no role. So-called lifestyle drugs, such as erectile dysfunction (ED) medicines, are generally not paid by insurance companies nor subject to PBM rebates. In what was clearly a well-executed and rehearsed example, Miller pointed out that the prices of the three most common drugs (Viagra, Levitra, and Cialis) have increased more than nine-fold since their introduction. Moreover, the price increases tended to occur within hours of one another, which suggests the unlikeliness that "these drugs either have the same costs or is evidence of collusion." He went on to indicate a similar phenomenon arising with the price of insulin, even though it is a lifesaving drug, essential to more than 7 million Americans according to a November 7, 2019, article in *U.S. News and World Report*.[15] So, both lifestyle and vital medicines are subject to such upward and potentially collusive price pressures.

In response to this statement, Eric Pachman of 46brooklyn cited examples where PBMs have gamed the system by taking advantage of the fact that some drugs can be used for different indications when given at different doses. In the case of sildenafil (the generic name for Viagra),

PBMs have placed lower dosage pills on specialty drug lists, which allows the PBMs to charge much higher rates than the comparatively inexpensive form used for ED.[16]

Miller also pointed out that while PBMs have been subject to criticism about the transparency of their dealings, a similar demand for transparency has not been placed upon the pharmaceutical industry to defend their pricing decisions. Rather than suggesting that both industries be required to do so, Miller indicated that "the easy solution" of transparency would solve nothing. He proceeded to pose a rhetorical question about the costs of manufacturing and distributing a bottle of Coca-Cola and why those costs are not subject to transparency inquiries. He concluded that when consumers are satisfied, they only care about the final price. Miller was essentially asking why his industry should have to reveal its inner secrets when others are not asked to do so.

Some of Dr. Miller's points are understandable, but misguided. Consumers are not satisfied with the price of medicines. Indefensible price increases have tainted the reputation of the pharmaceutical industry for decades, even before the rise of PBMs. In addition, two wrongs do not make a right with regards to transparency. If PBMs are required to operate in a transparent fashion, so should pharmaceutical manufacturers. Both should be required to be fully transparent in their pricing decisions. As pointed out by biotech pioneer Wayne Hockmeyer, the profit margins associated with pharmaceuticals are quite substantial (estimated to be in the range of 25–45 percent for drugs as compared to low single digit percentages for consumer products).

As such, the Coke analogy falls apart a bit for other reasons. Consumers are not satisfied with the price of medicines and failure to procure the product does not result in a lack of satiation on a hot day, but an increased likelihood of death or additional pain and suffering from debilitating disease. Furthermore, the costs of a Coca-Cola is necessarily constrained by its competition with Pepsi and other products. Were the price of Coke products to be inflated at the rate of pharmaceuticals, consumers would likely migrate to other less expensive competitors.

Like representatives from virtually all the other players in the drug development game, Miller pointed outward to other components of the bloated pharmaceutical enterprise. Even pharmaceutical industry executives agreed that their products captured exceedingly healthy margins when compared to nearly every other industry. But these admissions were followed by the claim that such profits are needed to offset regulatory risks and short period of market exclusivity (due to patent expirations). After stating a belief that manufacturers indeed deserve a healthy profit margin to offset the considerable risks of that industry, Miller questioned whether the present levels are excessive, even when considering risk. In particular, he pointed out that a dozen large pharmaceutical companies capture 50 percent of overall drug profitability.

Beyond merely targeting drug manufacturers, Miller identified yet another component of the ever-expanding pharmaceutical enterprise. Specifically, he fingered the consultants and brokers of pharmaceutical contracts (middlemen who work with large employers to help them select the best PBM contracts). Indeed, companies such as Marsh and McLennan and Willis Towers Watson that broker such deals play a role in the drug pricing conundrum. Miller emphasized that they "overwhelm customers with spreadsheets" and undermine attempts to curtail drug costs. In particular, Miller argued these organizations "hate value-based contracts as they are more complicated." For example, he pointed out that Express Scripts will reimburse two-thirds of the costs for a drug if the patient decides to cancel or change the drug within the first ninety days. Miller stated that "no consulting company can figure out how to build this [reimbursements] into their contracts."

PBMs are not a phenomenon unique to the United States, but this relatively new industry and its mighty lobby has a particularly powerful hold on this nation. Looking beyond our shores, we will now highlight some of the problems and solutions other nations have explored or implemented to identify a way out of the drug pricing morass.

CHAPTER SEVENTEEN

American Exceptionalism

A s we noted at the very beginning of our story, Americans spend vastly more for prescriptions medicines than our counterparts around the world. According to the Organization of Economic Cooperation and Development (OECD), a club of rich-world countries, the average American spent more than $1,000 on medicines in 2016.[1] In comparison, the average in France, the United Kingdom, Australia, and virtually all other wealthy nations was less than half of that. Even the average Swiss, who almost seems to take pride in the fact that everything is pricier in their native land, spent more than twenty percent less than an American. But keep in mind this is not because Americans consume more medicines, they just pay more. In fact, the rate at which Americans and Europeans take pills, tablets, and injections are indistinguishable.

The exceptional spending by Americans certainly does not reflect a demographic disadvantage. Quite the opposite. It is generally accepted that as we age, our dependence and financial outlay for medicines increases steadily. According to statistics compiled by the American Central Intelligence Agency (yes, the CIA), the average age of a citizen of the European

Union is nearly 43 years, five years older than the average American.[2] While the average German boasts an age of 47.3 years, they can trumpet that they pay a mere $685 per person per year for medicines as compared with $1,011 for their American brethren, who are a full decade younger.

The price differential is not due to Americans preferring brand name drugs. In fact, it's quite the opposite. The United States consumption of medicines is disproportionally skewed toward low-cost generic medicines, which comprise 84 percent of the prescribed medicines.[3] This places the United States in a tie with the United Kingdom for the use of low-cost drugs. In contrast, only 33 percent of the medicines taken by the Swiss, whom you may recall have the second highest drug costs, are generics.

Eric Pachman from 46brooklyn pointed out an Australian study that revealed Australia and New Zealand were by far and away getting lower drug prices than much larger developed countries like Canada and the United Kingdom.[4] Spain was the only country that even came close to the United States in terms of pricing. Recalling Munos's costs of scale argument, this would seem to be applicable to countries as well; the larger you are, the higher the price you pay.

Simply put, Americans pay far more for their medicines than their counterparts around the world.[5] Why is this the case? For one thing, the practice of discounts, which we discussed in the previous chapter, is rather unique to the United States. A 2015 study of six top-selling drugs conducted by Bloomberg News revealed the absurdity of drug discounting. The nondiscounted sales price for Lantus, a form of insulin, was $372, whereas discounts reduced the price by 50 percent (for those who qualified and utilized the discount). Although this may seem promising, even the discounted price of $186 paid by the American consumer was exorbitantly high when compared with the prices paid in Europe and Canada, which ranged from a low of $45 in Norway to a high of $67 in Canada. Similar findings were observed with other popular drugs used to manage diabetes, cholesterol, and asthma. Also, bear in mind that the discount can expire or shrink, leaving drug-dependent customers to pay full freight for their medicines.

At the end of the day, a study conducted by the University of Southern California (USC) in partnership with the Brookings Institute concluded that American consumers are responsible for 64–78 percent of pharmaceutical profits despite the fact they account for only 27 percent of global income.[6] Part of the reason for this disparity is a tendency for Americans to use newer and more expensive medicines that come with higher profit margins; the rest of the reason is that the same drugs cost less in other countries. Moreover, Americans pay more for medicines because they are not protected by their government from doing so.

Before conveying a successful example of how one European country addressed skyrocketing drug prices, let's take a look at how the world might look if European countries paid prices at a level comparable to the United States.

The same Brookings/USC study pointed out that an average price increase of 20 percent for Europeans would increase revenues to pharmaceutical companies, which would in turn invest more into new research and development.[7] The study maintains that new products would improve the welfare of Americans by $10 trillion through the introduction of new medicines to combat infectious, neurodegenerative (e.g., Alzheimer's and Parkinson's) and other diseases. Stated another way, our planet, which is warming, favors the release of deadly new pathogens (like SARS-CoV2) on a more regular basis. Compounding the problem, the world's population is now older on average. Together, these issues will require new medicines and vaccines to prevent diseases that are ever more costly, both in terms of financial outlays as well as preventative illnesses and deaths. This same study further conjectures an overall savings of $7.5 trillion to Europeans given this population is likewise aging more rapidly than their American counterparts.

The premise that European prices should increase to match America's to help promote innovation is a bit perplexing. Certainly, the branded pharmaceutical industry has a long and distinguished track record of investing heavily in innovative new drugs (despite or perhaps because of Eroom's Law). However, one would argue that fairness dictates not that the Europeans be required to match the exorbitant prices of the United States but rather that the Europeans pay their fair share (i.e., higher Europeans prices to offset lower prices to the American consumer, bringing them closer to parity based on income levels).

In asking why Americans pay so much, a common complaint from patient advocacy groups is that American regulators (i.e., those at the FDA) are pricklier than their European counterparts. This assertion is not supported by the data. Europeans generally roll out and accept new medicines at a comparable pace to the United States. The difference, it seems, is that European governments control drug prices more aggressively, and frankly more practically, than the law allows their American counterparts to do.

As an example, look no further than Germany. In 2011, the German government introduced legislation with the rather intimidating name of *Arzneimittelmarktneuordnungsgesetz;* with the slightly shorter but no less guttural acronym, AMNOG.[8] Roughly translated into English as the Act to Reorganize Pharmaceutical Markets for the Health Insurance System, the new law rewarded innovative new medicines that provide clear medical benefits while controlling the prices of less innovative or nonbeneficial drugs.

The government had been pressured to take action after mounting evidence that the Central European nation was paying more than a quarter more for medicines than other European nations (though barely half of what's paid by Americans).[9] Using an approach predicated upon "value for money," the new law allowed drug pricing in Germany to reflect the benefits realized by patients. In doing so, this law would actively discourage "fast-follower" and other medicines that convey little, if any, clinical benefit relative to existing medicines.

The core of AMNOG is a requirement that drug manufacturers produce a dossier that conveys the benefits of a new therapeutic entering the German market. This document is evaluated by a nonprofit commission, which is granted six months to assess the medical benefit (who benefits and how many patients are expected to use the drug), price, reimbursement considerations (i.e., whether the drug will be restricted to certain patient populations based on price), and overall cost-effectiveness. If no additional benefit is conveyed (such as often arises with fast-follower drugs), the maximum price of the new medicine is defined by the costs of existing medicines that convey comparable safety and efficacy.[10] The manufacturer can charge a higher rate but will not be reimbursed by insurance companies beyond the determined price. If a consumer still decides they want a medicine that is priced higher than the cap, then the consumer is required to pay out of pocket to make up the difference.

If a new medicine is determined to convey a therapeutic benefit, a period of public negotiations between the insurance organization and pharmaceutical manufacturer begins to assign a maximum price for the drug. This negotiation must be concluded within six months and binding arbitration is invoked if an agreement cannot be reached. All the while this is occurring (i.e., the first year after the drug is approved but before a maximum price is negotiated), the company is permitted to sell the drug at whatever price they choose.

The AMNOG model is widely viewed as successful, saving German consumers more than a billion dollars in 2015 alone. Paradoxically, the AMNOG example might suggest that additional bureaucracy (oversight of drug prices) might improve the efficiency of drug pricing. In particular, more attention could be placed upon the proliferation of industries within the larger pharmaceutical enterprise that now seem to exist only to increase costs. Although there had been concerns that some manufacturers might choose not to market their products in Germany, these concerns proved unfounded. Perhaps most importantly, the German system for insurance more closely resembles the situation in the United States, with multiple payers (including government and private sector insurance companies), which obviates concerns about adopting measures taken by government-run, single-payer systems in other European countries or Canada.

To look at an example of how an AMNOG-like system might improve current practices in the US we examine a recent case where modifications in chemical composition led to a new, easier-to-consume liquid-formulated drug that was found in clinical trials to be medically as good as an existing remedy only available in tablet or powder form. The original innovator company developing the liquid formulation decided the enhancement deserved premium pricing because it substantially improved patient compliance, leading to better long-term outcomes.

Ravicti (glycerol phenylbutyrate) is a liquid oral drug used to treat urea cycle disorders (UCDs), which are rare genetic conditions that result in high levels of ammonia in the blood. If left untreated, urea cycle disorders can lead to confusion, coma, or even death. Historically, a majority of those who suffer from UCDs were children, as few struck with the conditions would live into adulthood. Prior to Ravicti's approval by the FDA on February 1, 2013, the only product available to help in controlling ammonia levels was Buphenyl (sodium phenylbutyrate), a chemically similar drug approved in 1996 to control UCDs that is most commonly dispensed in tablet or powder form.[11] While both products are dosed according to a patient's weight, patients taking Buphenyl were faced with consuming a large number of very foul-smelling tablets, an extreme challenge for parents desperately trying to encourage their children to take a medicine that could save their lives. Comparatively, Ravicti is an odorless liquid requiring a patient to consume substantially less to control their UCD.[12]

As it was considered a treatment for an unmet medical need, Ravicti was granted orphan drug status and a fast-tracked review. The major study supporting Ravicti's safety and effectiveness involved forty-four adults who had been using Buphenyl.

The blood results from the pivotal study showed Ravicti was as effective as Buphenyl in controlling ammonia levels. Up to this point this story sounds like a great advancement, but then we get to the pricing considerations. Once approved, Ravicti was priced considerably higher than Buphenyl. In March 2015, the innovator company that developed Ravicti, Hyperion Therapeutics, was purchased by Horizon Pharmaceuticals for $1.1 billion amid a flurry of pharmaceutical takeovers for that year. Within months, Horizon increased the price for not only Ravicti, but also Buphenyl (which it also got as part of the acquisition), making the original tablets less attractive as an inexpensive alternative. A month's supply of Buphenyl (250 tablets) is more than $7,000, according to the website Drugs.com. And according to a 2020 analysis by GoodRX, Ravicti currently has a list price of $55,341 for a thirty-day supply, making it one of the most expensive drugs on the market today.

In reviewing the Ravicti story, it appears that the process improvement was a major step forward, especially as improved compliance in the real world could lead to substantial enhancements in patient outcomes. In fact, it did "demonstrate[s] FDA's commitment to providing treatments for patients suffering from rare diseases" as Donna Griebel, MD, director of the Division of Gastrointestinal and Inborn Errors Products in the FDA's Center for Drug Evaluation and Research was quoted as saying at the time of Ravicti's approval. However, one could also consider the pricing decision to be exorbitant for a drug that needs to be taken for the entirety of a person's life to ward off the devastating effects of a life-threatening, inherited, rare disorder affecting a very small patient population. As such, one can imagine the potential outcomes for Ravicti if run through an AMNOG-like process that could both reserve the incentives for an innovator truly interested in advancing patient outcomes by allowing them to recoup some of their development costs in the year following the product's launch—the time period that AMNOG allows developers to price their product as they see fit. Thereafter, the assessment by the commission evaluating the new drug's benefits would be used in determining the maximum price allowed, which in Ravicti's case would come down to how much value was conveyed by a liquid formulation showing equivalent medical outcomes in pivotal trials, but which provided real-life compliance benefits that could result in better long-term patient outcomes.

While there is no shortage of examples of how the German model might be applied, other countries, like Canada, also have ideas worth investigating. And indeed, it is to our neighbors to the north that we will now turn, as this nation has powerfully influenced American awareness of drug prices and policies meant to begin correcting the system.

Oh my, Canada . . .

Anyone comparing the United States and Canada faces an uphill challenge. Although the two neighbors share much history, some language, and the longest undefended border in the world, the demographics and political structures of the two nations are quite distinct. Nonetheless, Canada has consistently featured prominently in discussions about drug pricing. Yet the current idyllic view that many have of Canadian drug pricing is the consequence of a cauldron of attempts, most of which failed, to improve healthcare affordability. As a result of these changes, many of which were rather tumultuous, consumers in Hamilton, Ontario, pay considerably less for medicines than their counterparts in Hamilton, Ohio. A brief review of history is required to understand the various experiments conducted in Canada, many of which might be informative to improving the situation south of the border.

Canada experienced a remarkably challenging history in terms of struggling with the subject of intellectual property, especially patents. The nation gained self-governing authority from the British government in 1867 but was acknowledged as a coequal only in 1931. An early act of independence was the creation of the first Patent Act in 1869. The original act provided exclusivity for fifteen years and this was extended first to eighteen years in the late 19th century and finally to the international standard of twenty years after being compelled to do so by the World Trade Organization (WTO). Along the way, other changes were enacted, some of which specifically targeted the pharmaceutical industry.

In 1969, the nation felt the prices of medicines were being manipulated by its powerful southern neighbor, which held a firm grip on both the branded and generic pharmaceutical sectors.[13] In an effort to spur the creation of a Canadian pharmaceutical industry, the government amended the Patent Act to allow domestic generic medicine companies to manufacture and market medicines that were still under patent. Innovator companies were forced to grant a "compulsory license" to Canadian firms and were reimbursed with a 4 percent royalty on sales made in the country.

This scheme proved successful and facilitated the creation of a lucrative generic and specialty pharmaceutical industry that prospers today. This ecosystem would soon facilitate the creation of the company ICN, which after a series of scandals would be renamed Valeant, and rebranded yet again as Bausch Health (after Valeant incurred even more scandals and purchased Bausch and Lomb). As detailed in *A Prescription for Change*, Bausch Health and its precursors adopted aggressive (and occasionally illegal) business practices, ranking it among the most prominent villains responsible for the price increases capturing headlines around the world.

With the adoption of continent-wide free trade agreements, such as the North American Free Trade Act (or NAFTA), the practice of "compulsory licenses" eased with legislation passed in 1987 and was finally abolished altogether in 1993. Despite conforming more to the American system of intellectual property protection, the Canadian experience still differed from that in the United States. For one thing, the 1987 revisions introduced into the Canadian system created the Patented Medicine Prices Review Board, a federal agency of about three dozen employees who review the prices paid in other countries for patented drugs. This information is then analyzed to negotiate a maximum price for drugs to be sold within Canada. As a sop to branded pharmaceutical companies, still resentful about the period of "compulsory licenses," the legislation also created a waiting period of seven to ten years before which an innovative new medicine would be subject to generic competition.

The Canadian legislation also created a complex and layered litigation system that triggered a myriad of lawsuits and thereby enriched attorneys throughout the nation. One estimate suggests that these changes in litigation cost hundreds of millions of dollars in legal expenses to both innovator and generics companies (which were undoubtedly reimbursed by consumers through higher prices).[14]

A 1992 assessment of the Canadian system by the United States General Accounting Office (GAO) for the US Senate concluded the changes had restrained the prices of prescription drugs by as much as one-third. The GAO report was split as to a question of whether the reduced prices had stifled innovative tendencies by pharmaceutical companies to pursue new medicines. Frankly, this outcome is not surprising, as one could argue rather forcefully that reimbursement issues in Canada likely do not convey the most compelling decisions for corporate boardrooms to invest in new research and development activities. The United States is the largest single market for new medicines, followed by the European Union. As we have already seen, the higher prices paid by American consumers offsets the savings enjoyed in Europe and Canada.

Despite the clear benefits of the 1987 law to its citizens, the complexity of the Canadian pharmaceutical patent system created its own set of problems, particularly as it pertained to the abundant litigation. These concerns compelled the Canadian Parliament to reform the system yet again in 2019.[15] This time, the Patented Medicine Prices Review Board was directed to exclude the United States and Switzerland from their pricing analyses. This acted to significantly lower the average rate to be negotiated with pharmaceutical manufacturers, much to the chagrin of international pharmaceutical companies, and represent even more monies that would have to be compensated by American consumers.

The new law would go even further, requiring pharmacy benefit managers and companies to disclose confidential rebates. However, the boldest piece of the legislation is a power granted to the review board, which can allow it to declare that high prices are illegal and could be remedied by stripping away the intellectual property of the innovator organization.

With its passage, the Canadian government proclaimed the legislation would translate into nearly 10 billion US dollars (13 billion Canadian dollars) in consumer savings.[16] Needless to say, the new law was opposed by the pharmaceutical and pharmacy benefit manager industries, which, as of this writing, had successfully lobbied to delay its implementation.

Despite all the resources devoted to lobbying and lawsuits, Canadian prices are still substantially lower than those in the United States. This fact, you may recall, compelled high-profile pharmaceutical tourism by Bernie Sanders and other politicians. The Canadian example has created domestic turmoil in the United States as well with lawsuits and political finger-pointing surrounding issues such as importation of drugs from Canada.

As one example of the political turmoil as reported July 2019, the Trump administration declared it may base the prices Medicare pays upon Canadian benchmarks.[17] As we will now see, this was not the first time these stresses had forced lawmakers to look to the north for guidance.

CHAPTER EIGHTEEN

A Stomach-Churning Story

A decade after the creation of Canada's Patented Medicines Prices Review Board, the American government began to consider reforming how it pays for certain medicines. As we have seen, the GAO had submitted a report that extolled the virtues of the Canadian model while leaving open the question of whether the price restrictions had stifled innovation.

These views were emphasized by many American consumers, who began crossing the Canadian border solely to purchase lower-cost medicines. The idea of allowing Medicare to provide a benefit to reduce the prices of prescription medicines was championed by Congresswoman Nancy Pelosi of California and Senator Thomas Daschle of South Carolina, who initiated legislation in their respective chambers. The cause was then championed in 1999 by outgoing President Bill Clinton. The fact Clinton hoped to champion a form of healthcare reform just days following his failed impeachment, combined with the reality he was a lame-duck president, scuppered any chance that he would be able to sign drug pricing reform into law.

As is too often the case, a combination of technology and tragedy was needed to affect meaningful change. The technology was the commercial potential of the internet, which had captured the public's imagination in the 1990s. As with all new technologies, some seized upon opportunities to abuse the system and the headlines were filled with stories of fake medicines sold online. The practice of selling adulterated medicines was certainly nothing new: the titular character in Graham Greene's 1949 novella (and later Academy Award–winning movie), *The Third Man*, portrayed a villain who profited from selling watered-down penicillin.[1] Similarly, the print and airwaves rang with real-life stories of watered-down cancer drugs and forged medicines, many of which were manufactured in untraceable Chinese laboratories. Indeed, that nation suffered an estimated 192,000 deaths attributable to fake drugs in 2001 alone.[2]

As suspicions grew about the reliability of medicines, including both purchases made over the internet or in Canadian pharmacies near the border, American concerns grew and President George W. Bush picked the cause to champion, much as Clinton had done. The Republican Congress, which had quashed the Pelosi-Daschle legislation in 1999, suddenly favored the bill, now known as the Medicare Prescription Drug, Improvement, and Modernization Act. The bill barely passed the House with a vote of 216 to 215 but then sailed through the Senate and was signed into law on December 8, 2003.

The legislation created an entitlement benefit for prescription medicines, known widely as Medicare Part D. The passage of the law was not assured, but many provisions were baked in to appeal to the Republican-controlled houses of Congress and to key constituencies. Driven by lobbyists from the American Association for Retired Persons (AARP), the benefit included a subsidy for large employers to prevent them from dropping private prescription coverage for retired employees. Much of the opposition to the final bill in the House reflected the fact that the law prohibited the federal government from negotiating discounts with pharmaceutical companies and from creating a formulary of approved medicines. Both provisions were understandably favored by the pharmaceutical industry. Notably, the Louisiana Republican who championed the legislation, Billy Tauzin, would leave the House of Representatives to serve as the chief lobbyist for the Pharmaceutical Research and Manufacturers of America (PhRMA) weeks after passage of the critical legislation.

Aside from the controversies and apparent conflicts of interest, a key point of our story is that the Medicare Part D law adjudicated claims based on a geographical basis, with fifteen jurisdictions created to cover all fifty states and various territories. In response to Freedom of Information Act requests, the Center for Medicare & Medicaid Services (CMS) published a report of the monies paid by each of these states; a report that returns us back to the work being done by our associates at 46brooklyn.

As you may recall, this Ohio-based nonprofit is devoted to shedding light upon the factors involved in drug pricing in general and Medicaid and Medicare in particular. The nonprofit is a labor of love, and its members earn their living running a consultancy known as 3 Axis Advisors. In late 2019, the consultancy published an illustrative example of the need for transparency.[3]

The example we will use in this chapter is the Purple Pill (not to be confused with the blue pill or any other colors of the rainbow, for that matter). However, one could be forgiven for some confusion as there have been two purple pills—different but intimately related to one another and reflective of rather unseemly practices that were made possible by the flawed system that oversees drug pricing in the United States.

A Queasy Feeling

Stomach ulcers have plagued our species for much of human history. Ulcers are simply perforations of the stomach lining that allow the powerful acids that aid digestion to leak out and spawn infections as microorganisms in the stomach gain access to the warm and gooey tissues in the abdomen. Notable sufferers who have died from complications of ulcers and gastric bleeding include the scientist Charles Darwin, the author James Joyce, the Ayatollah Khomeini of Iran, and, controversially, Napoleon Bonaparte of France.[4]

Treatments for the disease have varied over time and were mostly ineffective. For example, an oft-used remedy of drinking warm milk actually triggered higher levels of gastric secretion, worsening its symptoms. Thus, the disease ran rampant for centuries and represented a lucrative opportunity for the pharmaceutical industry. Scientific advances in the late 1970s had fingered a set of futuristic-sounding proteins known as proton pumps, which were essential in allowing the stomach to produce acid. These findings triggered a race to block stomach acid production as a means of alleviating peptic distress.

The race would ultimately be won in 1989 by a Swedish company named Astra AB, which would introduce the first commercial proton pump inhibitors, a drug with the generic name of omeprazole. Originally branded as Losec, the name would have to be changed due to FDA concern that physicians or patients might confuse "Losec" with "Lasix," a popular medicine used for heart failure. The revised name resulted from adding a few letters to the original one and became "Prilosec."[5]

Prilosec was a commercial blockbuster, quickly bounding to the top of the league charts for commercial sales. The number of purple-colored pills downed by patients exceeded all expectations, generating five billion dollars in annual revenues. Although Astra AB executives were made giddy by the revenues, the pharmaceutical treadmill rendered their elation into concern as Prilosec sales climbed, ultimately accounting for 40 percent of commercial sales. While fantastic in the short term, these revenues would soon be doomed to generic competition.

Astra AB (which would become AstraZeneca in 1999 through a merger with the British Zeneca Group) faced two looming crises that threatened to destroy the drug upon which the company had become addicted. Predictably, the blockbuster revenues would be lost starting in 2001, when omeprazole sales would succumb to rival generic manufacturers.

Worse still, two renegade Australian scientists, Barry Marshall and Robin Warren, had become convinced that the underlying cause of ulcers was a bacterium living in the stomach. Moreover, they had demonstrated that this organism gone bad, *Heliobacter pylori,* could be readily treated with conventional antibiotics. This treatment opportunity would be proven in a most unusual way when Marshall performed a high-profile experiment upon himself by intentionally infecting himself by swallowing the contents of a fetid beaker full of the obnoxious bacterium. The resulting gastrointestinal distress was then reversed with a course of antibiotics. Beyond compelling the warning that one should not try this at home, the scientific duo had discovered cheap antibiotics to provide a low-cost way for the medical community to eliminate stomach ulcers. Marshall and Warren quickly rose from crackpots espousing a crazy idea to receiving the Nobel Prize (albeit more than a century later than Alfred Nobel, a prominent ulcer sufferer, might have liked).[6]

Given these concerning developments, company officials at AstraZeneca initiated a series of activities to mitigate their risks. Lucky for them, a hallmark of modern society is the ever-accelerating amounts of psychological stress. One beneficial manifestation of this stress (at least from the perspectives of stressed-out AstraZeneca officials), is that anxiety has a tendency to push the stomach contents from their intended location up into the esophagus. The resulting burning of esophageal lining by concentrated acids is not only a source of discomfort but can cause lasting damage and even cancer. Thus, at the same time that Prilosec was losing one market due to the causal link between bacteria and stomach ulcers, another was created by ever-increasing rates of indigestion (known in the medical community as gastro-esophageal reflux disease, or GERD, an acronym whose pronunciation nicely captures the manifestation). Thus, Prilosec was opportunistically repositioned from a treatment of ulcers to GERD.

The piles of cash generated by Prilosec helped Astra AB underwrite the aforementioned corporate merger. With an eye constantly upon the patent clock for Prilosec (due to expire in 2001), the combination provided a more promising pipeline of products to ensure future stability. The AstraZeneca merger would prove a bellwether of sorts, being an early catalyst for waves of industry consolidations that continue today.

Beyond the corporate merger, the management at AstraZeneca were not content merely to let revenue streams from Prilosec go. They tasked a team of executives, that was given the nickname "Shark Fin" since the shape of the dorsal fin nicely captured the revenue projections presumed for Prilosec (an accelerating rise followed by a steep, nearly vertical, drop-off once generic competition had been baited by the chum of expired patents).[7]

As beautifully conveyed by a report commissioned by Arnold Ventures and executed by 3 Axis Advisors, the Shark Fin team came up with a list of five options to keep Prilosec alive. The company eventually chose what many considered the daftest option, a seemingly amateurish strategy that 3 Axis Advisors appropriately labeled with a cheeky B-movie title, "Son of Prilosec."[8]

Just like people, some chemicals can have right or left-handedness,[9] which one can think of as mirror images of a structure. In the case of Prilosec, the handedness arose at roughly equal proportions. However, only one hand was primarily responsible for the effectiveness of the drug (the other conveying neither harm nor help). What AstraZeneca elected to do was to isolate the version (the handedness) responsible for the benefits of Prilosec. The company would then protect this "Son of Prilosec" with patents to provide additional decades of exclusivity. This new version of the drug would be known as Nexium, a name conflating "next" and "millennium." Likewise, the generic name was esomeprazole, which reflects the handedness (the S-form) of omeprazole. As an aside, the term S-form refers to the Latin term *sinister* (meaning "left-handed"), a coincidence that seems somehow applicable to our story.

A reasonable person might concede that a strategy to introduce Nexium, an expensive new drug, to compete with a cheap generic medicine was destined to fail. However, AstraZeneca accompanied the launch of Nexium with a rather extraordinary strategy. First, the company petitioned to release Prilosec as an over-the-counter (OTC) pill. This audacious decision effectively deterred generic manufacturers, who recognized that if an OTC drug is on the market, many insurers will refuse to cover the generic medicine, which would reduce the incentive for would-be generic competitors to enter the market. Recognizing that the company did not have a strong presence in consumer products (especially in the United States), AstraZeneca had partnered with Procter & Gamble (P&G) to launch Prilosec OTC coincident with the expiration of the patents. AstraZeneca would continue to manufacture the medicine but grant the industrial giant the rights for the marketing and distribution of a product branded "Prilosec OTC." Moreover, the FDA granted P&G a three-year period of exclusivity for their new OTC drug, ensuring that no other competitor could encroach upon their sales.

In parallel, the company launched Nexium claiming it was better than Prilosec and hence should command a higher price tag (even than full-price Prilosec, not to mention generic or over-the-counter versions). The drug was "technically" better in that half of Prilosec (the wrong handedness) did nothing whereas Nexium eliminated the noneffective forms of the molecule. The company took the quite clever approach of gaining approval by directly comparing the strengths of Prilosec and Nexium. Impressing no one but the regulators it seems, Nexium out-performed Prilosec when the two drugs were compared side-by-side at the same strength. This was obvious since 20 mg of Nexium contained twice as much active ingredient as 20 mg of Prilosec. Other studies that compared 40 mg of Prilosec revealed, unsurprisingly, no relative benefit of the pricey Nexium.

Although one could achieve the same effect by swallowing two Prilosec pills, AstraZeneca began a campaign to convince the FDA, physicians, and pharmacists (including PBMs) that Nexium (at $4 per pill) should be considered superior to Prilosec.[10] This attempt would be an uphill battle in light of opinions such as that of an executive at Kaiser Permanente, who stated, "Nexium is no more effective than Prilosec. I'm surprised anyone has ever written a prescription for Nexium."[11] Yet AstraZeneca pulled off the strategy brilliantly.

The company began a sales and marketing effort to convey the idea that Nexium provided "superior clinical efficacy" as compared with Prilosec. This audacious statement was constantly reinforced by a saturation campaign of advertising in all forms of media. The advertisements disingenuously continued to refer to Prilosec as "the purple pill" but distinguished Nexium as "the healing purple pill," which was suggestive of improved efficacy (when the only difference was dosing levels).

Another rather odd situation arose when, as noted by the *New York Times*, Prilosec OTC began to disappear from the store shelves.[12] These absences were not the result of increased sales but insufficient production. Procter and Gamble and AstraZeneca pointed fingers at one another while industry analysts smiled and pondered the fact that consumers had little other choice than to turn to AstraZeneca's more expensive Nexium product.

AstraZeneca broke records in the days after the launch of Nexium, spending more than $260 million on advertising in the first year alone.[13] Nonetheless, this strategy paid off nicely as Nexium generated over $14 billion in net revenues, placing Nexium in the pantheon of pharmaceutical product launches—despite the fact it conveyed no better benefit than Prilosec OTC. The result was a coup for AstraZeneca, which saw revenues from Nexium exceed even Prilosec in its heyday (not to mention the profits generated by OTC Prilosec). Indeed, the work by 3 Axis Advisors revealed that by 2006, four years after its launch, generic omeprazole only accounted for 7 percent (one in fourteen doses) of Medicaid sales, sandwiched between and effectively asphyxiated by a sandwich composed of Nexium and Prilosec OTC.

Nor does the story end there. A decade after its record-shattering launch, Nexium faced imminent patent expirations and cannibalization by generic medicines. Having learned from its prior experiences, AstraZeneca again decided to take a creative approach to the looming deadline.

As you may recall, the first company to file an abbreviated new drug application (ANDA) with the FDA for a generic drug is granted a six-month period of exclusivity. This provision had been included in the Hatch-Waxman legislation as an inducement to promote generic manufacturers but instead has been a persistent source of abuse, as we will now see.

The Indian generic manufacturer Ranbaxy filed an ANDA in October 2005 and was promptly sued by AstraZeneca for patent infringement, as were two other generic manufacturers who similarly filed ANDAs later that year. Given Ranbaxy's edge in terms of the 180-day period of generic exclusivity, AstraZeneca negotiated a multiproduct agreement with its competitor, which had the effect of Ranbaxy delaying its launch of generic esomeprazole in exchange for a cash payment and the granting of certain rights to market or manage other AstraZeneca drugs. The value to Ranbaxy was estimated to be roughly $700 million, whereas AstraZeneca, you may recall, was bringing in many times that amount each year in Nexium sales.[14] Similar deals were later struck with other generic companies threatening to market generic esomeprazole. These deals are increasingly commonplace and referred to as "reverse payments" or more colloquially, "pay to delay."

In frustration, a $20 billion federal lawsuit was launched against Astra-Zeneca and Ranbaxy, claiming reverse payments were a violation of antitrust regulation. The case made its way through the courts but was struck down both by the Circuit Court and Appeals Court when the judges ruled a precedent from a 2013 Supreme Court decision upheld the use of "reverse payments."

Ranbaxy also proved to be the type of competitor that every company dreams of. In the midst of all this wheeling and dealing, Ranbaxy pled guilty to multiple charges of drug adulteration. The charges singled out the manufacturing plant where generic esomeprazole was intended to be manufactured, thus further sidelining Nexium's primary competition.[15]

Meanwhile, AstraZeneca turned back to a strategy with which it had negated generic competition with Prilosec. In 2012, the company announced an agreement with Pfizer to market Nexium OTC. They also revealed that the over-the-counter version would be released on the same day that the first generic versions of esomeprazole were scheduled to hit the market.

Keep in mind this new consumer product would not only be competing with generic drugs, but with Prilosec OTC. Although Nexium OTC would be priced at $0.50 per dose, store-brand omeprazole could be found by that time at nearly a tenth of the price. Indeed, physicians around the world began sounding an alarm that the price of store-brand omeprazole might be too low, thereby encouraging the overuse of these proton pump inhibitors.[16] Indeed, these drugs were not without their side effects (no drug is), which can include kidney damage and polyp formation.[17]

Whereas information about over-the-counter medicines are not readily available to physicians, these primary care providers do monitor prescription medicine. In this context, AstraZeneca partnered with major pharmacy benefit managers to launch a mail-order program to deliver prescribed Nexium to a patient's home. As detailed by the report from 3 Axis Advisors, this scheme served to enrich AstraZeneca (which obtained a premium price and did not lose sales to generic manufacturers) and PBMs (through the negotiated yet confidential rebate program as detailed in the previous chapter). The losers in the scenario were employers, who were left paying more.[18]

Because of these types of schemes, branded Nexium remains in the formularies of most Medicare and private insurance providers. This fact is particularly stunning given not merely that Nexium long ago became subject to generic competition but works no better than branded, generic, or OTC omeprazole. Moreover, the inability of Medicare to negotiate (by law) means that the organization continues to pay more than three dollars per dose despite the fact that generic drugs cost a fraction of that and, as we have seen, over-the-counter omeprazole retails for pennies a dose.

The Nexium story was closely watched by industry analysts and pharmaceutical executives around the world. The myriad strategies successfully deployed by AstraZeneca were replicated whenever possible and continue to the present. A recent example was the 2019 approval of esketamine. This left-handed version of ketamine, a drug first approved by the FDA for use in 1970, entered the American market as a nasal spray for treatment of depression. The drug garnered an average price tag of $5,000 for the first month of treatment and $3,000 every month thereafter. Although its sponsor,

Johnson and Johnson, had no evidence that the drug was more efficacious than its older parent compound, it garnered a price tag manifold higher.

The stories of Prilosec, Nexium, and esketamine are symptoms of a wider disease consumers face in dealing with a combination of pharmaceutical manufacturers, insurers, and PBMs, all of whom, because of the complexity of the system responsible for gaining an FDA approval and producing, distribution, and reimbursing medicines (while maximizing their profitability), are able to point their fingers at one another in conveying the blame for who is responsible for escalating drug prices.

CHAPTER NINETEEN

Views of an Archaeologist

N ow that we have witnessed an example of the dysfunction propagated by our current system of drug development, approval, and pricing, it is important to review the components of the system that failed and, more optimistically, that offer opportunities for future improvement.

We appreciate that the breadth and depth of the subject matter presented in this book is dense and, at times, may seem convoluted. Therefore, we present in this chapter examples and brief summaries of the array of inefficiencies and blinders that have simultaneously discouraged innovation and yet magnified the costs of new medicines over the past few years. Consistent with the title of this chapter, we will take a position that the old ways of developing drugs and vaccines were already in decline and merely expedited by the sudden shock presented by the recent COVID-19 crisis.

It seems reasonable to anticipate that in the not-too-distant future we will look back upon the overly complex and inefficient means by which medicines are discovered, developed, and distributed to seem as ancient and foreign as the diggings of Carthage are to an archaeologist or that a rotary dial telephone is to a contemporary American teenager.

Two of the primary drivers of the dysfunction that have plagued drug development, and thus have contributed to the accreting price of medicines, are unique to the industries involved. The first is Eroom's Law, which reflects the ever-increasing costs needed to develop a new medicine. Were this not sufficient to be problematic, Eroom's Law is coupled with the pharmaceutical treadmill, the idea that even the most innovative and impactful products have a short shelf life and will inevitably succumb to generic competition.

In spite of these profound hurdles, the modern pharmaceutical era, which spanned the period from the end of the Second World War until the 2008 economic downturn, provided a myriad of wonder drugs, which immeasurably improved the quality and quantity of health available to the public. The last two generations have witnessed millions of lives saved by penicillin and other antibiotics that it inspired. This true wonder drug allowed our species, for a time at least, to conquer many infectious diseases, which had historically been the major causes of human mortality.

Looking back, the era of antibiotics, which began in the 1940s and lasted through the first few decades of the 21st century, may be reaching an end (some indeed already insist we already live in a post-antibiotic world).[1] Resistance to many, if not all, conventional antibiotics has flourished among our bacterial adversaries and this is a fight we are destined to lose because unrelated bacteria have the capacity to circumvent even the most recent manmade anti-infective and, more worryingly, to communicate this capacity from one deadly bacterial species to another through the transmission of highly mobile genetic elements known as plasmids. These plasmids allow two utterly different pathogens across the globe, species, and environments, as distant and foreign as any two that can be imaged, to share the same ability to resist even the most recent weapon in the antibiotic arsenal and at the speed of a plane, train, or automobile. Indeed, humans are not even necessary for this transmission as revealed by studies of antibiotic resistant bacteria in remote Siberian lakes, hundreds of miles from the closest vestiges of humans.[2]

If we were merely to restrict our story to infectious agents, we would see another extraordinary series of unprecedented successes by the pharmaceutical industry in the form of the many vaccines that save countless lives worldwide. Starting with the first vaccine against smallpox, enabled by a humble but perceptive farmer by the name of Benjamin Jesty toiling in the verdant countryside of southeast England and later popularized by Edward Jenner, our species was able to utterly eliminate a scourge that had blended the infectiousness of COVID-19 with the lethality of Ebola and that had terrorized people for centuries.[3] Likewise, the past two generations have benefited from the elimination of a host of diseases including diphtheria, pertussis, measles, mumps, and rubella. Indeed, one of the greatest, unsung successes of the vaccine age was the introduction of a vaccine to prevent rotavirus, a diarrheal disease that killed a half-million children worldwide each year prior to the approval of a safe and effective rotavirus vaccine in 2006.[4] Likewise, entire cancers, including many malignancies of the liver, cervix, anus, head, and neck can be entirely eliminated with safe and effective HPV vaccines.

Yet vaccines have fallen out of favor, perceived by many in the pharmaceutical industry as not conveying sufficient revenues to be worth the effort. In truth, the price of vaccines are relatively low as compared to other medicines, although not necessarily any cheaper or less challenging to develop. Work by Dr. Kinch's team at Washington University in St. Louis demonstrated that the net number of vaccine-preventable infectious agents has not changed in a quarter-century. You might (correctly) counter this assertion by stating, "Didn't you just say we developed high-profile vaccines for human papilloma virus and rotavirus?" At roughly the same time we were celebrating this success, a vaccine meant to protect against Lyme disease was quietly withdrawn from the market amid questions about its safety and reliability. Consequently, the number of vaccine-preventable infectious agents stood at twenty-six in 1995 and twenty-seven in 2020 (figure 7).

As the attraction of the revenues to be earned from vaccines waned, so did the number and capabilities of organizations that had historically participated in vaccine development. In effect, we let our guard down and thus were caught largely flat-footed for the COVID-19 calamity that began in rural China starting in late 2019. A warning had been sounded years before when a related virus, SARS, broke loose in China in 2003 and quickly spread around the world, killing at least 774 of the 8,098 people known to be infected. Although fear of pandemic triggered frenzied interest in developing a vaccine in 2003, our memories are notoriously short and interest in a SARS vaccine died away as quickly as the epidemic had. This would prove to be a fatal decision given the genetic identity SARS shared with the agent responsible for COVID-19 (known as SARS-Cov2).

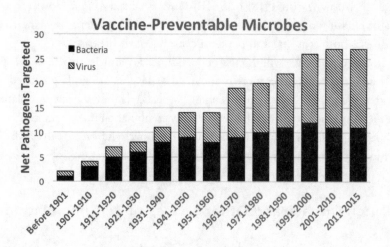

Figure 7. Vaccine Preventable Infectious Agents
The number of vaccine-preventable pathogens has remained stagnant since the 1990s, reflecting the lack of financial attraction of these vital medicines (results reproduced from data provided by CRIB).

As of this writing, the first vaccines for COVID-19 are gaining approvals, both in the United States and internationally. Yet it remains unknown whether these will remain safe and effective over months and years to prevent SARS-Cov2. Nonetheless, the unprecedented speed at which these early vaccines were discovered and developed reveals the amazing capabilities of the pharmaceutical enterprise when it works in close coordination with its regulators, such as the FDA. Thus, one can imagine that the horrific tragedies of COVID-19 might usher in a new era of mutually beneficial cooperation among those who discover, develop, regulate, and distribute new medicines and vaccine. Learning from the past, we might identify efficiencies that will finally make it possible to get away with breaking the law—Eroom's law that is.

The lessons taught in 2020 can potentially enable further improvements and preparations for the next plague, which is most certain to come. Pandemics are a natural phenomenon and, on average, occur every decade or two. Indeed, we are overdue for an influenza pandemic and are as unprepared for this still today (even after COVID-19) as we were with the Spanish Influenza (in 1918) or SARS-Cov2 a century later. However, we might regain footing by emphasizing a "universal" influenza vaccine that addresses both seasonal and pandemic strains of the disease.

In this chapter, we will discuss opportunities for anticipating such events, both infectious and other more mundane diseases that are easily predicted to shorten lifespans and human potential. For example, our society and planet are growing older, fatter, and hotter, a deadly combination that guarantees, at a minimum, an increase in Alzheimer's and metabolic syndrome, both of which already thrive and will merely grow in number and disease severity.

Dutch Disease and Other Causes of Self-Immolation

Despite, and we will argue because, of the extraordinary achievements afforded by successful development of drugs to treat or prevent infectious diseases, cancer, and cardiovascular diseases, the century since the Long War (an amalgamation of both 20th century world wars) was characterized by accelerating complexities and inefficiencies in drug development. Most of these barriers and setbacks were self-inflicted and purposely done in an attempt to stem an affliction that was undiagnosed in almost all those afflicted.

Financial success has a rather rude habit of creating a bit of a mess of things. The chronic malady afflicting the industries involved in the discovery, distribution, and payment of pharmaceuticals seems awfully similar to "Dutch disease." This term was apparently first applied by *The Economist* magazine in a 1977 article to describe how newfound wealth arising from a gas field in the northeast part of The Netherlands two decades before had effectively doomed the manufacturing capacity of the entire nation.[5] The revenues from fossil fuels drove up the price of the Dutch guilder and thereby rendered other Dutch exports uncompetitive. This was indeed not the first time this tidy, northern European nation had suffered such a calamity; the "tulip mania" period in the early 17th century temporarily spurred massive inflation and then wrecked the small nation's economic prospects once the bubble burst. Likewise, Dutch disease is implicated in the paradoxical economic failure to thrive in countries that have suffered the good fortune to find natural resources (think Middle Eastern, Russian, and Venezuelan oil or African blood diamonds).

Bearing in mind that neither author is an economist, the situation afflicting the pharmaceutical sector bears a close resemblance to Dutch disease. The rise of blockbuster drugs (those earning a billion dollars or more in annual revenues) created a paradox of good news prompting bad news as we have already seen with the saga of Eli Lilly's Year X and later Year Y/Z. Beyond that single company, the industry has been saddled with a form of the disease that is worsened by the fact that a blockbuster product has a very short life span, rarely exceeding a decade. This causes a scramble to find another blockbuster to replace it, which in the end, will only be a temporary fix for a longer-lived drug addiction problem.

Add to this already dismal scenario and complications arising from Eroom's Law, the ever-increasing costs and risks needed to develop a new medicine. Indeed, one might argue that Eroom's Law is both a cause and consequence of success. The escalating revenues that can be extracted for hot new medicines generate real and perceived value, creating a form of inflation and currency influx (e.g., a soaring stock price).

The pharmaceutical industry (and now biopharmaceuticals, factoring in the biotechnology sector that has been assimilated as a consequence of consolidation trends) has done remarkably well. Despite the fact that Eroom's Law and Dutch disease have been eating away at the industry, it has until recently continued to thrive. As we have already seen, like Moore's Law, which will ultimately be halted by the laws of physics, Eroom's Law will ultimately either be broken or will hollow out the industry's ability to continue making new medicines. The evidence suggests the latter outcome is more likely.

Conscious of Eroom's Law and Dutch disease, the biopharmaceutical industry responded to their symptoms in ways that were completely rational and defensible at each stage throughout time. Nonetheless, these actions worsened the situation, compelling the need for even more radical measures. In each case, these activities drove up the prices of medicines and thus it is worth a brief review.

Eroom's Law Revisited

In retrospect, we now know that Eroom's Law had begun in earnest coincident with the rise of the pharmaceutical industry in the years following the Second World War. Early signs of stress included a trend that began modestly in the 1980s and quickly accelerated thereafter. Dr. Kinch's team at Washington University has analyzed pharmaceutical mergers and acquisitions over the years, revealing a rather extraordinary finding. Whereas mergers and acquisitions would sporadically occur in the four decades from 1945 through 1988, the annual number of mergers in a given year could be reliably counted with one hand and never entered double digits. Nineteen eighty-nine was the first year of double-digit mergers, and this rate has steadily risen ever since. The next milestone would occur in 2008, when the number of mergers reached three figures in a single year and the rate has never dropped back down to double digits (figure 8). In science, there is a term known as autophagy, which literally translates from Greek into "eating oneself." This seems an appropriate term to capture the behavior of the pharmaceutical industry. It seems that while Eroom's Law has driven the hunger behind consolidation, high prices are a sign of unpleasant indigestion.

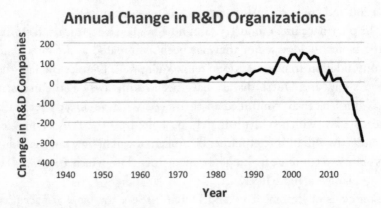

Figure 8. Rate of Loss Graph
Consolidation has triggered a rapid contraction in the number of companies performing research and development. 2019 witnessed the loss of nearly 300 companies, leaving fewer than 2000 remaining R&D companies (results reproduced from data provided by CRIB).

In the latest year to be analyzed, 2019, more than three hundred companies were lost in a single year, mostly to consolidation. Fewer than 2,000 companies remain. Looking at this another way, there are only six to seven years of losses left in the reserve of companies performing pharmaceutical research and development. This includes a subset of "big pharma," but the majority of these are the "small fish," too few and small to satiate the top-level predators.

Compounding or alleviating the situation (depending upon your viewpoint) is the growing reliance upon outsourcing. While the practice of outsourcing is well-known within the software development and technical support call centers, the pharmaceutical industry was an early adopter and took this to an extreme. More and more of the day-to-day drug development activities are increasingly performed by outside vendors, known as contract research organizations (CROs). These activities include everything from clinical trial management to even the most fundamental tasks of chemistry and biology, which historically had been the lifeblood of innovative biopharmaceutical companies.

As such, the outsourcing trend has created yet another layer (and industry) seeking to maximize profitability. As the dependence of both start-up, and established pharmaceutical companies upon CROs has grown, so have the costs charged by this comparatively nascent industry. This practice has thus merely kicked the can down the road a bit and ensured continued adherence to Eroom's Law.

Drug developers have taken the practice of outsourcing to an ever higher extreme, outsourcing even the basic ideas for new products. This abdication manifests itself in the form of start-up biotechnology companies, which have become ubiquitous and now dominate the earliest stages of drug discovery and early development. On one hand, it could be argued this makes logistical sense. Early-stage discovery activities are the furthest from revenue generation and the risks are highest at these nascent stages of drug development. On the other hand, the risks are nonetheless reflected in drug pricing as two additional industries (discovery-based biotechnology companies and the venture capital organizations behind them) must be sated.

Consequently, the ever-rising costs of research and development will inevitably be paid by the large pharmaceutical competitors, be it in the form of the internal staff and funding required to develop their own products or in the fees required to rent and buy the works of other companies and, indeed, industries. The industry has largely opted for the latter, driven almost entirely by the short-term (quarterly) need to remain in the good steads of Wall Street investors.

Given what we have described, please remember that a decision to merge or acquire another company arises when the larger (or more highly capitalized) company management concludes that their internal business strategy or pipeline does not meet their future expectations. Stated another way, if one's own ideas and innovations are not sufficiently valuable, then they are required to pay for someone else's ideas and products.

Over time, the use of mergers and acquisitions has evolved from a one-time opportunity to a constant crutch. Like a tale of gothic vampires, old companies needed the lifeblood of the younger, more vibrant entity to survive and, more importantly, to avoid the risk of failing to keep up with the ever-accelerating velocity of the pharmaceutical treadmill. As the doomed shots on goal approach burgeoned, failure not only became an option but an expected write-off. The key was to minimize the number of high-profile failures (those that might disappoint short-term minded investors) or to eliminate risk altogether by paying a large premium for products that had already successfully run the gauntlet and achieved a nod from the FDA. Further, this strategy is often used for a quick means to gain access to a hot new market when the acquirer's pipeline is sorely lacking.

Other symptoms of Dutch disease included risk avoidance strategies such as fast-follower drugs. These products did not contribute meaningfully to public health but have proven to be highly lucrative, albeit ultimately punitive to the actual consumer, as it causes prices to rise. As we have seen, pharmaceutical representatives avow that fast-follower approaches are a remnant of an ignorant past. Yet our research has put the lie to such claims. Although it is true that we are developing fewer statins than in past ages, the number of immune oncology drugs targeting the exact same molecule and in the exact same way has skyrocketed over the past ten years. And one can safely assume that an influx of new fast-follow drugs will presage neither lower prices nor orthogonal improvements in patient care.

Likewise, the incentives conveyed by the Orphan Drug Act proved successful, though arguably too much so. The loopholes provided in a legislation meant to help the sufferers of rare diseases have instead provided a gateway for drugs to enter the market in a more lucrative manner and to justify inordinate prices. In reality, most of these same medicines are then repurposed for wider use without lowering the price, thereby implicating this well-intended legislation with much of the responsibility for drug price inflation and further Dutch disease.

Adding to the costs of new medicines was a form of drug repurposing; creating new life for old medicines. One example of this trend is the rise of specialty pharmaceutical companies. These organizations generally create new formulations, such as a means of delivering a drug to a particular site in the body (i.e., a topical or ocular form of a drug for a skin disease) or in prolonging the residence time that the drug remains in the body. While these achievements are clearly improvements of existing medicines, they rarely represent the types of medical breakthroughs that will revolutionize patient care. Nonetheless, these repurposed medicines tend to command hefty price tags that have contributed to price increases.

A variation on this theme of increased prices despite minimal improvement over conventional medicines is exemplified by the rise of fast-follower (me-too) medicines. By modifying, ever so slightly, the active component of a tried-and-true medicine, motivated primarily by the desire to circumvent intellectual property (patent) claims rather than to effect substantial medical improvements, fast-follower drugs have added considerably to the costs of new medicines (recall that later-generation statins could charge a higher price and commanded a larger audience that the pioneering drug). Yet, a decision to advance such medicines was embraced in many corporate boardrooms because following a known (and successful) medicine equated to a substantially lower risk of new product development (and the ability to leverage existing commercial assets) while simultaneously banking upon the greater commercial success too frequently enjoyed by fast-follower drugs. Despite the protests of many executives who acknowledged the problem after being called out for the approach, our work suggests this approach is alive and kicking.

Perhaps the most egregious example of a fast-follower tendency conveying minimal, if any, clinical benefit, arises from a bit of chemical sleight of hand. As exemplified in the story of "the purple pill" that we described extensively in the last chapter, the development of drugs that contain a preferred left- or right-handedness provides a defensibly new product that commands a very high price and yet is essentially no better than its predecessor in terms of safety and efficacy. To be certain, esomeprazole (the S-form of omeprazole, better known as Nexium) is not alone, being joined just in the past few years by escitalopram and esketamine, to name but a few. Although legally defensible from the standpoint of patent protection and subject to regulatory approval, the overuse of this loophole simply to game the system rather than improve patient outcome leaves a bad taste in the mouth and a rumble in the gut (which drives Nexium sales further upward).

As a consequence of all these actions, the manifold medicines churning out of the conventional biopharmaceutical industry became affordable to fewer and fewer customers. Those lucky enough to have gold-plated insurance plans provided by their place of employment faced skyrocketing co-pays while their employers were increasingly burdened with rising insurance costs. And those buying their own insurance through the Affordable Care Act were burdened by not only the escalating co-pays but ever-more exorbitant premiums.

In parallel with the changes in research and development of new medicines, other components of the system were undergoing ever greater tectonic changes. An emphasis upon generic medicines led to a race to the bottom in terms of drug pricing. This was indeed the intended outcome. However, the race to the bottom would discourage many generics companies from marketing low margin drugs. All too often, the downward pricing trends abruptly reverse when only a handful (and sometimes just a single supplier) are the only ones left to meet market demand. This lack of competition results in a rapid price rebound as we have seen with the EpiPen and the many exploits of industry charlatans like Martin Shkreli. Even more tragic is the example of certain pediatric oncology drugs, where all the manufacturers have left the market, resulting in a patient population desperate for already proven medicine.

Another unintended consequence is that generic and branded pharmaceutical companies would emphasize the formation of "creative" deal structures. Among the most notorious of these new structures was bundling, in which a company or distributor would require that a suite of medicines be included in a deal, most of which were loss leaders for the manufacturer. This structure almost invariably ended up increasing the overall price of medicines even though one high-profile component of the bundle might be less expensive.

Deal-making overall has been a major contributor to escalating drug prices. Often, these deals were intended to keep down the price of new drugs but had the opposite effect. Nowhere is this more apparent than in the creation of the pharmacy benefit manager industry. This industry, which began innocently enough, has added to drug prices by evolving into a powerful component of the pharmaceutical enterprise that seeks to maximize its own profitability, often at the expense of both its suppliers (i.e., pharmaceutical companies) and customers (insurance companies, employers, and individual beneficiaries).

The pharmacy benefit manager industry is admittedly an easy "bogey man" that has been distorted and magnified by their many detractors. However, the industry has left itself exposed to these criticisms due to the sheer opacity in which they operate. In the course of researching this book, we were surprised at the abject hostility conveyed by both its upstream and downstream partners. Upstream from PBMs, pharmaceutical manufacturers resent receiving most of the blame for high drug prices while they unconvincingly plead their innocence. Such claims tend to fall on deaf ears as confidentiality agreements prevent manufacturers from revealing how much they receive from PBMs for medicines. The downstream payers (private-sector and governmental insurance) likewise encounter customer backlash from resentful policy holders, facing ever-increasing insurance premiums and deductibles.

The End of Blockbuster Deals

Such hostility raises questions whether the pharmacy benefit manager system might be susceptible to disruption by an entirely new business model, such as a modified return to direct-to-consumer or direct-to-payer transactions for prescription medicines. Paradoxically, the intense dislike of PBMs, described by one senior venture capital professional with whom we talked as "an industry impossible to defend" has spawned waves of new PBM creation.

The reasons for the new wave of entrepreneurship simply boils down to money, which has driven both cynical and constructive responses. On one side, there are great profits to be made and PBMs seem to be sprouting everywhere one looks. A notable example was the launch of Amazon's Pill

Pack, which is marketed as a way to merge all your medicines into a single pouch but in reality is rebranding of the standard PBM role. This is not necessarily a bad thing as more competition should drive down prices. Yet if Amazon replicates its strategy of conquering the pharmaceutical benefit manager industry in the same way it has come to dominate bookselling, then it seems likely that many PBMs will be driven out of business. And decreasing competition is unlikely to compel lower prices.

More optimistically, the fundamental concepts that gave rise to the PBM industry, namely a desire to lower costs, may be returning. With increased access to information about which medicines work (and do not), a new wave of PBM-like services are being launched by insurance providers and companies responsible for providing healthcare for their employees. A key feature driving these homegrown PBMs is the desire and increasing ability to generate their own formulary (a list of medication that will be underwritten) tailor-made for a particular population. Such trends are being adopted by larger organizations, but as the technology and access to information (i.e., pricing transparency) improves, it seems likely that customized formularies will better serve companies and other collections of people, large and small. Consequently, it seems feasible that the original PBM industry may be destined to go the way of shopping malls and video-rental stores.

A Different Relay for Life

The result of many changes is that the pharmaceutical enterprise, from the conception of a new product to the final delivery to the patient needing the medicine, involves an ever-larger number of organizations and industry types, each seeking to optimize its profitability. Using an analogy of a relay race, many additional runners have been added to each stage of the competition. In the beginning, the race begins with early stage discovery and research activities, often performed by royalty-driven universities and venture-backed biotechnology start-ups, which discover new medicines (and the investors seeking strong returns). This first wave of handoffs eventually requires better capitalized partners (often established pharmaceutical companies), who then finish the first lap by gaining an FDA approval. Strangely enough, this race may not be run by the company staff themselves, but by outside contractors paid to do so.

The second lap begins with manufacturing, sales, and marketing activities, which have captured an ever-larger fraction of company budgets and attention (recalling that this is a race with many teams of competitors). The types of drugs and technologies being made are ever more complex, and thus expensive to discover, develop, and manufacture. These products are likewise burdened by stacks of patent and royalties to be managed. Worse still, all these rising costs seem to have been matched by the costs needed to advertise the product to direct to consumers and to entice key opinion leaders (high profile specialists in the field) to adopt their shiny new object.

Eventually, the race will witness a handoff to pharmacy benefit managers, who play the role of a not-always-so-friendly competitor, negotiating the best costs of goods they purchase and prices they charge to consumers or insurance companies. This final leg of the relay race is rather unusual, as the PBM may decide it is in their best interest to drop one baton and instead pick up the baton of a competitor, sticking with whichever runner seems to be the most lucrative at the time.

Each handoff detailed above involves multiple parties and legal agreements, which are often subject to the tightest of confidentiality standards, thus rendering it virtually impossible to fully comprehend who benefits the most from the higher prices of medicines. This opacity cannot hide the fact that the behemoth system is unsustainable. Evidence that the current system is faltering can be found in the constant finger-pointing among the organizations in response to an increasingly irate general public and threats for regulations from their elected officials. The finger-pointing might allow the individual units of the system to protest their innocence, but such behavior has undermined the credibility of the entire pharmaceutical enterprise. Rather than turning inward and asking how the system might be improved, it is far easier to simply complain and bet that the status quo will carry on.

Even if we eliminate the complications and profiteering from specialty pharmaceuticals, distributors, and pharmacy benefit managers, a combination of Eroom's Law and the pharmaceutical treadmill alone seem to presage a slow-motion train wreck for the entire drug development enterprise. It seems nearly certain that there will soon be a disruption in our ability to develop and distribute new medicines. Some of the more pessimistic among us might argue evidence is already at hand in support of this notion, invoking antibiotics and vaccines as exhibits.

With this in mind, we now spend some time explaining how we might innovate our way out of these dilemmas. We begin by returning to the federal government, the alpha and omega of drug discovery, development, and utilization.

CHAPTER TWENTY

All Roads Lead
to Washington

T he title of this chapter betrays the fact that when considering the discovery, development, prices, and availability of medicines many aspects of the problem arise from and might be addressed by our elected lawmakers, especially when seeing how the governments of other countries like Germany and Canada have interceded to keep drug prices down. As we will see, some of these roles are obvious, others less so. Yet appreciating the enormous and diverse roles not to mention the power of the federal government are crucial for understanding the opportunities to improve drug pricing efforts in the future.

The most prominent role for the federal government is its role as the primary regulator of drug development and distribution. These functions largely (though not entirely) reside in the venerable Food and Drug Administration (FDA). Earlier in our story, we briefly reviewed the historical precedents that drove the evolution of the FDA into its current and vital role as both a facilitator of innovation and a watchdog to prevent potential dangers.

The FDA is tasked with oversight of the interstate marketing, manufacturing, and distribution of most medicines. There are a few exceptions: The Centers for Disease Control and Prevention control a subset of medicines meant to treat exotic diseases while the Federal Trade Commission has oversight control for some over-the-counter drugs. However, the vast majority of government regulation of medicines in the United States falls under the FDA mandate. As such, the FDA has the ability to tighten or loosen restrictions on the needs for safety or efficacy, which occasionally rises to the public's attention as it did during the HIV/AIDS and the COVID-19 outbreaks.

Unlike the situation in other countries to be discussed below, the FDA does not have a direct say in pricing questions. However, the chief pharmaceutical regulator in the United States certainly plays an indirect role. Revisiting a past topic, one can argue that the rise of FDA-mandated Phase IV clinical trials has contributed to rising research and development costs. The FDA also plays a key role in the oversight of the intellectual property needed to hold off generic medicines, for example by extending the period of exclusivity for certain medicines such as orphan drugs, and thus holds a potential to utilize this power to help address drug pricing.

One might ask, "If drug pricing is so important, why doesn't the FDA play a greater role?" The blunt answer is that the agency is utterly swamped with the tasks for which it has already been assigned. Recall that a relatively small staff of 15,000 people is already overwhelmed with ensuring the safety and reliability of products that, in aggregate, account for nearly a quarter of every dollar American consumers spend every year. These products span the range from the obvious (food and all forms of legal drugs) to less conspicuous articles, such as microwave ovens and bottled water.

The responsibilities of the FDA entail not merely the approval of a new product but oversight of everything from manufacturing to advertising and distribution. Nor does the enforcement of these activities end at the US border, as many medicines (not to mention food and microwave ovens) are manufactured around the world and FDA staff are tasked with ensuring that the quality, safety, and efficacy of these products meet American standards with a staff of fewer people than Walmart employees in the state of Kansas alone.[1] Indeed, FDA employees have quietly conveyed to us that a popular intramural conspiracy theory is that the government intentionally under-staffs the agency to prevent it from too closely regulating the bio-pharmaceutical industry.

What might the agency do without being accused of over-regulating or micromanaging? Well, we have already seen the impact of deploying incentives such as the Orphan Drug Act (ODA) or changes in PDUFA charges. Therefore, they might consider deploying a similar incentive, perhaps even more lucrative, to address unmet public health needs. Using recent events as an example, enticements could be wielded more surgically, for example, to encourage new anti-infective agents or vaccines for SARS Cov-2, pandemic influenza, or any number of drug-resistant microbial pathogens to name but just a few potential targets.

To help guide important decision-making, we will briefly expand upon the idea of a QALY. Originally conceived in the late 1960s, the quality-adjusted life year is a measure of disease burden that could be used to prioritize incentives.[2][3] Disease indications that impact the most QALYs could be given the greatest incentives and, in so doing, overcome the current prioritization schema based on emotional impact. Yet QALYs bring their own issues, as the QALY will vary among different communities (based upon income, race, or social factors) or regions (given diversity in diet and environments). To arrive at a fair QALY, the Bill and Melinda Gates Foundation has been working with investigators around the world to establish and apply objective QALYs to different diseases.[4] This work, largely involving the University of Washington in the Gateses' hometown, has begun a Herculean task that may nonetheless help to prioritize those diseases that take the greatest toll on society.[5] Referring to the outcomes with the slighted modified language of DALYs (disease disability adjusted life years), these investigators are evaluating the impact of disease not merely in the United States but around the world. Such data could be used both to create federal incentives for basic and applied research and also to help prioritize efforts at FDA.

Similarly, the FDA could identify ways to prioritize their efforts to deprioritize efforts on less impactful indications (e.g., hair loss treatments). Likewise, the QALY/DALY could help assess potential misuse of the provisions of the Orphan Drug Act. The goal in reviewing and amending this well-intended legislation is not meant to dissuade research or treatment of rare and deadly afflictions but rather to prevent companies from abusing the system by taking advantage of a loophole to get to market quicker and demand a high price for a drug that is ultimately intended to be marketed to additional markets beyond the initial orphan indication.

As part of such changes, the FDA could appoint a non-partisan, non-government body (such as the National Academy of Sciences, a respected organization that has historically been tasked to help address large questions pertaining to science and innovation). A standing taskforce could define existing or anticipated diseases that could qualify for incentives (such as those provided by the Orphan Drug Act) and perhaps modify these to encourage even more robust responses in periods of dire need, such as arose in early 2020 with COVID-19. Likewise, this body would be required to review past activities and to eliminate incentives that are no longer needed or subject to abuse.

Another means of providing incentives could be tied to the requirements needed to obtain FDA licensure. Most of the costs needed to develop new medicines, which can soar far north of a billion dollars, are tied up in the largest clinical trials (pre-approval Phase III and post-approval Phase IV trials). Therefore, a regulator could grant different forms of an approval dependent upon the data provided while capping what manufacturers charge for that medicine.

In the recent pandemic, we saw a variation on this theme with the emergency use authorization (EUA) granted to remdesivir (an unapproved drug) to treat COVID-19. An emergency use authorization is unique to unexpected medical situations arising from chemical, biological, radiological, or nuclear calamities. Enacted in the days following 9/11 and the anthrax attacks, this legislation allows unapproved drugs to be used in times of emergency. Although deployed infrequently and temporarily to address hazards such as Ebola, Zika, and H1N1 influenza, its use was invoked multiple times in 2020 to expedite the means to detect and treat SARS CoV-2. In a controversial announcement, the FDA stated that while it would approve the emergency use of remdesivir, they left it up to the company to decide how much to charge.[6] Using QALY-like approaches, the values cited for the drug by external opinions ranged from one dollar to $4,460.[7][8][9] Gilead elected to charge $3,100. This high price was particularly difficult to defend as more patient data revealed that the benefit of remdesivir was marginal at best. Indeed, the WHO ultimately elected to recommend against the use of remdesivir, as there was no evidence of any survival benefit. Yet the high price tag persisted.

One might consider allowing for different levels of an FDA approval and linking these to different drug price ceilings. An experimental medicine might be approved based on strong safety evidence (at least equivalent to what is required for a conventional FDA approval) and at least one peer-reviewed report of efficacy study (i.e., a large Phase 2 clinical trial). This mechanism could only be invoked if the indication addresses a high-QALY disease with an unmet medical need. Moreover, this medicine would not be allowed to be advertised or marketed using direct-to-consumer techniques. Finally, data would be collected from patients and their caregivers to further assess the safety and efficacy of the newly approved drug, an expansion of current pharmacovigilance monitoring for safety purposes. These data would be reviewed on a regular basis and the drug re-approved at these intervals, much as Congress currently does as an oversight measure for PDUFA and other legislation. In the event that any drug approved through this alternative process would ultimately be found to not be effective after broader usage (or if safety issues arose), the approval would be withdrawn. Given that fewer resources would have been expended to gain approval and because advertising costs would be precluded, the pricing of this medicine would necessarily be capped at a lower level than a drug approved utilizing the conventional approval process.

At the other extreme, drugs approved with extensive post-approval requirements, such as expensive Phase IV clinical trials, could be allowed a higher price point, which would relate directly to the additional amount required by the regulator for approval and be capped at a percentage of those additional costs. Of course, the drug sponsor could refuse the approval, repeat Phase III investigation, and resubmit rather than accepting the revised Phase IV trial methodology. Such a flexible approach might allow the regulator and drug sponsor to balance unmet medical needs with pricing restrictions for the betterment of the patient.

Another means to encourage good behavior (i.e., addressing low-incidence diseases or products that don't inherently have a large return on investment) is a more liberal use of creative ways to incentivize the development of needed medicines. As has been well-established and conveyed (though to little benefit) for decades, antibiotics act as a type of canary in the coal mine, reflecting an imbalance between public health needs and products advanced by the pharmaceutical industry. A perfect example of this is vancomycin, an antibiotic approved in 1954 and on the World Health Organization's List of Essential medicines. While the creators of vancomycin developed a much-needed tool, they were essentially and unintentionally punished for doing so as the revolutionary antibiotic was held back as a "drug of last resort," crippling its ability to generate revenue sufficient to pay for its own development. Flash forward a few decades and vancomycin resistance is increasing at a rapid clip, but the lessons learned by the pharmaceutical industry have remained just as durable. The bottom line they learned: antibiotics are money losers.

How might we change such well-worn assumptions?

Such outcomes might be reversed with incentives such as patent term extensions, expanded periods of exclusivity, and bounties placed upon unmet needs. The experience with the Orphan Drug Act teaches us that change is possible and can lead to new behaviors and investment strategies. For example, extensions of exclusivity might be deployed for drugs that would otherwise "sit on the shelves" while the patent clock continues to tick.

Even these incentives may not be enough, particularly if the company has a choice to discover and develop some other medicine that could generate greater and/or more immediate revenue. Therefore, additional out-of-the-box thinking might be needed to inspire innovation. One model might be derived from the social sciences. A mechanism first conceived by Ronnie Horesh, a New Zealand economist, envisioned the creation of social policy (or impact) bonds, an investment vehicle meant to deploy market incentives to affect societal advances. The mechanism provides a reward to those able to successfully meet a stated challenge. For example, the government of the United Kingdom announced in 2020 it would offer a five-billion-pound reward for approaches that could decrease prisoner recidivism by at least 7.5 percent.[10]

A similar bounty could be placed upon a transformational new antibiotic (not merely a new incremental improvement upon an existing agent) that meets defined criteria (e.g., safe and effective against drug-resistant bacteria). The amount of the bounty would need to be sufficient to incentivize investigation and could include back-payment of all or part of the research and development costs. Proper incentives placed upon front-end outcomes (i.e., approval and deployment of a new medicine) could then offset later revenues and profits that are generally reaped on the backend, namely by charging a high price. Were the incentives sufficient to do so, one could imagine that the product (i.e., a desired drug or vaccine) could be acquired by the bond issuer, who could then manufacture and distribute it thereafter (though greater efficiency generally resides with these activities being performed by the private sector). Another advantage of this approach is that the payer (e.g., the government or a philanthropist) only expends its limited resources after they have achieved the specific goal that they had desired and priced accordingly. Likewise, a well-constructed program would create enough incentive to motivate not only the entrepreneurial scientist but also the venture investors backing their programs. Although such a practice has not yet been applied to medicines, this example reveals that fresh ideas outside of conventional pharmaceutical research and development practices could help address both the need for continued medical innovation and to help restrain high prices.

A Sticky Proposition

The FDA holds the potential to wield not merely a carrot but also the proverbial stick. Whereas incentives can encourage good behavior, the chief regulator could be deployed to discourage activities that do not benefit the public. Within its current mandate, the FDA could impose a moratorium on broadening the use of a drug approved under the provisions of the Orphan Drug Act to nonorphan indications, at least for a period of time. To be clear, under this approach we do not envision that a wider use of the drug for a different orphan indication would be restricted (such as compendium-expansion strategies for cancer drugs.) Rather, the goal would be to send a strong signal to drug developers to end their abuse of loopholes that are a part of current incentive structures.

In an action presently beyond its purview, the FDA could be given the power to require that a subsequent approval for an orphan drug to a disease indication with a wider applicability be required to submit an altered price model that reflects the broadened market. In other words, the pricing would have to be adjusted downward to account for the new economics of a drug's expanded use that is well beyond its original small target population. Such an approach is already used by many European countries and is one reason why medicines have lower prices on one side of the Atlantic than the other. Indeed, this model is not simply restricted to orphan drugs but is applied across the board. The danger in such a model is that it could discourage a potentially useful drug from being expanded to meet an unmet need. Therefore, such a system would have to be created in a manner that does not actively discourage broadened use. An independent oversight board could be engaged to help finely balance such an equation.

Another action could be to discourage fast-follower ("me-too") drugs. The FDA could be tasked with disincentivizing and deprioritizing its approval of drugs that do not convey significant benefit over existing medications, since we have well established in this book that, unlike other industries, having a number of similar drug products do not lead to lower prices. Such a proposal is not meant to prevent such drugs from being approved, but to place fast-follower drugs at the bottom of the pile to be reviewed. Building upon the idea put forth in PDUFA, a particularly high fee could be charged for applications reviewed for fast-follower compounds, ideally in a manner that excess funds could be used to hire staff to expedite the approval of drugs to address unmet needs for high-QALY diseases or underserved populations.

It is crucial to understand that the FDA does not have the authority to undertake such drastic changes on its own. Rather, it would require new legislation to provide such authority and, like PDUFA, it would be essential that such rules be reviewed periodically (every five to ten years) to ensure they are applied and enforced as intended. The powerful pharmaceutical lobby would be expected to embrace the aforementioned carrots and oppose the sticks. Consequently, the legislative courage needed to enact such changes has heretofore been woefully lacking. However, the high-profile awakening of public health concerns in the wake of COVID-19 might pry loose some of these restraints. It is the opinion of your authors that Americans must evolve merely from hoping for such outcomes and instead initiate grassroots movements to see them through.

Public Venture Capital

While it is widely appreciated that the federal government underwrites much of the basic science research performed in the United States, the implications of this funding are often less obvious. Research from Dr. Kinch's team at Washington University has revealed the central role of one organization, the National Institutes of Health (NIH), as a crucial facilitator of drug development. The NIH alone provides over three billion dollars annually in research aid, with additional healthcare-focused monies provided by the Department of Defense, Department of Agriculture, and other federal mandates.

An assessment of the hundred most prescribed medicines showed NIH funding alone contributed to the approval of almost all (94.4 percent).[11] For drugs approved in the past decade, the number rose to 96.7 percent, a suggestion that drug discovery has become even more dependent upon NIH funding. Even if we restricted our analysis to look at situations where the NIH funded work on a drug or mechanism at least ten year before that drug was approved, 82.9 percent of the most prescribed medicines in the United States were enabled by NIH funding. Stated another way, absent NIH funding, the discovery of nearly every drug on the market today, or the fundamental understanding of how those medicines operate, would have been substantially delayed or precluded altogether. (And keep in mind that all these NIH-funded activities are made possible because of the US taxpayers.)

Under a system that has proven to be one of the more efficient means by which federal dollars are expended, the NIH has largely worked under a "push" mechanism. In general, the ideas for grant proposals arise from academics and are pushed to NIH to be funded. This has proved quite successful, being responsible for many advances in medicine as detailed below. However, the NIH also has the ability to invoke "pull" mechanisms to incentivize research in particular areas. Notable examples include extra funding added to the agency to address the COVID-19 crisis.[12] Likewise, other agencies, most notably the Department of Defense, have specialized programs to encourage new ideas in areas ranging from protection of the warfighter to novel ways to diagnose and treat breast cancer.

For an example of a successful pull system that the NIH already manages, look no further than grants directed to support small businesses. Amid the challenging era of stagflation in the early 1980s, the Small Business Innovation Development Act, which created Small Business Innovation Research (SBIR) grants, was signed by President Ronald Reagan to divert a small percentage of the NIH budget to create a grant mechanism for small start-up businesses.[13] This law has proven both successful and popular, being reauthorized every few years. Learning from success, the NIH budget could be bolstered with additional dollars to create an SBIR-like fund devoted to high-QALY diseases that are deemed insufficiently addressed by existing mechanisms.

This critical importance of NIH involvement should not merely be considered solely a beneficent act. The United States has held a dominant position in the biotechnology revolution. The number of conventional pharmaceutical endeavors (herein defined as companies that opened their doors before 1970) was almost evenly divided between Europe and the United States. In contrast, six of seven biotechnology companies founded since 1971 have been located in the United States, with the remaining divided between Europe and Asia.[14] This fact underscores the reality that the biotechnology and pharmaceutical industries have been responsible for millions of high-paying jobs and trillions of dollars in taxable revenue.

The location of these companies is revealing, not necessarily because Americans are more entrepreneurial than other nations, but instead because this reflects an impact of NIH funding. Specifically, the vast majority of successful biotechnology companies have been clustered around American universities in general and NIH-funded laboratories in particular. The biotechnology industry is largely centered around current biotechnology powerhouses such as the Bay Area (e.g., Stanford and UCSF) and Boston (around Harvard and MIT). Moreover, upstart biotechnology communities are emerging in Austin (home of the flagship state university), Raleigh-Durham (and a Research Triangle defined by three world-renowned schools), as well as the Maryland suburbs surrounding the NIH headquarters itself.

A primary driver for the burgeoning domestic biotechnology industry is a piece of congressional legislation that nearly did not occur. As outlined in greater detail in *A Prescription for Change*, two Rust Belt senators, Evan Bayh of Indiana and Robert Dole of Kansas, came together amid the stagflation era in the late 1970s with a bill to help promote American entrepreneurship. Prior to this key law, all intellectual property developed using federal resources fell into the hands of a federal organization, where it generally tended to gather dust rather than generate new ventures. The Bayh-Dole Act of 1980 granted this intellectual property back to the universities and other research institutions. A key provision, known as "march-in rights" was included to assure that the universities themselves would not sit on a crucial invention and instead work to satisfy the "health and safety needs" of the American public. This clause would allow the government essentially to take over a patent and grant it to another organization that would develop the invention. In this way, academic entrepreneurship was launched and has been a relatively sustained success since that time with the thriving American biotechnology industry as the evidential outcome.

Yet there is no evidence that the biotechnology and drug development industries will continue to be dominated by the United States. Dr. Kinch had the great fortune to attend the University of North Carolina in Chapel Hill for a postdoctoral fellowship in the laboratory of Keith Burridge, one of the greatest cell biologists of our ages. This English-born and Cambridge-educated researcher had established his career at UNC following his own postdoctoral studies under the famous (and occasionally notorious) James Watson, who solved the structure of DNA.

An early impression from the first day in Dr. Kinch's new position was a yellowed magazine clipping taped to the door of the main laboratory. The 1990 *Nature* headline read, "British Science Is Alive and Well as It Has Ever Been. It Is Just that It Is Currently Living in the United States." This is a concise summary of the diaspora triggered by economic and governmental decisions that caused many of the best and brightest of the United Kingdom to establish successful careers in their former colonies. A primary lure for the brain drain that helped establish the economic and scientific dominance of the United States in biotechnology was funding of and by the National Institutes of Health.

Over the past twenty years, American government's commitment to research has faltered. Starting immediately after completion of "the doubling" of the NIH budget between 1998 and 2003, allocations decreased in real terms, did not keep pace with inflation, and then suffered a precipitous setback following the 2013 budget sequestration. This latter legislation had been designed to be so draconian that lawmakers promised that reduced NIH funding would be avoided at all costs. That promise was not kept. Instead, the reduced funding levels have served as the starting point for future budgetary discussions. More recently, the Trump administration has continued to threaten the NIH budget with cutbacks of 20 percent.[15] Fortunately, those threats were countered by bipartisan action in Congress.

Such shortsightedness fails to recognize the impact of federal support on the economy and factors threatening the health of the nation. In the years following the Second World War, visionaries such as Vannevar Bush, who during that time headed the US Office of Scientific Research and Development, anticipated federal research funding would provide an engine to support innovative new enterprises. The nation's economic dominance in aerospace, software, and biomedical sciences exemplify how federal support served as public venture capital to power the "Engines of Innovation" as described by the current editor in chief of *Science* magazine, Holden Thorp.

But the US dominance is rapidly waning. In a 2016 paper published in *Cell Chemical Biology*, the Center for Research Innovation in Biotechnology warned that between 2000 and 2014, the industry lost more than half of all biotechnologies that had contributed to the approval of at least one FDA-approved medicine due to industry consolidation.[16] A disproportionate number of American companies were acquired by international firms, which will impact the geography of decision-making of the future. At the same time, the number of new companies entering the field was insufficient to offset such losses. At the present rate, we are on track to have no companies remaining within a decade.

The publishing of more than two dozen papers on the subject inspired and cajoled Dr. Kinch to write *A Prescription for Change* in 2016, which conveys a history of the biopharmaceutical industry and the looming crisis it faces. The stakes are high as witnessed by our recent inability to keep up with drug-resistant infectious diseases, not to mention the rising inevitability that we will soon enter a "post-antibiotic era," which witnesses a return of infectious diseases as the major causes of death all throughout the world.

As importantly, when we consider the impact of continuing to reduce federal commitments to biomedical research, we are not simply threatening the development of new medicines but the stabilization of a multitrillion-dollar industry that generates high-paying jobs and tax revenues. New medicines will continue to be developed, but perhaps not driven by Americans or consistent with our public health priorities.

This raises the inevitable but avoidable question of whether the door to our offices are fated to be covered with a newspaper headline stating, "American science is alive and well and living in. . . ."

The title of this section is a perspective nicely conveyed by the economist, Mariana Mazzucato in her book, *The Entrepreneurial State*, in describing NIH funding as "public venture capital."[17] This book convincingly advocated for government financing of research opportunities in a manner that provides outsized returns on investment, defined as financial benefits as well as improvements in public health. Indeed, the NIH itself reports a 43 percent return on investment for its funding.[18] More specifically, every dollar invested by NIH stimulates $8.38 of private sector research and development within eight years and $2.13 in pharmaceutical sales.[19] [20] Again, these numbers merely reflect investments by the NIH and do not include the National Science Foundation, the Pentagon, and other sources of federal research support.

Another quite refreshing perspective on this form of public venture capital came from one of the most well-known and successful private venture capitalists, Mark Cuban. The comment was triggered amid a conversation about the efficiency of NIH spending. Responding to a concern of inefficiencies arising from the fact that NIH mandate prevents them from taking a monetary position for products developed by academics using tax dollars, Cuban stated succinctly, "Looking out for the people and their welfare should be part of every agency mandate."

Any way you look at it, the federal government must be viewed as a crucial source of venture capital. Indeed, the number cited above undoubtedly underestimated its impact as the NIH tends to support the earliest, and thus most risky, stages of research. With rare exceptions, NIH funding is not product-focused and the government earns these high returns by funding what is mostly ad hoc basic research. Specifically, the NIH operates by funding small- to modest-sized projects that are submitted by academics. While there are occasional "requests for proposals" emphasizing areas of particular needs, most grants are funded based on what is on the cutting edge of science. This contrasts with the "big science" research projects, such as billion-dollar campaigns to develop new medicines by the private sector. The NIH conveys its funding in relatively small packets (typical research grants are less than a hundred thousand dollars; rare grants exceed a million dollars annually). Despite this, the gross impact of this highly dispersed funding is not insignificant and has proven crucial for nucleating later and much larger financing from the private sector.

An example of the impact of NIH funding was confirmed when Mark Cuban asked teams at Washington University and 46Brooklyn to analyze the impact of the NIH on drugs approved by the FDA from 2017 through 2019. For this analysis, we relied upon disclosures of key patents conveyed to FDA for 93 medicines approved between 2017 and 2019. Such records are required to notify the FDA (and the world) when patent coverage is likely to expire and thus allow for competition from generic manufacturers.

As these drugs were all conventional chemicals from pharmaceutical companies (known in the drug development community as "small molecules"), it was presumed we would find few, if any, that included NIH-funded academic inventors. This view dominated because pharmaceutical industry chemists are usually the sole inventors for mature biomedical products. These chemists in turn are nearly always industry employees who are putting the finishing touches on molecules in-licensed from academia or other companies. Therefore, it seemed too high a bar to think that NIH-funded laboratories would meaningfully contribute to these key patents.

To our considerable surprise, this presumption proved to be flat wrong.

Eleven of the ninety-three drugs approved in that three-year period listed academic inventors on key patents who were funded by NIH.

Beyond reiterating the fact NIH funding is the foundation for new cures, high-paying jobs, and American dominance in drug development, there is another interesting, and potentially explosive, implication of these findings. As you may recall, the Bayh-Dole Act provided the government with reach-in rights if the invention fails to satisfy the "health and safety needs" of the American consumer.

Given the high prices of medicines, which are unaffordable for many, one might ask whether the health and safety needs of the American consumer are being satisfied. Although march-in rights have never been successfully practiced, one potential example of where this might be useful is the drug nusinersen (trade name: Spinraza). This drug was approved in 2017 as a much-needed treatment of spinal muscular atrophy, a form of muscular dystrophy. Although initially celebrated by disease advocates, they were shocked to learn the price. According to 46brooklyn, the price for a single vial of nusinersen, which contains 12 milligrams of drug (0.0004 ounces), will set back a consumer $127,000. This number raises the question of whether a drug, which was developed with federal funding, truly meets the "health and safety" needs of the American public. This could be an interesting question and would undoubtedly precipitate considerable political and legal turmoil. Nonetheless, this option might provide one way, albeit an extreme one, to address the rising prices of some medicines.

The Biggest Customer

We will now turn to the fact that the United States federal government is not merely the investor and regulator of new medicines, but also the largest customer for the biopharmaceutical industry.

Less obvious is the fact the federal government is the primary consumer, being a direct employer for 2.1 million people in the non-postal workforce and 1.4 million people in the military, not to mention their dependents. Add to that the nearly 65 million people covered by Medicaid and 44 million beneficiaries of Medicare and one arrives at the fact that the federal government is by far responsible for the healthcare of more people than any other single organization (or even industry).

Despite this heft, most of the federal government is unable to negotiate with PBMs or pharmaceutical manufacturers.[21] As we have already seen, lawmakers caved into pressure from pharmaceutical lobbyists and refused to allow Medicare to utilize its heft to negotiate prices.[22] [23] To these authors, this decision reflects a profound dereliction of duty and has garnered warranted criticism. In this context, one must also be wary of seeming quick-fix provisions such as "Medicare for All," as extensions of these fatal flaws would simply increase the magnitude of the drug pricing question.

Might the "D" Stand for Dumb?

Medicare Part D is a well-intended program to help seniors gain access to much-needed medicines. However, the means by which it was crafted created loopholes that actively contributed to the rising prices of medicines. Here we will cite an example identified by the team at 46Brooklyn. In an outstanding report, these investigators identified a class of drugs they refer to as "zombie brands": medicines that are subject to generic competition and yet just keep plodding along, earning outsized revenues.

Glatiramer acetate (brand name: Copaxone) was approved in 1996 to treat multiple sclerosis, a deadly autoimmune disease. Despite the fact the drug had gone off patent years before, it still captured 82 percent of Medicare sales in 2018, amounting to a whopping $1.2 billion in revenues for the drug maker Teva in that year alone. Looking further, the team at 46brooklyn discovered that while Medicare Part D had been crafted to minimize patients' out-of-pocket spending, it instead encouraged branded pharmaceuticals to increase their prices. The complexities of this bureaucratic program are substantial, but it suffices for our purposes that the program began with a conventional deductible, with the patient paying 100 percent of costs up to an annual maximum of $435, after which the patient was responsible for 25 percent. Once out-of-pocket costs reached $4,020, one would encounter the so-called "donut hole," where the patient was again on the hook for 100 percent until finally reaching a point (at $6,320), known as the "catastrophic phase," in which the patient only had to cover 5 percent. The donut hole was politically contentious and, in 2011, the Affordable Care Act (ACA) closed the donut hole, ostensibly to help consumers, but was executed in a way that it unintentionally drove up drug prices.

In what 46brooklyn cleverly refers to as "the Race to Catastrophic," the ACA legislation required manufacturers of branded (but not generic) pharmaceuticals to pick up 50 percent of the costs to close the donut hole (this was later increased to 70 percent). This approach sounds reasonable enough, but the catch was that consumers could count the full 100 percent of the branded drug price in their race to reach the catastrophic phase (when the prices for most drugs would be picked up by the insurance plan). Consequently, consumers were induced to select branded pharmaceuticals, leaving the manufacturers of less expensive generic medicines discouraged and scratching their heads as to why their sales were shrinking. Worse still, these loopholes sent signals to the manufacturers of branded drugs (even those subject to generic competition) that they should raise their prices even further because it would allow consumers to reach the catastrophic phase more quickly, obviating their need to supplement costs and forcing Medicare to pay the full price. This experience was not unique to Copaxone and indeed a Vanderbilt University study revealed that overpayments to branded drugs covered by Medicare Part D ranged from \$869 to \$1,072 for each drug in 2019, thereby contributing even further to the rising price of medicines.[24]

There are other comparable stories but rather than piling onto the failures of Medicare Part D, as so many others have rightfully done already, we will turn instead to convey a promising outcome, where a federal government agency has been able to utilize its heft to lower healthcare prices, and can be a model for the future.

Unlike Medicare, the Veteran Health Administration (VA), has been allowed to negotiate prices and to establish its own formulary of preferred prescription medicines and centralized purchasing authority to leverage its considerable size. Mandated by the 1992 Veterans Health Care Act, this provision set a ceiling for drug prices and thereby allows 22 million military veterans access to less expensive medicines.[25] The VA is also guaranteed a 24 percent discount off the nonfederal average manufacturer price and can negotiate further cuts. Notably, the prices paid by VA recipients are fully transparent and published regularly, providing much needed sunlight on otherwise opaque questions about how much drugs really cost to buy. Nonetheless, Steve Miller of Express Scripts pointed out that the negotiations leading to these prices are thoroughly opaque. He further stated that the VA has advantages that ordinary consumers lack: 1) pharmaceutical manufacturers often provide better pricing to the VA so they can be seen as patriotic and 2) the VA has a very narrow formulary (often only one or two drugs offered for many indications). Indeed, these provisions allow the VA to spend one-third the amount for medicines as compared with the national average. Interestingly, this spending level is roughly comparable to that spent by Australia.[26]

An open formulary is a unique feature of the VA system that helps overcome the opacity of most other government and private insurance groups. The drugs approved for a particular indication are transparently revealed, as are the prices paid for these medicines. To utilize the heft of the federal government as the largest customer, the formularies for all prescriptions paid using federal dollars (including its role as a direct employer and its indirect roles in Medicaid and Medicare) could be published openly, even if they are managed by contracted pharmacy benefit managers. Such an action would shed light on the price of medicines, disclosing information that would undoubtedly promote disinfection of some of its more contaminated elements. Ideally, the government could require private employers, insurers, and pharmacy benefit managers to do the same, but this would undoubtedly be shouted down as governmental overreach.

While the model enacted successfully by the VA provides an example of how a government-run entity can lower prices, we are reminded of an even more progressive and commonsensical model for pricing reform that exists across the seas in Germany.

Turn Your Head and Cough

In Chapter Seventeen we discussed in great detail an ongoing experiment that could prove to be a successful model for the United States that is worthy of highlighting again here as we consider options for change. You may recall that Germany has consistently ranked among the highest per capita pharmaceutical spending countries in Europe, and that through much of the 1980s and '90s its spending outpaced even American outlays for medicines.[27] Government after government became increasingly vexed by the problem. Unlike other European nations, which fixed prices for pharmaceuticals, such socialistic tendencies were anathema for many Germans. Therefore, pharmaceutical companies (and PBMs) continued to set prices at what the market would bear, which meant that the nation continued to spend more and more of their family and national budgets on medicines. In fact, on average, Germans paid nearly a quarter more for medicines than other EU citizens. Searching for a solution, German instead began experimenting with ways to balance the need to favor innovation while ensuring medicines would remain affordable.

The ongoing experiment they settled upon is called Arzneimittelmarkt-neuordnungsgesetz or AMNOG. In short, under the provisions set forth by the adoption of AMNOG in 2011, the practice of allowing pharmaceutical companies to set their own prices remained, but only for a year after their introduction.

As a reminder of how this works, the sponsors of a new drug must submit a standardized dossier at the time of their launch to a nongovernmental committee for review. This committee, named the Federal Joint Committee, is an advisory group of thirteen members reflecting the four pillars of the German healthcare system that has historically been tasked with overseeing strategic decision-making about disease management and planning. But under AMNOG, this committee is now also in charge of how to price new medicines.

Within six months of receiving a new dossier, the Federal Joint Committee will categorize the benefits of a new drug over existing treatments based on mortality, morbidity, and quality of life.

Once the benefit assessment for a drug has been established based upon pricing, negotiations begin between the drug sponsor and a board composed of representatives of the nations' major health insurance companies (both state and private sector organizations). If the new drug has been deemed to convey no benefit, then the sponsor cannot charge more than the existing treatment. If a drug does show benefit, the magnitude of a price premium is guided by the extent of the improved benefit. All decisions are made within a one-year window after the product is launched, after which the original, sponsor-defined price is changed to the negotiated price.

Although widely viewed domestically in Germany as successful in keeping drug prices in check, AMNOG has unsurprisingly not resonated with drug manufacturers. Major complaints include concerns about choices of comparator treatment and the fact that decisions for more than half of the new drugs rated as providing "no benefit" were based upon data that did not conform to peculiarities of the AMNOG system.[28]

However, even with these complaints we would deem AMNOG to be a successful experiment. Many aspects worked and yet there remain opportunities for future improvement. A similar means to catalog the relative benefits of medicines, both to one another and to new drugs being introduced into the marketplace, has been adopted in Canada, France, and the United Kingdom. Were such a system to be used here, we might learn from the German experience and make periodic tweaks aimed at constant process improvement. We would recommend testing such a system within a well-understood and transparent community to provide both its supporters and critics the opportunity to assess its merits and fallibilities. Given the leadership displayed by the VA in the past, this might provide a logical place to start.

In defending PBMs against such requirements, Steve Miller of Express Scripts stated that transparency would result in everyone being charged the same mediocre price. He further asserted his contention that the total spending on medicines would not change. After conveying a view that larger organizations should benefit from their heft (as compared with small businesses), he dropped a bomb, declaring that charging everyone the same price for a drug would be a form of socialized medicine.

To be clear, the authors do not support the use of socialized healthcare. Instead, we interpret such name-calling as a desperate attempt to instill fear rather than a constructive goal of addressing the widely recognized problem of unaffordable medicines. Indeed, we approached the project of writing this book with an assumption of sunshine being the best disinfectant. Demanding transparency for transactions that are vital to the health of American citizens is not a socialist tendency. Demanding that everyone pay the same price for the same product might be construed as leaning in that direction, but even this is a substantial stretch when one throws the word "socialism" about. Instead, we maintain that the opacity of the present enterprise, including both manufacturers and distributors, contributes to the dramatic overcharging of American consumers and, in tragic cases, their inability to receive lifesaving medicines.

Does Cost = Price?

Do the costs of developing and delivering medicines actually relate to the prices paid for medicines? As we have seen, this is a challenging question because, despite popular opinion, there is not a simple pharmaceutical industry but rather a much larger, more complex and ever-expanding pharmaceutical enterprise. Each component of this enterprise seeks to extract the largest amount of profit. Yet an answer to the question seems apparent. Escalating costs are not unique to newly minted medicines but apply to old drugs, well-past the time of investing in research and development and period of patent exclusivities. The high-profile debacles associated with the pricing of the EpiPen and seemingly every drug touched by Martin Shkreli provide but a few examples of products developed decades before.

Even the most well-intentioned actions, such as the need to address orphan diseases, have become the new "in" targets for companies seeking both high profits and to game federal incentives. As we discussed, the Orphan Drug Act has been used and arguably abused as many companies discovered they could charge substantially more for those drugs.

In discussions with Bernard Munos, Charles Muscoplat, and others, we heard mention that pricing now has less to do with the cost to research, manufacture, or distribute the drug, but more to do with what the market will bear. But one has to wonder, is it really? Or does it reflect the demands of Wall Street masters?

Early stage discovery is not limited to the confines of a few large industry players, but a flood of start-up companies funded first by venture capitalists and later by more conventional investors after they ring the bell and join the ranks of the publicly traded. Once traded, the need to worry about day-to-day stock price rises remains a constant as raising money for product development and marketing can require several rounds of fundraising and new issuance of shares. The higher the price of a company's stock the more money the company can raise.

Early in Ms. Weiman's career, she worked at a company whose focus was rare diseases in oncology and immunology. Wall Street at the time didn't care much for such companies, as the prevailing view was they would never make much money even if they succeeded in delivering a drug to the market. Simple mathematics was at play. The revenues from a particular medicine are the product of multiplying the number of patients who take a drug times the price of the medicine. Back then, the presumed price of a rare drug plugged into the projected spreadsheets was substantially lower than today. Since rare diseases have fewer patients, the final tally was thought not to be lucrative enough to waste their time.

But then the prices of drugs approved through the incentives of the Orphan Drugs Act rose sharply. The multipliers used in the spreadsheets throughout Wall Street started adding zeros to prior assumptions, creating outsized ambitions long before the benefits of a drug could be established in the clinic. By the time a drug had gained a nod from the FDA, Wall Street expectations had established a certain floor for the price.

Given the aforementioned example as the road most traveled, it raises the question of whether today's prices are more about "what the market will bear" or instead "what Wall Street's return on investment demands will be?" One must wonder what the price of these drugs would be if the companies were privately held, as they once were. How might the margins change? How would this impact decisions to invest in a product or kill it? What sort of marketing practices would be abandoned if quarter over quarter returns weren't constantly in demand?

As the old adage goes, if you want to answer a question, "follow the money." Increasingly, patients cannot afford their drugs while some in the pharmaceutical enterprise become exceedingly rich. Might the next step in the evolution of the pharmaceutical enterprise arise from shining more light on the flow of money and ask who is really benefiting from medical innovation? Pharmaceutical innovators, venture capitalists, contract research organizations, advertising agencies, and pharmacy benefit managers all must be scrutinized individually and in aggregate.

Beyond the question of how individual drugs are priced, we look to the future for ideas of how we might ensure a continued ability to develop new medicines. This question arises when looking at both long- and short-term trends in the organizations responsible for discovering and developing affordable new medicines that convey "extensive benefit" to high-QALY diseases.

To summarize, the federal government of the United States has a variety of means at its disposal to both ensure future innovation to protect against threats to individual and collective public health, as well as to lower the costs of the resulting medicines. Utilizing its role as regulator, the FDA could offer additional proverbial carrots. There is little argument that exploitation of the Orphan Drug Act has, to be generous, not met the expectations of its designers. However, these incentives have served a purpose: to demonstrate how to motivate a cumbersome pharmaceutical industry that tends not to be terribly nimble.

The intent of the Act was indeed noble: to stimulate development of medicines for long-neglected, low-incidence diseases. Instead, the ODA has been exploited both to capture its lucrative incentives and to justify high prices for drugs with a small initial market (despite the fact that these prices would remain high after the drug was expanded to larger markets). Rather than scrapping the Orphan Drug Act, as many have advocated,[29] [30] it could be deployed differently, such as to meet its original intentions and to address high-QALY unmet needs. These high-QALY needs include widely applicable diseases for which there are few clinical options (e.g., neurodegenerative, metabolic, and cardiovascular diseases), as well as emerging threats, such as drug-resistant infectious agents and vaccines.

Likewise, the FDA could wield the stick at times to discourage the overuse of incentives. For example, an ODA designation could be revoked or structured such that incentives must be reimbursed back to the government if the drug is applied too widely or priced at an egregious sum. In a different vein, the PDUFA program, which garnishes fees to expedite FDA review, could be modified to substantially increase fees upon me-too medicines. All this is within the current purview of the agency, but even more efficacious measures could be taken were the agency permitted to directly address pricing questions (like many European nations have already done).

Likewise, the NIH could build upon past successes to encourage more "pull" mechanisms to fund research into high-QALY indications that are presently under-served. In modifying the NIH, it would be essential not to break that which works, namely the small-scale grants conceived by experts seeking to advance knowledge using the more traditional "push" approach.

In light of lessons taught by the COVID-19 crisis, which demonstrated the extraordinary impact of public health issues, a research portfolio that blends and balances activities to address today's concerns while anticipating future problems versus reactive or fast-follow approaches seems a prudent and cost-effective means of moving forward.

CHAPTER TWENTY-ONE

Future Shock
Already Happened

The need for new medicines will truly never cease. New diseases are always on the rise and old foes, be it malignant cancer cells or infectious agents, too often return as a result of treatment resistance. Therefore, continued innovation will always be essential to ensure a better quantity and quality of life. Our ability to continue discovering and distributing new public health improvements over the past century, many of which we have taken for granted, are now fundamentally threatened by the failing business models that have led to ever-escalating costs to develop new medicine and prices that must be paid to benefit from them. In the previous chapter, we discussed ways that the federal government can help in its roles as an investor, regulator, payer, and consumer of medicines. Herein, we focus upon other key components of the system, including some rising stars that might reshape the entire enterprise.

A major source of concern presented throughout this story has been that the current manifestation of the pharmaceutical enterprise is unsustainable and inevitably will experience a major disruption (presuming one is not already well underway). The destruction of one way of doing things represents opportunities for the creation of another. Quoting a popular song, "Every new beginning is another beginning's end." In this final chapter, we convey some of the concepts being discussed and tested that could provide solutions for the range of problems that manifest themselves in symptoms such as Eroom's Law and price hikes. We believe therefore that the question of how new medicines will be developed and distributed is likely to change, and we will discuss how this might look and why the future may be quite promising.

As the conventional ways of developing medicines began to show signs of instability, we witnessed a progressive transition away from relying almost exclusively on large, established pharmaceutical companies to champion discovery activities toward the present strategy where such activities are left up to academia or start-up companies. Yet this transfer of early stage discovery to the academic sector is likely itself to contribute to further adherence to Eroom's Law. Frankly, academic organizations and their faculty are understandably not overly familiar with the nuances associated with drug discovery, which will inevitably decrease the efficiency of these activities. As one example, many universities and the start-up companies that they spin out tend to file intellectual property (patent) applications too early. This is often done to attract an investor or commercial partner but has the unintended consequence of decreasing the amount of time that a drug can be marketed with exclusivity. Consequently, the pharmaceutical sponsor will make up for the shortfall in timing by charging more during the limited time they can monopolize the market. As we have seen, a high initial price will likely trigger comparably high generic competition and thereby keep the high price set point.

The transition of early-stage discovery research to academia is neither complete nor irreversible. Some early-stage discovery still remains in large companies such as at Pfizer and Merck. This is not merely a smart approach to keep an innovation culture but ensures that the scientists within the organization remain cognizant of cutting-edge breakthroughs and the means to exploit these to improve health. At a minimum, such awareness of trends in science and medicine are necessary to ensure that licensing and consolidation activities are well-informed. In this light, we question the sustainability of an entire sub-industry, as exemplified by Bausch Health (formerly Valeant, formerly ICN), focused solely on last-minute acquisitions of companies about to receive their first approval. These predators rarely maintain an active research team and thus may not be as well-positioned to keep pace with fast-changing trends in science and medicine. Consequently, they may be forced to pay increasingly dear incentives to maintain their pipelines; ironically burdening them with the same "treadmill effect" that large, conventional pharmaceutical companies suffer.

Large pharmaceutical companies themselves are facing a choice: Do they maintain a forward-looking and vigorous research and development emphasis or build upon brands through sales and marketing and go the way of Coca-Cola? The Atlanta-based company was founded to market a pharmaceutical substance. Some might agree that the company has done rather well purveying this product over the years, primarily through a combination of superior execution in manufacturing, advertising, and distribution.

Indications of a looming Sophie's choice of sorts arises from some rather dramatic experiments being conducted around the world involving several of the world's best-known organizations. In 2013, the healthcare giant Abbott Laboratories announced a dramatic change, spinning out its research and development arm into a new company that would be known as AbbVie (the translation of *vie* in French is "life," so the name of the new company was intended to convey "life after Abbott").[1] This outcome allowed the parent company to focus upon its legacy products but it seemed inevitable that AbbVie would ultimately experience the same problems that its parent company had.

Given the herd mentality that tends to shape the industry, the Abbot/AbbVie transition proved tempting for a time, arguably reaching a zenith when Pfizer announced in 2015 its intention to merge with Allergan, a company most famous for its lead product, Botox.[2] Within hours, even more dramatic news arose with the company announcing that one-plus-one would equal three as the newly merged company would split into entities focused upon consumer products, established branded pharmaceuticals, and a development organization akin to AbbVie. Soon thereafter, it emerged that a major motivation for the transaction was the intention to domicile the new companies in Ireland, the headquarters for Allergan, given its lower tax status, allowing the companies to avoid paying more than a billion dollars a year in US taxes. While the practice of offshoring had been popular for years, Pfizer pushed it a bit too far when it emerged that the behemoth had not acquired the smaller Allergan but rather the reverse. This impressive David eats Goliath feat would be made possible after Pfizer loaned Allergan the money to purchase it. Without specifically naming Pfizer, the United States Treasury scuppered the deal, rendering such a transaction to be illegal.[3] Speculation remained for a time that Pfizer would simply try a 1+1=3 transition with another company (perhaps a large, domestic company). However, the old adage of "once bitten, twice shy" would predominate.

Pfizer is also an exemplar of another interesting trend, which suggests a tectonic shift in the strategies undergirding large pharmaceutical companies. After spending most of its history losing more and more revenues to generic manufacturers, the company seems to have taken the approach of "if you can't beat 'em, join 'em." The company had amassed experience in developing and manufacturing lucrative monoclonal antibody products and elected to deploy these capabilities to produce and distribute biosimilar medicines: generic biologics.[4] These actions were paradoxically paired with later announcements that the company would sell off its generic medicines business to Mylan and spin out its own consumer healthcare (over-the-counter medicines) into a new venture. Another pharma giant, GlaxoSmithKline, did virtually the same thing.

Meanwhile, many generics companies are moving in exactly the opposite direction. A "race to the bottom" has decreased both the margins and attraction of generic medicines, compelling many generics companies to consider developing branded medicines. Arguably the highest profile example, and cautionary tale, is Teva, the third largest generics manufacturer by revenue. Teva devoted ever more resources toward the development of branded pharmaceuticals, intent to cash in on the high revenues that can be earned on a patented product.[5] In a true use of the word irony, the aggressive business approaches used to build Teva's branded drug portfolio would come back to haunt it when its ability to pay off these debts came into question. It seems the primary revenue driver, the branded drug Copaxone, had succumbed to generic competition, forcing the company to enact massive layoffs and restructuring. You may recall that Teva continues to earn some revenues by exploiting loopholes in Medicare Part D but other payers (i.e., insurance companies) were not as foolish as the federal government.

The race to the bottom has also compelled consolidation within the generics industry. In an effort to save costs, mergers and acquisitions have been on the rise and there is no reason to believe that the outcome for generics companies will differ from that experienced by conventional branded pharmaceutical companies, who attempted to enact the same remedies starting in the 1970s.

Profitable Nonprofits

All the while that the grass seemed ever greener on the other proverbial pharmaceutical fence for both branded and generics companies, even greater tectonic changes began to erupt from a most unlikely source. Charities have become more sophisticated and even aggressive in their actions. A prominent example came from an announcement from the Cystic Fibrosis Foundation in the closing days of 2014. Since the late 1990s, the nonprofit had been underwriting many of the costs to develop a drug named ivacaftor (brand name: Kalydeco) for the treatment of cystic fibrosis. This drug was being developed by Vertex Pharmaceuticals and the foundation had expended more than $150 million toward this cause. However, this was not merely a charitable act, as the company had agreed to grant the foundation a royalty on revenues generated by the drug. Ivacaftor was approved by the FDA in 2012 and looked to be a major money maker. As a result, Vertex decided to buy out the royalty from the foundation (akin to a lottery winner deciding to take a smaller lump sum rather than wait out their winnings). The price tag: $3.3 billion.[6] With this windfall, the Cystic Fibrosis Foundation vaulted past better-known nonprofits (e.g., the American Cancer Society and American Heart Foundation) and doubled down on its investments, underwriting much of the costs to develop two more drugs: lumacaftor (brand name: Orkambi), which proved to be another winner, garnering FDA approval in 2015; and tezacaftor (brand name Trifakta), which got an FDA nod three years later.

In many ways, the Cystic Fibrosis Foundation is beginning to look and act like a pharmaceutical company advancing a portfolio of products. Like Dutch Disease, it will be interesting to see if and how these windfalls modify the outlook and actions of the nonprofit. From the perspectives of our story, the foundation looks perhaps a bit too much like the pharmaceutical industry. The windfall experienced by the Cystic Fibrosis Foundation was not merely paid by Vertex Pharmaceuticals because they were grateful to the charity, but because Kalydeco and Orkambi rank among the most expensive drugs available today. Orkambi costs a throat-clearing $258,000 per year while Kalydeco and Trifakta each list a price of $311,000 per patient each year.[7] It is not clear whether the foundation offsets these high prices (for drugs that are not all that chemically complex or expensive to manufacture) for patients who need them but can't afford them, which raises fundamental questions about affordability and the responsibilities that a charity has to its constituency. With the prevailing view that sunlight is the best disinfectant, it will be important that nonprofit and for-profit organization alike provide transparent information about pricing issues.

To be fair, the Cystic Fibrosis Foundation is not alone as many nonprofits have adopted an aggressive form of so-called "venture philanthropy." Chief among this new generation of philanthropists is the Gates Foundation, which demands intellectual property rights for inventions developed with its funding. The Gates Foundation does so to ensure global access, which roughly translates into the idea of ensuring affordability, especially in the developing world.[8] This compromise, which combines aggressive entrepreneurial spirit with assurances that the resulting products will be accessible, seems to strike a proper balance. Although the Gates Foundation has faced criticism about emphasizing one disease over another or placing too much value upon emerging technologies, it seems to have enacted a self-correcting approach focused upon constant improvement.

Such successes are by no means unique to the United States and, indeed, some of the most progressive and successful forms of venture philanthropy have been practiced overseas for many years. A venture with ties to both the United States and the United Kingdom is the Wellcome Trust. Earlier in our story, we met Henry Wellcome, the American founder of the eponymous Burroughs Wellcome & Company (now part of GlaxoSmithKline).[9] Unlike his business partner, who died at a relatively young age, Burroughs would live on to a ripe old age of eighty-two. In his will, Burroughs established a trust containing his shares in the company, directing that their revenues be used to improve animal and human health. Since 1936, the Wellcome Trust has invested billions of dollars (technically British pounds), primarily into biomedical pursuits, championing causes such as the need for medical improvements in sub-Saharan Africa and Southeast Asia and seeding research into the discovery of new medicines. Its American arm, the Burroughs Wellcome Fund, likewise supports biomedical research and, interestingly enough, is one of the primary funding mechanisms for the rising subject of regulatory sciences, which seeks to improve the impact and efficiency of the FDA and other regulatory agencies.

Another successful example of a nonprofit that could prove instructive to developing and conveying affordable medicines is Cancer Research UK (CRUK). This nonprofit has its roots in two early 20th-century charitable funds, the Imperial Cancer Research Fund and British Empire Cancer Campaign. Spending nearly a half billion pounds (roughly three-quarters of a billion US dollars) per year, the fund contributed to the development of a large number of successful cancer drugs, including platinum-based therapies and tamoxifen, a widely used treatment for breast cancer. More recently, CRUK commissioned a study on cancer drug pricing, which concluded that outcome-based payments, essentially allowing the price of a drug to reflect its efficacy, would serve both to incentivize new drug development while keeping prices at a reasonable level.[10]

The example of CRUK might provide some guidance to foundations in how to balance their missions to help discover new medicines with the focus that these drugs remain affordable to those who need them most. This balance of facilitating innovation with price advocacy was sadly absent in the well-meaning, but ultimately destructive actions of the Cystic Fibrosis Foundation in supporting the science of Kalydeco (and their medicines) yet allowing the drug to be priced so high.

Learning from this combination of success and failure, we turn to a subject with a rather oxymoronic name: nonprofit drug companies. A new generation of charitable organizations are being explored to address unmet needs in patient care and to assure that these drugs are widely available. An early experiment is taking place in the form of Civica, a nonprofit formed by philanthropic funds and supported by a network of healthcare systems.[11] Focusing on generic medicines that are overpriced or in short supply, Civica seeks to be a reliable and affordable source of vital medicines, avoiding the sorts of shortfalls that we witnessed in our discussion of the availability of pediatric oncology drugs. Backed by a consortium of philanthropic nonprofits, such as the Gary and Mary West Foundation, Peterson Center, Arnold Ventures, SSM Health, Trinity Health, and the Mayo Clinic, Civica is determined not to be squeezed out of the market by generic rivals, who might seek to underprice their products in the short term to drive out competition (an approach that has proven successful previously). Such a model is innovative and yet somehow obvious and indeed already widely deployed. Unlike their for-profit counterparts, many hospital systems run using a nonprofit model (including some of Civica's backers). Their founders were simply working together and applying the business approach to produce generic medicines. Some of these same founders will provide reliable customers for the lower cost products being manufactured and distributed for Civica.

A logical next step, which carries far more risk, is the concept of creating a nonprofit pharmaceutical focused upon proprietary, patent-protected medicines. The risks return us to Eroom's Law, reflecting the many years and billions of dollars needed to develop a new medicine. Although we remain as faithfully adherent to Eroom's Law as ever, some early and ongoing experiments could lead in that direction.

In the hallowed hallways of some Ivy League universities, a new opportunity to incentivize medical entrepreneurship is being tested. Leonard Blavatnik was born in the Ukrainian city of Odessa, but emigrated to the United States, where he finished college, obtained an MBA from the Harvard Business School, and started an investment business focused on opportunities in the former Soviet Union.[12] The company, Access Industries, increased its influence around the world, leaving Blavatnik as one of the wealthiest individuals in the world (number 27 in February 2020, according to *Forbes*). Blavatnik has invested some of his earnings into a foundation, which has endowed scientific and governmental causes around the world.

In 2018, Blavatnik announced a $200 million gift to Harvard University and a $15 million gift to Yale. Although sizable, such news might have simply blended into the news of other major gifts given to such organizations.[13] However, this was different. The money given to both organizations was to be dedicated to addressing the "valley of death" in drug development that too often prevents good ideas for medicines from reaching a point of maturity, where they can be commercialized. In essence, Blavatnik provided seed capital to help inventors realize opportunities for advancing new medicines.

Although not necessarily intended in this way, the Blavatnik gifts could represent the type of early capital that could underpin the creation of a nonprofit pharmaceutical company to develop proprietary medicines. Such structures could minimize, if not outright eliminate, the need for venture capital and, if properly managed and coupled with incentives provided by the federal government (see Chapter Twenty), convey opportunities to address high-impact diseases with low-priced solutions. They could theoretically avoid some aspects of the pharmaceutical treadmill and not be unduly influenced by the quarterly need to appease demanding investors looking for ever-increasing returns on investment. The race to pioneer such an accomplishment has admittedly not yet begun but, if it could be achieved, a demonstration of success could provide a precedent that allows for other similarly designed organizations to emerge.

With this in mind, there is certainly no shortage of capital available to try out such an approach. The Giving Pledge, a campaign to secure philanthropic gifts from ultra-wealthy individuals, is one potential source, as are other advocates of venture philanthropy such as the Chan-Zuckerberg Initiative.

There will be many challenges and keys to success required to develop a successful nonprofit pharmaceutical company with a mission focused upon proprietary medicines that are widely affordable. Among the challenges will be strong management, focused on picking projects that are likely to succeed in terms of their science, product impact, and availability. Such challenges are never easy but are particularly intended for companies hamstrung by a nonprofit motive (and thus not attractive to conventional, return-based venture capital).

Another key hurdle to be overcome involves the old nemesis, Eroom's Law. To be successful, a nonprofit pharmaceutical will need to avoid the temptations that often drive up the cost of research and development, especially large and cumbersome clinical trial costs (including Phase IV trials). To accomplish this, our imaginary nonprofit pharmaceutical company could work closely with regulators at the FDA and seek support from nondilutive sources, including governmental and philanthropic endeavors with shared goals.

Managing the Managers

The greatest opportunities for improving the price of medicines are arguably the easiest. However, these will require considerable courage, leadership, and selflessness from actors not always known for these traits. If one believes the information arising from pharmaceutical companies, the majority of revenues and profits are captured by pharmacy benefit managers. Everything about the increasingly influential PBM industry seems paradoxical. This industry was specifically created to decrease the price of medicines and instead seems to be the greatest contributor to the problem (too closely reminiscent of the children's song about the old woman who swallowed a fly).

The fundamental issue preventing us from addressing the paradox of PBMs is the sheer opacity of their operations. Consequently, alleviating the problem must necessarily begin by eliminating that core issue. The utter inability to address the problem of PBMs resides fundamentally in the secrecy that pervades contracts made with both their upstream pharmaceutical providers (manufacturers) and their downstream customers (insurance companies and governmental groups).

Many opportunities exist to change this lack of transparency. At the most fundamental level, one could envision that both upstream and downstream customers, especially those who feel abused by the system, could require their contracts to be transparent, open to the public they serve. This idea might sound promising but, in practice, the PBMs might simply choose not to work with those customers. Thus, it would be important that such transparency be the demand of the largest partners.

As we have seen, there is no larger customer on the downstream end than the federal government. Were lawmakers and the executive branch to require open sourcing and pricing information for the massive customer base they represent (civil service, acting and former military, and entitlement recipients), then the opacity might be overcome. Ideally, PBMs should fully disclose their formulary information: what drugs are covered, what they pay for these medicines, and the amount they pay to pharmacies providing the drug. A disclosure about the composition of the formulary (which drugs they will or will not represent) could provide an opportunity for advocacy groups to determine opportunities for improvement and to avoid the types of shady deals reflecting in the "purple pill" saga. The difference between the costs paid to them by the insurer and the amounts they pay for medicine, known as spread-pricing, would similarly provide opportunities to prevent potential abuse.

Importantly, the goal of such practices is not to advocate for socialized medicine or to rail against the free market but instead to point out that the opacity that has allowed secret deals to lead to price increases for medicines, which are essential for improving the quality and quantity of healthy lives for all Americans, are unhelpful and a perversion of constructive capitalism. Although PBMs would undoubtedly feel targeted and resist such actions, they too would likely benefit from such scrutiny. At present, the utter opacity of PBMs causes their industry to suffer a reputational likeness akin to the South American kingpins of the illegal drug trade. Going back to the idea of sunshine being the best disinfectant, greater transparency could drive best practices that improve the reputation of organizations, many of which were sincerely created in an effort to hold down drug prices.

Other even more drastic efforts have been discussed in statehouses around the nation. Legislation is pending in many states, but Illinois could serve as a bellwether to gauge reform. Propelled largely by advocacy from pharmacies and more quietly supported by pharmaceutical companies, the state of Illinois passed a bill in late 2019, signed into law by Governor J. B. Pritzker, which not only intended to increase transparency but set out-of-pocket maximums and prevented gag clauses that restrict pharmacists from recommending lower cost alternatives.[14] It is too early to predict whether this law will alter drug pricing trends or alter PBM behavior; but it is safe to assume that PBMs will seek out every opportunity to avoid these new mandates.

A Solution: Transparency of Costs and Pricing Decisions

Many may argue that having more transparency into the pricing decisions of drugs, or even into the costs associated with making drugs, could have a chilling effect on innovation—or lead to (aghast) socialized medicine. Providing greater insight into pricing decisions is certainly not a means to socialize medicine nor even part of a slippery slope. It is simply that: providing information to the public.

Rather than being portrayed as the death knell of a market-driven economy, such actions could instead serve to be the end of the beginning of the steep decline in consumer trust for the entities responsible for the creation, production, and distribution of new medicines. No less a figure than the billionaire investor Warren Buffett declared, "Healthcare is the tapeworm eating the US economy."[15] This tapeworm can be cleared, potentially rescuing both the American economy and providing a renaissance for the ailing pharmaceutical enterprise in general and the many zombie pharmaceutical manufacturers in particular.

Many of those involved in what we have called the pharmaceutical enterprise believe we use this term in a derogatory manner, with the full intent of discouraging further discourse on the subject. However, public sentiment is drowning out their complaints and calls from both the left and the right of the political spectrum are asking—nay, demanding—that something be done with excessive pricing of drugs.

As we have throughout this book, we can look to history to find many instances where a groundswell of public sentiment has led to regulations that address the needs of the US consumer and make for a more vibrant and sustainable nation.

Take for instance the Clean Water Act (CWA), which is the primary federal legislation governing water pollution. Its objective is to restore and maintain the chemical, physical, and biological integrity of the nation's waters. Its laws and regulations are primarily administered by the US Environmental Protection Agency (EPA) in coordination with state governments. The Federal Water Pollution Control Act (FWPCA) was first enacted in 1948 but took on its modern form when its mandate was overhauled in 1972.

The EPA first opened its doors in 1970, but conveyed little authority, lacking the ability to establish guidelines and limited to a narrow remit to regulate secondary treatment from industrial dischargers. A high-profile event that triggered the formation of the EPA had occurred weeks before in downtown Cleveland.[16] On June 22, 1969, firefighters received calls that the downtown area was engulfed in thick, acrid smoke. In searching for the cause, first responders tracked the blaze to the Cuyahoga River. The flames were rising not from a warehouse near, or a boat upon the river, but from the river itself. The foul water was burning, triggered by a spark from a train passing over a nearby trestle that ignited chemicals floating on the water.

At its peak, the blaze reached more than five stories in the air. Nor was this the first time the Cuyahoga River, which we will remind you is composed mostly of water, had ignited. Indeed, the river had similarly been afire no fewer than thirteen times since 1868.

The water burned because the detritus from various industrial and petroleum wastes and the Cleveland incident sparked national outrage in a public beginning to awaken to the damages caused by environmental pollution. The Cuyahoga flows into Lake Erie, which would be declared "dead" in 1970, lacking the oxygen needed to support both fish and microscopic life. Likewise, fish and wildlife populations had been devastated across the country as people and organizations had been treating waterways as open sewers for decades.

The overwhelming public outcry demanded action, compelling Congress to debate the Clean Water Act of 1972. Yet public outrage continued to escalate, with monumental devastation recorded from sea to shining sea: ranging from the collapse of aquatic life in the polluted Chesapeake Bay to the near extinction of America's symbol, the bald eagle, in Alaska.[17][18] Despite this outcry, an array of industries opposed the legislation, successfully lobbying President Richard M. Nixon to use his veto pen. Congressional leaders could sense the change in the air (or perhaps became irritated by the acrid smell of the same air), ignoring the big money that opposed the CWA and other environmental measures and handily overriding Nixon's veto in the process.[19]

The CWA introduced the National Pollutant Discharge Elimination System (NPDES), a permit system for regulating point sources of pollution for industrial facilities, governmental municipalities, and some agricultural facilities, such as animal feedlots. These changes meant these organizations had to obtain a permit before they could dump wastes into the waterways and they had to be transparent about what they were dumping. Importantly, some wastes were excluded from dumping altogether.

Passage of the CWA helped to dramatically improve water quality and is now largely regarded as an essential part of the effort to restore the Great Lakes and waterways throughout the United States, including streams and wetlands, as well as health. Attempts by corporations to whittle back the provisions of the CWA reminded us of the damages caused by poor water quality (e.g., the Flint, Michigan, water crisis).[20] However, the commitment to high standards has mostly held and water quality in many parts of the United States remains far better today than it was when both authors were growing up in the agricultural and industrial Midwest.

Recent history provides other constructive examples of legislation that have grown out of public demands for transparency and the need to keep pace with technological changes. For instance, Regulation Full Disclosure (known as Reg FD) was put in place in August 2000 by the US Securities and Exchange Commission (the SEC) in response to demands by individual investors to have equal access to the information that was provided by publicly traded companies to professional investors, brokers, and analysts. Regulation FD provided that when an issuer (meaning a company that issues shares of stock) discloses material nonpublic information to certain individuals or entities who may well trade on the basis of that information, then that issuer must make public disclosure of that information.[21] In short, this law sought to eliminate the practice of what was regarded as "selective disclosure," which put some investors at a significant disadvantage to others in having access to information on which to either buy or sell stocks of publicly traded companies.

In truth, Congress had originally enacted the federal securities laws to promote fair and honest securities markets, with a critical purpose of those laws being to promote full and fair disclosure of important information by issuers of securities to the investing public. The Securities Act of 1933 (Securities Act) and the Securities Exchange Act of 1934 (Exchange Act), as implemented by commission rules and regulations, provided for systems of mandatory disclosure of certain material information in securities offerings and in periodic reports. In enacting the mandatory disclosure system of the Exchange Act, Congress sought to promote disclosure of "honest, complete, and correct information to facilitate the operation of fair and efficient markets."

Despite this well-recognized principle, the federal securities laws on their own did not generally require an issuer to make public disclosure of all important corporate developments as soon as they occurred, rather they encouraged issuers to do so in a timely manner (via an 8-K filing) or through quarterly and annual reporting requirements (10-Q and 10-K filings). Further, the issuer retained control over when and to whom some important disclosures were made.[22]

During the 1990s, the SEC became aware of a number of cases of selective disclosure, as reported through lawsuits, by the media, or complaints by individual investors. These complaints were fueled by the rise of the internet, computer technology, and online trading opportunities increasingly utilized by individual investors. Examples cited by the SEC in their Proposed Ruling Release in December 1999 included stories about selective disclosures made by companies during conference calls or meetings that were open only to analysts and/or institutional investors, and excluded other investors, such as members of the public and media. The information shared during these situations often involved the company's upcoming quarterly earnings or sales figures—data that could have a major impact on the market price of the company's stock price. In making its initial Reg FD proposal, the SEC stated that it was "troubled by the many recent reports of selective disclosure and the potential impact of this practice on market integrity."[23]

The public was allowed to comment on the proposed regulation until March 2000 and an outpouring of public sentiment flooded the SEC. Nearly 6,000 comment letters were received, the vast majority of which came from individual investors who urged (almost uniformly) for the adoption of Regulation FD. These frustrated investors believed that selective disclosure put them at severe disadvantage in the stock market and expressed surprise that existing SEC laws did not already prohibit such practices. Commenters also pointed out that self-directed, online investors didn't rely on the research and analysis performed by professionals as much as in the past. Highlighting advances in technology, online individual investors had a greater demand, expectation, and need for direct delivery of market information equal to that of the traditional professional analyst or investor. At the same time, the new technology made it more practical and affordable for companies to allow all investors to listen in.

As you might suspect, while the SEC's proposed Reg FD was largely hailed as an important step in transparency and fairness by individual investors across the United States, support for the new regulation was not unanimous. Large institutional investors, accustomed to benefiting from selectively disclosed material information, fought vigorously against the proposed regulation. They argued that fair disclosure would lead to less disclosure (a fear tactic that has not materialized). At the end of the debate, the SEC chose to move forward toward the goal of fairness and transparency and on October 23, 2000, Regulation FD took effect.

As the head of investor relations and corporate communications for two different biotechnology companies over this span of time, Ms. Weiman personally experienced the transitions caused by implementation of Reg FD ruling. As a member of the National Investor Relations Institute (NIRI), an industry group for investor relations professionals, she remembers talking with the president of NIRI about the SEC's proposed regulation prior to its promulgation. A particular question centered upon whether a company would be following the basic tenets of the new Reg FD legislation if it had already adopted NIRI's "good IR practices." Indeed, the use of preexisting transparent procedures meant these companies could carry on as usual. In contrast, more opaque practices had to change. The president of NIRI concurred, adding it was disconcerting that so many organizations seemed to be in a panic over needing to alter their practices, which had allowed them to selectively disclose information to certain preferred investors.

Twenty years on from the introduction of Reg FD, it has become common practice for all publicly traded companies to provide equal access to the disclosure of material information, improving the transparency and fairness of information to all consumers and investors. Companies adjusted their investor relations practices to meet the demands of the broader group of investors, utilizing a wider array of communications tools and channels (that have in some cases led to updated guidance on the rule for using websites and social media).[24] And, by and large, Reg FD is perceived as having achieved its goal of leveling the playing field and providing more transparency.[25]

The examples of the Clean Water Act and Reg FD demonstrate how changes in public opinion can compel legislators and regulators to affect fundamental improvements that benefit all. While those benefiting from the status quo cried foul, an improved outcome (cleaner water and transparent investing information) benefited both the American environment and economy. Companies adjusted to the new reality and carried on.

The same positive outcomes might be possible were transparency to reveal the costs associated with drug development and distribution, as well as pricing decisions of approved medicines. Understandably, members of the pharmaceutical enterprise would prefer not to disclose the secretive deals that seem to benefit all but the American consumer. We have already seen the oft-repeated claim that any legislation leading to greater transparency will damage innovation or lead to "socialized medicine." Yet the truth is, nine in ten US adults are concerned about rising drug costs, according to a May 2020 study conducted by West Health and Gallup. Such an overwhelming unity arose in a period when the nation seemed divided in nearly all other aspects of day-to-day life. Indeed, virtually all Americans were united by a belief that the pharmaceutical industry would leverage the COVID-19 pandemic to raise drug prices even further.[26] Obviously, public sentiment is strongly in favor of doing something about drug pricing, regardless of fear mongering by industry lobbyists and executives.

Change That Is Easy to See

As part of his daily responsibilities, Dr. Kinch is tasked with promoting innovation and entrepreneurship in a major American university. Although the work of scientific researchers tends to be inherently innovative, entrepreneurship can be a bit more challenging for the ivory tower crowd; even intimidating or threatening. Experience suggests the more fundamentally academic an individual professes to be, the more suspicious they are of the perils of rapine capitalism. Indeed, Dr. Kinch has been told to his face, quite sincerely and without blinking, that he had clearly "sold his soul to the devil" when he gave up tenure early in his career and worked for more than a decade in the biotechnology industry.

Consequently, Dr. Kinch has worked hard to create many ways at Washington University in St. Louis to demonstrate entrepreneurial opportunities to his more questioning colleagues. One means of doing so is introducing the subject of entrepreneurship to a room full of researchers, who range from inherently suspicious to the inevitable few who are overconfident in their abilities. He begins a talk about innovation and entrepreneurship with a simple statement: "On my person and in clear sight is the most innovative medical product I have ever seen; something with the ability to revolutionize healthcare." While speaking these audacious words, he conspicuously fumbles around with a snazzy Fitbit on his wrist, a misdirection that nearly always delivers the desired responses. He then points out that is not the case and instead takes off his glasses; handing them to the closest engaged audience member. For those interested, he explains that he is near-sighted with slight astigmatism. The glasses, all agree, are rather boring and usually quite smudged.

He then points out that these glasses are truly extraordinary for one simple reason: they cost him $5.95. The pair of glasses replaced a $600 pair of glasses and yet have the exact same capabilities and style (or arguably lack thereof). The revolution, he points out, is not the technology deployed to make them (they are not the product of 3D printing or some other whiz-bang technology) but rather the consequence of a strategic approach by the manufacturer to produce a customized pair of glasses for less than a cheap pair of drugstore sunglasses. He then discusses that the primary innovation was a fundamental rethinking of why we have been willing (even desirous) of spending hundreds of dollars for a product that can clearly be produced for far less. He then challenges the audience to think about other areas of human medicine (or for that matter, anything else) where we simply take for granted paying high prices for something that might be innovated. The advantage of this approach is rather than advocating for the millions of dol-lars to be made (which might appeal to some in the audience), one can do good by rethinking everything, especially opportunities to improve public health and address underserved health disparities.

As we near the end of our story, we propose the same challenge. If we look objectively at the ways that drugs are discovered, developed, manufactured, distributed, and paid for, what might we be missing? Why do we, often with little hesitation, simply accept the high prices without considering alterna-tive approaches? We are not advocating "alternative medicines" or going without, but rather would suggest there are great opportunities for future improvement. More fundamentally, the data suggest the current system is on a slow-motion course toward self-destruction. Thus, we must as a society find new ways to discover, develop, and fairly make available new medicines to all who need them.

We must therefore question the fundamentals of each aspect of the current model, from discovery to payment, and ask if this makes sense. How might we do it better? A quick look at the headlines shows no lack of complaints, but such conversations need to evolve to stimulate new ways of thinking. The complicated system for developing, approving, and paying for medicines is like the tax code, with new layers all the time, some of which did not value but did contribute to considerable bureaucracy. Many questions need to be posed and answered, including: Can we strip away destructive regulations or enact incentives, both to discover new medicines and to make sure that these are affordable and accessible for all? Who would pay for their discovery, development, and deployment? Does advertising help or hurt medicines? Are PBMs protecting the public from price gouging or contributing to it?

We certainly do not claim to know the answer to these questions. Herein, we have pointed out a few nuggets that might serve as the beginning of the opportunities for improvement, including rethinking how we regulate medicines, the relative costs and benefits of direct-to-consumer advertising, and the bloated system for drug distribution and reimbursement. There are undoubtedly many other opportunities for improvement, some of which will be driven by necessity as we now close out our story. Many of these challenges and opportunities, like Dr. Kinch's $5.95 prescription glasses, are solutions to problems we didn't even realize we had. What else is out there?

A key talking point from the industry, bordering on a defensive excuse, is that high prices are needed today to deliver tomorrow's innovations. This goes without saying and the primary challenge facing innovators is Eroom's Law, a hurdle that must be overcome that also represents an opportunity for open-minded entrepreneurs seeking to disrupt and take over a struggling multitrillion-dollar industry. We have no doubt that successful disruption will take place soon and like glasses that cost less than ten dollars, will soon emerge, perhaps as a result of the overall need to rethink virtually every aspect of our lives that arose with the COVID-19 pandemic.

At the same time, we might not have to wait very long to witness dramatic changes in the price of most pharmaceuticals, one of the last subjects we will address.

Coke—Pushing (Legal) Drugs

The argument that innovation demands high prices holds no water when we consider the price of older drugs, well past patent exclusivity and with no further need for R&D. The world is full of examples, including insulin, childhood leukemia drugs, and antibiotics. We've documented each case earlier in this book and will not repeat them except to point out that there may be an opportunity to remedy the disease of escalating drug prices.

Harkening back to our discussion with Steven Miller from Express Scripts, you might recall that he derided the idea that all consumers should pay the same price, declaring this to be a form of socialized medicine. Miller further argued that manufacturers and distributors should not be compelled to disclose the costs of their products any more than we would demand of the manufacturers of Coke or Pepsi. Miller's argument got us wondering: Might he have unintentionally been onto something?

Might there be an opportunity for a private sector, for-profit company whose mission was to focus upon an off-patent, yet overpriced medicine, and to manufacture and distribute it safely and reliably?

Once again, we should go back to insulin.

A lean model could allow the company to efficiently manufacture and distribute insulin, provide industry-comparable employee compensation, and yet seek profit margins no better or worse than Coke or Pepsi. You might argue this is exactly the role that the generic pharmaceutical industry is supposed to play. In some cases you would be right. Yet, the example of constantly rising insulin prices show that the generics industry has fully embraced the what-the-market-will-bear pricing model/mentality even though it certainly does not cost more to manufacture insulin today than it did five or ten years ago—and yet the price keeps rising.

We've described how ongoing experiments are exploring nonprofit pharmaceuticals while others advocate that the government should play the role of a manufacturer, but both have a tendency to favor bureaucracy over efficiency and customer service. Instead, we retain faith in market-based solutions. Our idea is to blend the efficiency of the private sector with a goal to remain marginally profitable (enough to ensure continued survival, attract and retain talent, and introduce new products) but not driven by the need for continued growth as demanded by Wall Street investors.

Stated another way, the company would need to remain private and not publicly listed. Indeed, Michael Dell decided in 2013 to buy back his eponymous computer manufacturer in recognition of the damage done to publicly listed companies by investors constantly insisting upon short-term performance rather than long-term value creation.

Just as importantly, this hypothetical company would be fully transparent in what it costs to make and distribute its product, as well as what it charges (i.e., the drug's price), thus removing the veil of secrecy that allows many current manufacturers and distributors to claim such disclosure is prevented by confidentiality agreements allowing each party the opportunity to point fingers at the other mysterious components of the pharmaceutical enterprise to assign blame.

Our proposed model would require start-up capital but a low-risk, high-impact opportunity might even prove attractive to conventional sources of capital, especially now that dull but safe investments (such as commercial real estate) are fundamentally riskier in a post-COVID-19 world. Alternatively, initial investments might come from philanthropy or investment vehicles with declared goals of making medicines affordable and available to the public. It is also possible that a crowdfunding approach could be deployed.

We are not talking about the billions of dollars needed to develop and test a new product, but a far more modest, efficient, and focused organization targeting insulin manufacturing and distribution. The company could expand its product line to include other similar off-label products, such as pediatric oncology drugs or antibiotics, but only after the insulin franchise has broken even.

Such efforts could be boosted with a bit of regulatory assistance akin to that provided by Reg FD and the Clean Water Act. Mandatory cost and price transparency by the FDA might be required for ANDA licenses for off-patent drugs and thus might motivate manufacturers and distributors to charge more reasonable prices themselves or to off-load such products to our imagined low-margin, for-profit entity. Were the competition to lower its prices to avoid losing market share, one might argue that one goal had been met.

Imagine the benefits of such a company: every diabetic would be able to afford their insulin; pediatric oncologists would never have to tell desperate parents there was a shortage of the drugs that could keep their child alive; and the United States would have an adequate supply of antibiotics, removing the current threat caused by Chinese domination of this market space.

Should such an entity come to fruition, we must remember to thank Miller for seeding the concept—perhaps the latest unintended consequence of this long saga of the pharmaceutical enterprise.

As we conclude this story, it is important to realize that pharmaceuticals, while expensive and highly visible, reflect a mere 10 percent of the dollars spent each year on American healthcare. As we begin to address problems associated with prescription medicines, some of which we have highlighted herein, it will be important to ask if these might be general problems affecting the remaining 90 percent of healthcare costs, which, if true, could amplify even further opportunities to increase the efficiency of healthcare, an issue that will be increasingly important for an aging nation and indeed planet.

Ending at the Beginning

We end our story with an event that will sadly capture headlines for years to come: the COVID-19 crisis. The pandemic revealed the crucial need, for the sake of both public and national economic health, for nimble and goal-driven biopharmaceutical enterprises, able not merely to respond to the next pandemic, but to anticipate and provide solutions beforehand. The economic tumult that began in early 2020 provided clear evidence that active support of such mechanisms is in the best interests of even the most capitalistic societies. The fundamental emotions of hope and fear have triggered conversations about the most effective way to identify new therapeutics and vaccines meant to combat the disease. Some of these ideas were a bit off-balanced, but it is likely that new innovations will arise. As outlined in *A Prescription for Change*, a direct cause and effect can be mapped out for how the Spanish flu in the early years of the 20th century directly led to the biotechnology revolution of today. Likewise, the agonizing death toll of the HIV/AIDS crisis starting in the 1980s spurred innovations that allow afflicted individuals suffering from many other diseases to enroll in clinical trials of experimental treatments.

We therefore conclude with the idea of blending state and venture philanthropy to develop drugs and vaccines that target not merely future coronaviruses but inevitable pandemic influenza strains and other infectious outbreaks that arise quite naturally every few decades. Although the returns on an investment into a universal influenza vaccine might not be realized for years, perhaps even decades, the trillions of dollars in losses, not to mention the millions or billions of lives affected, would be well worth the cost. Indeed, it is impossible to put a price on it.

As a consequence of having our collective eyes opened by COVID-19, we are optimistic and bullish about the future and eager to usher in a new era. However, like with other diseases, recovery can only begin when we admit to the underlying causes of our problems. The systems to discover, develop, distribute, and pay for pharmaceuticals has become excessively complex, with too many mouths to feed and too much temptation for profit-seeking. All of these problems come at the cost of public health. Symptoms of this societal disease include Eroom's Law and skyrocketing drug prices.

A primary issue is that it is not in the direct interest of any of the contemporary key players to change a system from which they profit so much. For example, many executives at major pharmaceutical companies realize their industry is not sustainable, but a focus upon quarterly revenues compels them to continue propagating a fallible system. As a first step toward this much-needed recovery, we must open our eyes and take a long, hard look at the problem and how to move forward. Accomplishing this task, both as individuals and as a nation, is the motivation and measure for this book. Let us begin . . .

AFTERWORD

by Lori Weiman

In the summer of 2019, Dr. Michael S. Kinch was traveling the country (when time permitted from his regular full-time job) to promote his most recent book, *The End of the Beginning*. His travels would bring him to a bookstore in Washington, DC, where I would attend one of his readings, along with another of our former MedImmune colleagues. After the reading, Mike and I shared a couple of cocktails and caught up on life and work, as it had been several years since we'd walked the same halls and sat in the same meetings for what was then one of the largest and fastest-growing biotech companies.

Michael Kinch is a perfect example of why I came to love working in the biopharmaceutical industry. He's intelligent, passionate, hard-working, ethical, kind, and generous. He exemplifies 95 percent of the people that I've had the great privilege to work alongside and represent since starting in the industry on April Fools' Day 1990. I've not only respected the brilliance that my colleagues brought to work every day, but also their devotion to helping people. In truth, their passion was infectious, and I wanted to do my best in telling their stories, and the stories of the drugs they were developing.

From the beginning of my career I would eat lunch with scientists, doctors, regulatory experts, patent attorneys, and accountants. I would interrogate them about the science they were working on and what made it different. I wanted to know about the processes of developing drugs, getting them approved, and how patients would benefit from our products. I would take this information to my expanding roles of responsibility overseeing investor relations, corporate communications, product public relations, employee communications, public policy, government affairs, patient advocacy, and corporate philanthropy. As a result, I like to say that I rarely worked a day over these many decades—although I tallied twelve-hour work days, six or seven days a week—because for most of this time I flat-out loved my job.

But something started to happen in the late 2000s that was unsettling for me. The prices of drugs continued to escalate at alarming rates, without good reason in my opinion. The CEO of our company (a person whom I hold in the highest esteem) would most likely roll his eyes at me for this opinion. You see he will forever think me a bit of a goody two-shoes, but it's also one of the reasons he liked me and several other colleagues he would most likely tag with the same label (including Mike Kinch). One day during a period where headlines of untoward behavior between Wall Street and a healthcare company were dominating news outlets, he promised me that I would never have to worry about such missteps from him. And I believed him. It was easy to do, as the team of people I worked with that he personally hired had an agreed-to mantra when deciding what to communicate about the development of our drugs: first, we decided what we HAD to communicate (i.e., what was required by law), and, second, what we SHOULD communicate. This is what I would put in the draft texts for press releases, quarterly conference calls, and annual reports sent to senior management for review and approval. Don't get me wrong, serious debates and fights took place about certain topics before we delivered the content (and after it was reviewed), but at the end of the day I could look at myself in the mirror and in the eyes of my friends and family without guilt or shame.

But, as I said, something changed, and for me it centered most on the question of escalating drug prices. Story after story broke in the news about companies taking advantage of opportunities to escalate prices. New drugs coming to market were priced at seemingly nosebleed levels. I even experienced group ridicule and scorn from doctors, nurses, and therapists when attending a writers' conference at the University of Iowa College of Medicine once they learned I worked for the industry. One pediatrician even took aim at the very product that had put MedImmune on the map, stating: "I love Synagis, but your pricing is ridiculous and your annual price increases are unwarranted."

I had left the company not long before that experience. The eyes looking back at me became too much to bear.

Fortunately, in recent years, I've been able to put my experience to use working for nonprofit organizations that have in some part renewed my faith in good work being done outside the confines of the quarterly results treadmill, beholden to Wall Street masters. And then Mike Kinch reentered my life and proposed we work on this book together. The result of that effort is that I have remembered how much I love this industry. The intellect and passion that fuels mind-blowing advances in medicine is awe-inspiring. And the theme that runs throughout this book—unintended consequences—has renewed my belief in the primary focus of the biopharmaceutical industry to do good things. To help people. To be creative. To move beyond the status quo and develop a new solution to the current crisis that has brought us all to a healthcare breaking point. The industry must embrace change—as it has in the past—for the good of itself and for the very people it exists to serve.

I will forever be indebted to Mike Kinch for this gift.

LEARNINGS FROM
A MODERN-DAY PANDEMIC

On New Year's Eve 2020, Donald J. Trump, the President of the United States, unexpectedly flew back to Washington DC from his glitzy resort in Florida and recorded a five minute video in which he claimed, among other things, that he had lowered drug prices for the first time in fifty-one years. He also took full credit for accomplishing what had seemed impossible merely weeks before: creating and distributing new drugs and vaccines to prevent or treat the novel coronavirus (SARS-CoV2).

The sudden departure of Trump from Mar-a-Lago before his treasured New Year's Eve bash was precisely because he was under attack for making claims that weren't quite accurate. Specifically, the Trump administration was failing miserably in the roll-out of vaccines (a series of breakthroughs arising from a remarkable combination of academic and private sector collaboration). As the wealthy partygoers at Trump's Florida retreat nursed their hangovers on New Year's Day, Mitt Romney, a Republican senator from Utah and a former GOP presidential candidate, would decry the failure of the vaccine roll out to be "as incomprehensible as it is inexcusable." With hundreds of thousands of Americans already dead, and public health experts predicting far worse yet to come, it was hard to argue with Senator Romney's conclusion.

Once again, the development and delivery of new medicines and vaccines had become front and center in the lives of every American as 2021 commenced. Promising solutions to the COVID-19 tragedy were becoming reality and new hiccups and missteps were foreshadowing even greater challenges to follow. In addition to the threats posed by the ongoing COVID-19 pandemic and the development of related new perils, the world was also struggling with numerous healthcare issues resulting from a planet that is steadily becoming hotter, fatter, and older. Beyond the next infectious contagion, the world is facing comparable challenges to its economic and public health caused by diabetes and other metabolic diseases, as well as progressive neurological degeneration, evidenced by rising levels of Alzheimer's disease. Concern over these better known and more common maladies have not captured the headlines as their steady rise has occurred slowly and quietly, a clear contrast with the eruption of COVID-19 in 2020. Yet the funding needed to adequately discover, develop, and distribute new medicines to halt these diseases will soon eclipse the resources already devoted to the novel coronavirus. Equally disconcerting is that all trends suggest the prices to obtain these future remedies will be out of reach for an increasing segment of the American population—unless fundamental changes are made in the way drugs are priced and paid for in the United States.

So, we are ending this book as we started it: with a discussion of the dystopian world that we endured in 2020, experiences characterized not merely by the plague itself, but its accompanying social isolation and economic despair.

As of January 1, 2021, at least 80.8 million people around the globe had become infected with COVID-19, causing 1.7 million deaths. The United States alone accounted for approximately 20 million cases of the virus and 350,000 deaths. Many a reporter and public health official noted that while the U.S. accounts for only 4 percent of the world's population, the nation had suffered one-fifth of the total global deaths from the novel coronavirus. This abysmal outcome was ironic given that drugs and vaccines were immediately more readily available in the US than in other places, primarily because the US had invested substantially more of its taxpayer-funded resources in medical solutions, which is typical for all disease states.

Indeed, our research has shown that the US government has enabled more therapeutics and vaccines, not merely for COVID-19, than any other government or philanthropic organization in the world. Yet, availability does not necessarily translate into usefulness, or better health outcomes, if these medicines cannot be afforded by those who need them.

When our wonderful editor, Jessica Case, suggested we write this postscript, we agreed that having an extra few weeks before the book went to print could provide an interesting vantage point to see how the pandemic might impact the future of drug development and drug pricing. And while many things had changed since we finalized writing the main components of the book, the ground beneath our feet has continued its relentless shift, which includes the emergence of more infectious variants of the virus across the world, that may result in a continual mutation of the virus which will require development of updated vaccines for years to come. Though neither author has a crystal ball, we thought it would be constructive to discuss potential ways the pandemic may impact areas pertinent to the topic of this book.

First, the race to find cures, treatments, and vaccines against the novel coronavirus over the last year has served as a unique opportunity for the general public to gain a glimpse behind the curtain. The world is better informed as to the challenges and risks undertaken by the pharmaceutical enterprise in discovering life-saving medicine and vaccines, as well as the risks associated with bringing these products to consumers. The pandemic has shown us what can go right when adequate resources are brought to bear in the fight against disease. This same calamity also showed what can go wrong when competing political forces use public health as a field for combat. The number of deaths and infections experienced thus far, particularly in the United States, emphasized the need for improved regulations, public policy, transparency, and clear communications. These features are necessary to facilitate and coordinate all aspects of discovering and delivering scientific breakthroughs to improve the safety and lives of people all over the globe. The pandemic has also reminded us of the very real need to maintain a healthy pharmaceutical enterprise capable of addressing everyday medical concerns, as well as future pandemics that cause periodic panic and pandemonium. We believe Dr. Wayne Hockmeyer said it best when we last connected with him in early December 2020: "Thank God for all the scientists and companies bringing us these incredible new COVID-19 vaccines."

We are all grateful to the expertise and dedication of an army of pharmaceutical and biotechnology scientists, from basic researchers to manufacturing experts and supply chain gurus. They and their employers set aside other priorities to focus on SARS-CoV2. Yet it is important to remember that these organizations did not take on this burden solely out of beneficence. Billions of dollars have already been funneled into these companies to conduct this work. As of December 2020, the US government alone had invested somewhere in the neighborhood of $20 billion to develop therapeutics and vaccines against COVID-19. In exchange, the US had secured approximately one billion vaccines from six companies, two of which had gained an FDA authorization by the end of 2020.

These dollars also procured hundreds of thousands of doses of a new monoclonal antibody therapy, though this example revealed some of the dysfunctions of current drug development and pricing mechanisms. This drug, remdesivir, was given an EUA by the FDA for the treatment of patients with COVID-19, despite limited evidence that the drug provided meaningful benefit. We discussed in the body of the book, how the manufacturer of remdesivir, Gilead Sciences, had come under great scrutiny for its pricing decisions for this drug. The new pandemic provided an opportunity to investigate whether remdesivir might impact SARS-CoV2 and these costs were underwritten by the American taxpayer. Despite this goodwill, as well as unexpectedly favorable considerations given by a pliant FDA, the company elected to charge American consumers (as well as federal insurance schemes) thousands of dollars per treatment. This exorbitant price did not reflect manufacturing costs, which were estimated at $10 per dose. From every vantage point, the sad story of remdesivir is reflective of good intentions gone bad and indicative that, as of 2020, many in the pharmaceutical industry were still struggling with understanding how their business practices were impacting public opinion.

The COVID-19 crisis may serve as an opportunity for some pharmaceutical executives and investors to open their eyes to the reputational realities of the industry. According to a *Barron's* article, co-written by a former institutional investor with knowledge of the pharma industry, the COVID-19 emergency could not only be a huge opportunity for pharma companies to generate revenues and be seen as valuable players in the vaccine market, but also be a catalyst by which to improve their reputations with the general public. Confirming our previously stated opinions, the *Barron's* article rightfully pointed out that prior to the pandemic, the skyrocketing prices of medicines had eroded the pharmaceutical industry's reputation in its largest markets in the US, Canada, the UK, and the EU. The article noted a 2019 survey across 78 countries that found only 9 percent of patient organizations thought the pharma industry had fair pricing policies. Overlooking the billions of taxpayer dollars these companies received, the article highlighted the potential benefits of participating in the exercise, but doing so without appearing too greedy.

Interestingly enough, the *Barron's* article also points out that investors continue to awaken to the financial benefits of companies being seen as "good corporate citizens." Specifically for the pharmaceutical industry, building goodwill among consumers who have been devastated economically over the last year could be critical for the future livelihood of the industry. Investors cannot have helped but notice that as the virus devastated the global economy, conventional pharmaceutical transactions were particularly impacted as people avoided visiting their doctors for routine medical care and as 14.6 million Americans lost their insurance. Further, widespread business disruptions negatively impacting supply chains and hampering normal production cycles were particularly devastating for regular lines of business in the biopharma sector. As such, investors are beginning to see that the healthier the general public is, the faster the global economy can recover in general, and the pharma sector, in particular.

We cannot move on without highlighting one ironic by-product of the exceptional investment made by the US government: That of the soaring stock prices of many publicly traded companies involved in the process to deliver solutions to the pandemic. Contrasting the devastating reality of the main street economy, these booming stock prices serve to highlight one of the more complicated and murky components of the drug development cycle. The unhealthy and disjointed relationship between Wall Street investors and publicly traded biopharma companies has created a Vegas-style atmosphere that has contributed to the skyrocketing prices of drugs. Serving again as a unique look into this relationship, the COVID-19 pandemic has unintentionally lined the pockets of biopharmaceutical executives, board members, and institutional shareholders (and some elected officials) with millions of dollars throughout 2020. In some cases, the COVID-19 pandemic has provided magical windfalls for companies who had never before successfully developed a vaccine or drug and had been teetering on closing their doors. This scenario is one of the many reasons the pharmaceutical industry continues to be incapable of eliciting much public sympathy, even with their truly amazing scientific achievements.

In truth, the single largest accomplishment in our combined realities since we closed the final chapter of this book is this: After appropriate vetting, the first vaccines from Pfizer/BioNTech and Moderna received EUAs in the US. By year's end, the Pfizer/BioNTech vaccine had been approved in 40 countries. On one hand, it is tremendous news that several vaccines have been developed and approved by regulators around the globe in less than twelve months, nothing short of a miracle and one most certainly to be hailed as one. A quick review of interviews with vaccine experts in early 2020 shows that very few (including Dr. Kinch) were optimistic that a successful vaccine could be completed by year's end. Thankfully, they were wrong.

Exceeding even our most ambitious expectations, the Pfizer and Moderna vaccines demonstrated breathtaking degrees of safety and efficacy. The level of protection predicted informally by various vaccine experts to be in the range of 50-60 percent instead proved to be in the range of 90-95 percent. Moreover, early safety data revealed a remarkably well-behaved vaccine in most recipients. As Dr. Kinch pointed out in various forums, interviews, and articles throughout 2020, rushing to get a vaccine approved could have had dire consequences for the entirety of the vaccine market were too many corners cut. Significant political pressure was put to bear on career officials at the FDA and on pharmaceutical executives. These stresses were amplified by the pandemic arising in an election year. Yet neither the FDA, nor the companies involved, seemed to put public health second to political desires. Even Dr. Alex M. Azar II, Trump's health and human services secretary, was reported by the *New York Times* on December 31, 2020 as having told West Wing officials pushing for a faster approval of a vaccine that "a vaccine that did not go through the usual, rigorous government approval process would be a 'Pyrrhic victory' – or a shot no one would take." We agree with Dr. Azar in this regard and are grateful to those public health experts that stayed true to the safer course of drug development.

In short, the science worked remarkably well and for a year that seemed so cursed, luck arrived at the right time, delivering outstanding results with a tricky new technology deployed on the fly to intervene against an unknown virus. Yet, challenges remain, primarily in public trust. The naming of the campaign "Operation Warp Speed" unexpectedly conveyed a sense of rashness to many, deepening skepticism about the safety of vaccines. While we remain optimistic by the clinical results announced to date, we encourage regulators to demand additional study and data collection to ensure long-term safety of the vaccines as they are administered to the general public. We also encourage all pharmaceutical companies, not just those developing vaccines, to pay particular heed to their communications practices and embrace a policy of transparency, reinforcing the benefits of simultaneous, open dialogue to avoid the impression (intended or otherwise) that they are being less than forthcoming.

As we have seen throughout this book, much of the pricing of medicines (as well as the profits to be gained) result from distribution. In this light, the COVID-19 vaccines represent a bit of a departure as their dissemination are largely mandated by governments, rather than conventional distributors and pharmacy benefit managers. Nonetheless, the stumbles encountered in the early days of the vaccine distribution have reflected inadequate logistics. As the proper distribution of medicines is a major component of the pharmaceutical enterprise, and major contributor to costs, it seems reasonable to anticipate that the pandemic could disrupt current and increasingly inefficient models for the proverbial "final mile" for medicines to reach their consumers. New entrants, smelling blood in the water from customer dissatisfaction with the current system, include Amazon, who purchased PillPack in 2019. It thus seems reasonable to expect that the online behemoth will, at a minimum, seek to dominate the sector and drive out the less efficient or unpopular pharmacy benefit managers.

Amazon's presumed future dominance of drug development may ultimately prove illusory or transient as the entire pharmaceutical distribution industry appears to suffer from a shared and fundamental dysfunction. There is past precedence for this, as when small pharmacist-owned stores would be disrupted by chain stores and mail-order pharmacies. Much as the source of this modern system of pharmacy benefit managers arose out of the blue from an exceptional pharmacist in Cincinnati, the next Cora Dow may soon disrupt today's drug distribution structures.

As we await the emergence of the next iconoclast, we hope their actions and strategies will be driven in a more transparent manner. A major take-away from the research into this book is that growing public mistrust and dissatisfaction with the entire drug development enterprise (from discovery through product delivery) arises from the sheer opacity of the system. Remembering the "disinfecting power of sunshine," it will be crucial to gain the trust of both regulators and customers by eliminating this excessive secrecy. Indeed, we maintain that increased visibility of what works, and what does not, will allow future entrepreneurs to disrupt all aspects of the pharmaceutical enterprise, enabling new ideas to facilitate the discovery and distribution of affordable medicines.

A key theme of this book has centered upon "unintended consequences," which was once the working title for this project. It seemed to both authors that, throughout the decades, many advancements in science and new attempts by policymakers to protect consumers led to breakthrough achievements, but invariably resulted in unintended outcomes. As we watched the COVID-19 pandemic scenario unfold, one unintended consequence was a revelation that layers of the regulatory process can be safely eliminated or modified, rendering a faster and potentially less expensive means to develop future medicines. Much like the burgeoning tax code, many regulatory requirements have been added over the years, with some amounting to nothing more than mere box-checking exercises or steps not applicable to each and every drug being developed. Perhaps the COVID-19 vaccine experience will allow us to eliminate a few of those boxes and potentially lower the cost of developing some drugs. This hope of course presumes that drug developers and manufacturers will pass along some or all of these savings to the consumer.

And lastly, it needs to be stated again that for change to happen in the development, delivery, and pricing of drugs and vaccines in the US, politicians and policymakers must be bold, work collaboratively, and embrace the opportunity at hand. The COVID-19 pandemic showed that bipartisan progress can occur if enough members of both parties focus on the long-term and address real problems. Improvement will require leadership. Elected officials must not forget the lessons offered by the COVID-19 pandemic, but rather work together to bring about real change for the development and affordability for future drugs and vaccines. History has shown us this is possible. It is for us to decide.

ACKNOWLEDGMENTS

We are so very much indebted to a large number of people who helped us put this project together. The subject of drug pricing was so enormous, so overwhelming, as to seem insurmountable. Paradoxically, that complexity represented the genesis of this project.

Having just completed *The End of the Beginning,* Michael Kinch was contemplating his next project and was deep in thought about whether there were any other untapped subjects about medicines that might be of public interest. His wife, Kelly, looked at him incredulously, stating the obvious fact that other than perhaps the opioid epidemic, no other subject pertaining to the pharmaceutical industry has captured more headlines in recent years than drug pricing. Yes, he acknowledged, "This is an important subject, but I don't know anything about it."

"That," countered Kelly, "is exactly why you should do this. You won't come in with preconceptions. Just see how the story unfolds." This proved a pivotal point and Michael is so grateful to Kelly and to countless others who helped us put together this comprehensive but admittedly focused (and thus imperfect) history of the twisted system that has evolved to discover, develop, and distribute lifesaving medicines.

Other inspirations behind this book include Holden Thorp, who recruited Michael to Washington University and helped found its Centers for Research Innovation in Biotechnology and Drug Discovery. Although Holden has since moved to another Washington to become editor in chief of *Science* magazine, his influence and inspiration continues to be felt on a daily basis. Likewise, we have been inspired throughout this effort by Bill Bryson, who has masterfully been able to bridge the chasm between scientific thought and "the real world" and whom we have sought to channel in this book, balancing the need for facts interspersed with humor. Although we take very seriously the subject covered in this book, we hope the reader was able to smile and perhaps even laugh (at the right times, of course).

In putting together this story, we have called upon many past and present colleagues from our shared days at MedImmune, as well as trusted colleagues with whom we have had the pleasure to interact before and after that pivotal experience. We apologize in advance for those we have forgotten to list and ask for their forgiveness.

Former MedImmune colleagues include (in alphabetical order): Wayne Hockmeyer, Jonathan Klein-Evans, David Mott, Linda Peters, and Lota Zoth. We would also like to thank Andrew Dahlem (formerly of Eli Lilly and Company and now at Indiana University), Kevin Love (from Arnold Ventures), Kristi Martin (Arnold Ventures), Steven Miller (Express Scripts), Bernard Munos (FasterCures), Charles Muscoplat (University of Minnesota and formerly of MGI Pharma), John MacDonald (from Ridge Road Consulting and formerly of PepTx, Azano Pharmaceuticals, MGI Pharma, and Warner-Lambert), and Rachel Sachs (Washington University in St. Louis). All of these individuals helped widen our perspective.

A special thanks goes to Eric Pachman, the founder of 46brooklyn, who spent a ridiculous amount of time guiding us through the thicket of opacity surrounding pharmaceutical distribution and pricing issues. Eric also meticulously read through the manuscript, identifying opportunities for improvement. Eric's contributions also include an introduction to Mark Cuban, who has generously supported both 46brooklyn and Washington University's Center for Research Innovation in Biotechnology and was kind enough to write a foreword for this book. Mark has been a valuable source of inspiration and insight as our story progressed.

We would also like to thank our agent, Don Fehr at Trident Media, and Jessica Case at Pegasus Books, who both supported our vision to tackle a subject so important and yet so opaque. We hope that this book not only meets their high standards but helps to effect constructive conversations that lead to meaningful change.

We also thank current and past members of the Center for Research Innovation in Biotechnology at Washington University: Tyler Schwartz, Zachary Kraft, Mereith Herd, Rebekah Griesenauer, Constantine Schilebeeckx, Ryan Moore, David Maness, and Tom Krenning.

ENDNOTES

INTRODUCTION

1   Derek Hawkins and Marisa Iati, "'No way to spin that,' Romney says of U.S. coronavirus deaths, blaming Trump administration," *Washington Post,* August 15, 2020, https://www.washingtonpost.com/nation/2020/08/15/coronavirus-covid-updates/.

2 Michael R. Gilchrist, "Disease and Infection in the American Civil War," *The American Biology Teacher* 60, no. 4 (1998): 258–62, https://www.jstor.org/stable/4450468?seq=1.

3   Allison Guy, "How Modern Sanitation Gave Us Polio," Next Nature, accessed June 17, 2020, https://nextnature.net/2014/01/how-modern-sanitation-gave-us-polioa.

4   Linton Weeks, "Defeating Polio, The Disease that Paralyzed America," NPR, https://www.npr.org/sections/npr-history-dept/2015/04/10/398515228/defeating-the-disease-that-paralyzed-america.

5   "Jonas Salk," Salk Foundation, accessed June 17, 2020, https://www.salk.edu/about/history-of-salk/jonas-salk/.

6   Michael Kinch, *Between Hope and Fear* (New York: Pegasus Books, 2018).

7   Fred Leonard, "What My Polio-Stricken Mother Would Tell Parents Today About the Importance of Immunization," Stat News, April 19, 2019, https://www.statnews.com/2019/04/19/mother-polio-importance-"immunization/.

8   Michael Fitzpatrick, "The Cutter Incident: How America's First Polio Vaccine Led to A Growing Vaccine Crisis," *Journal of the Royal Society of Medicine* 99, no. 3 (2006): 156, https://www.ncbi.nlm.nih.gov/pmc/articles/PMC1383764/.

9   "Jonas Salk," Salk Foundation.

10   Alan R. Hinman, Walter A Orenstein, and Lance Rodewald, "Financing Immunizations in the United States," *Clinical Infectious Diseases* 38, no. 10 (2004): 1440–46, https://academic.oup.com/cid/article/38/10/1440/346900.

11   Bruce Y. Lee and Sarah M. McGlone, "Pricing of New Vaccines," *Human Vaccines* 6, no. 8 (2008): 619–26. https://www.ncbi.nlm.nih.gov/pmc/articles/PMC3056061/.

12   "Should I Get the HPV Vaccine," Planned Parenthood, accessed June 17, 2020, https://www.plannedparenthood.org/learn/stds-hiv-safer-sex/hpv/should-i-get-hpv-vaccine.

13   Teresa Carr, "Why Does My Shingles Vaccine Cost So Much?" *Consumer Reports*, accessed June 17, 2020, https://www.consumerreports.org/health/why-the-shingles-vaccine-cost -so-much/.

14   "ProQuad Prices, Coupons and Patient Assistance Programs," Drugs.com, accessed September 4, 2020, https://www.drugs.com/price-guide/proquad.

15   Christopher Rowland, "Taxpayers Paid to Develop Remdesivir But Will Have No Say When Gilead Sets the Price," *Washington Post*, May 26, 2020, https://www.washingtonpost .com/business/2020/05/26/remdesivir-coronavirus-taxpayers/.

16   Kyle Blankenship, "Gilead Asks FDA To Rescind Remdesivir Orphan Drug After Public Backlash," *FiercePharma*, accessed June 17, 2020, https://www.fiercepharma.com/pharma /gilead-asks-fda-to-rescind-remdesivir-orphan-drug-tag-after-public-backlash.

17   Dana O. Sarnak, David Squires, and Shawn Bishop, "Paying For Prescription Drugs Around The World," *The Commonwealth Fund*, accessed June 17, 2020, https://www .commonwealthfund.org/publications/issue-briefs/2017/oct/paying-prescription-drugs -around-world-why-us-outlier.

18   Paige Winfield Cunningham, "The Health 202," *Washington Post*, December 17, 2019, https://www.washingtonpost.com/news/powerpost/paloma/the-health-202/2019/12/17/the -health-202-congress-failed-to-pass-a-drug-pricing-overhaul-so-it-set-another-deadline /5df7c57a88e0fa32a5140777/.

19   Kinch, *Between Hope and Fear.*

20   Joey Garrison, "John Kapoor, founder of Insys Therapeutics, sentenced to 66 months in landmark fentanyl bribery case," *USA Today*, January 23, 2020, https://www.usatoday.com /story/news/nation/2020/01/23/insys-therapeutics-founder-john-kapoor-serve-66-months -prison-opioid-scheme/4552871002/.

CHAPTER ONE: THE LAW OF UNINTENDED CONSEQUENCES

1   Sydney Ember, "Bernie Sanders Heads to Canada for Affordable Insulin," *New York Times*, July 28. 2019, https://www.nytimes.com/2019/07/28/us/politics/bernie-sanders-prescription -drug-prices.html.

2   Emily Miller, "US Drug Prices vs. The World," *Drugwatch*, accessed June 17, 2020, https://www.drugwatch.com/featured/us-drug-prices-higher-vs-world/.

3   Steven Morgan, "What's Driving Prescription Drug Prices in the US?" *The Commonwealth Fund*, accessed June 17, 2020, https://www.commonwealthfund.org/publications/journal -article/2018/nov/whats-driving-prescription-drug-prices-us.

4   Ben Hirschler, "How the US Pays 3 Times More For Drugs," *Scientific American*, October 13, 2015, https://www.scientificamerican.com/article/how-the-u-s-pays-3-times-more-for-drugs/.

5   The roots of this stereotype likely reside in a derogatory statement made by Britons in referring to American troops as "oversexed, overpaid and over here."

6   Phill O'Neill and Jon Sussex, "International Comparisons of Medicines Usage," accessed June 17, 2020, http://www.lif.se/contentassets/a0030c971ca6400e9fbf09a61235263f /international-comparison-of-medicines-usage-quantitative-analysis.pdf.

7   Sarnak, Squires, and Bishop, "Paying For Prescription Drugs Around The World."

8   "Historical," Centers for Medicare and Medicaid Services, accessed June 17, 2020, www .cms.gov/Research-Statistics-Data-and-Systems/Statistics-Trends-and-Reports/National HealthExpendData/NationalHealthAccountsHistorical.html.

CHAPTER TWO: A HISTORY OF MEDICINE MEN (AND WOMEN)

1   Lesley Smith, "The Kahun Gynaecological Papyrus," *BMJ Sexual and Reproductive Health* 37 (2011): 54–5, https://srh.bmj.com/content/37/1/54.

2   Norman Gevitz, "Pray Let the Medicines Be Good," in *Apothecaries and the Drug Trade*, ed. Gregory J. Higby and Elain C. Stroud (Madison, WI: American Institute of the History of Pharmacy, 2001).

3   Bob Zebroski, *A Brief History of Pharmacy* (Milton Park, England: Routledge, 2015).

4   "Mendenall Order," US Metric Association, accessed June 17, 2020, https://usma.org/laws-and-bills/mendenhall-order.

5   Edward H. Niles, "The Massachusetts Pharmacopoeia of 1808," *Journal of Pharmaceutical Sciences* 25, no. 6 (1936): 542–3.

6   Alan David Aberbach, *In Search of an American Identity: Samuel Latham Mitchill* (Bern, Switzerland: Peter Lang, Inc., 1988).

7   James Alfred Spalding, *Dr. Lyman Spalding: The Originator of the United States Pharmacopeia*. (Boston: W.M. Leonard, 1916).

8   "To Thomas Jefferson From Lyman Spalding, 22 February 1802," Founders Online, accessed June 17, 2020, https://founders.archives.gov/documents/Jefferson/01-36-02-0412.

9   Glenn Sonnedecker, "The Founding Period of the US Pharmacopeia," *Pharmacy in History* 36, no. 3 (1994): 103–22, https://www.jstor.org/stable/41112555?seq=1#metadata_info_tab_contents.

10   S. Jarcho, "The United States Pharmacopeia of 1820 and Its Background," *Bulletin of the History of Medicine* 46, no. 4 (1972): 402-4, https://www.ncbi.nlm.nih.gov/pubmed/4562985.

11   Michael Kinch, *A Prescription for Change* (Chapel Hill, NC: UNC Press, 2016).

12   P. Roy Vagelos and Louis Galambos, *Medicine, Science and Merck* (Cambridge, UK: Cambridge University Press, 2004).

13   Chandrasekhar Krishnamurti and SSC Chakra Rao, "The isolation of morphine by Serturner," *Indian Journal of Anaesthesiology* 60, no. 11 (2016): 861–2, https://www.ncbi.nlm.nih.gov/pmc/articles/PMC5125194/.

14   Staci Larsen, "Morphine's Modest Origin," *The Hospitalist*, October 2006, https://www.the-hospitalist.org/hospitalist/article/123203/morphines-modest-origin.

15   James Harvey Young, "Three Atlanta Pharmacists," *Pharmacy in History* 31, no. 1 (1989): 16–22, https://www.jstor.org/stable/41111210?seq=1#metadata_info_tab_contents.

16   Metta Lou Henderson and Dennis B. Worthen, "Cora Dow (1868–1915)," *Pharmacy in History* 46, no. 3 (2004): 91–105, https://www.jstor.org/stable/41112217?seq=1#metadata_info_tab_contents.

17   "Martha Cora Dow. A Pioneer Druggist," *The American Woman's Magazine and Business Journal* (September 1895): 82–3, 6.

18   M. Cora Dow, *Once There was One Little Store 25th Anniversary Pamphlet* (Cincinnati, OH: Dow Drug Stores, 1910).

19   "Miss M. Cora Dow of Cincinnati," *The Pharmaceutical Era* (May 1910): 43, 449–50.

20   Wendy K. Bodine, "Grocery Store Pharmacists," *Pharmacy Times*, accessed, June 17, 2020, https://www.pharmacytimes.com/publications/career/2006/Careers_2006-09/Careers_2006-09_3915.

21   An overdependence on the just-in-time approach would also be responsible for the shortage of toilet paper widely reported in 2020, when the innovative inventory approach became but one more victim of COVID-19.

22   Henderson and Worthen, "Cora Dow (1868–1915)."

CHAPTER THREE: THE MORE THINGS CHANGE, THE MORE THEY STAY THE SAME

1   Spalding, *Dr. Lyman Spalding: The Originator of the United States Pharmacopeia*.

2   K. Jack Bauer, *The Mexican War: 1846–1848* (Lincoln, NE: Bison Books, 1992).

ENDNOTES

3   Walter R. Borneman, *Polk: The Man Who Transformed America and the Presidency* (New York: Random House, 2008).

4   Christian G. Meyer, Florian Marks, and Jurgen May, "Gin & Tonic Revisited," *Tropical Medicine & International Health* 9, no. 12 (2004): 1239–40.

5   Layla Eplett, "Quinine and Empire," *Scientific American,* August 20, 2015, https://blogs .scientificamerican.com/food-matters/quinine-and-empire/.

6   David. D. McKinney, "The Mexican-American War Brings Regulation on Drug Importation," *Frontline Magazine* 3, no. 2 (Summer 2010): 50–1.

7   "E. R. Squibb," Britannica.com, accessed June 17, 2020, https://www.britannica.com /biography/E-R-Squibb.

8   James Harvey Young, *Pure Food: Securing the Federal Food and Drugs Act of 1906* (Princeton, NJ: Princeton University Press, 1989).

9   Squibb's name remains a fixture today in the name of the international pharmaceutical conglomerate Bristol Myers Squibb.

10   Clayton A. Coppin and Jack C. High, *The Politics of Purity: Harvey Washington Wiley and the Origins of Federal Food Policy* (Ann Arbor, MI: The University of Michigan Press, 1999).

11   Upton Sinclair, *The Jungle* (New York: Doubleday, Page & Co, 1906).

12   Laura Schumm, "Food Fraud: A Brief History of the Adulteration of Food," History.com, accessed October 31, 2020, https://www.history.com/news/food-fraud-a-brief-history -of-the-adulteration-of-food.

13   James H. Cassedy, "Muckraking and Medicine," *American Quarterly* 16, no. 1 (1964): 85–99, https://www.jstor.org/stable/2710829.

14   Ross E. DeHovitz, "The 1901 St. Louis Incident: The First Modern Medical Disaster," *Pediatrics* 133, no. 6 (2014): 964–5, https://pediatrics.aappublications.org/content/133 /6/964.short.

15   Mark E. Dixon, "Why Nine Camden Children Died From Smallpox Vaccines in 1901," Mainlinetoday.com, accessed June 17, 2020, https://mainlinetoday.com/life-style/why-nine -camden-children-died-from-smallpox-vaccines-in-1901/.

16   Kinch, *Between Hope and Fear.*

17   Ludy T. Benjamin, Anne M. Rogers, and Angela Rosenbaum, "Coca-Cola, caffeine and mental deficiency," *Journal of the History of the Behavioral Sciences* 27, no. 1 (1991).

18   Coppin and High, *The Politics of Purity: Harvey Washington Wiley and the Origins of Federal Food Policy.*

19   Jeffrey Bishop, "Drug Evaluation Program: 1905-1966," *Journal of the American Medical Association* 196, no. 6 (1966): 496–8, https://jamanetwork.com/journals/jama/fullarticle /659482.

20   Gwen Kay, "Healthy Public Relations: The FDA's 1930s Legislative Campaign," *Bulletin of the History of Medicine* 75, no. 3 (2001): 446–87, https://muse.jhu.edu/article/4725 /summary.

21   Arthur Kallet and Frederick J. Schlink, *100,000,000 Guinea Pigs* (New York: Vanguard Press, 1933).

22   Kristin Jarrell, "Regulatory History: Elixir Sulfanilamide," *Journal of GXP Copliance* 16, no. 3 (2012): 12–7.

23   Carol Ballentine, "Taste of Raspberries, Taste of Death," FDA.gov, accessed June 17, 2020, https://www.fda.gov/files/about%20fda/published/The-Sulfanilamide-Disaster.pdf.

24   Jef Akst, "The Elixir Tragedy," *The Scientist,* accessed June 17, 2020, https://www.the -scientist.com/foundations/the-elixir-tragedy-1937-39231.

25   Paul M. Wax, "Elixirs, Diluents and the Passage of the 1938 Federal Food, Drug and Cosmetics Act," *Annals of Internal Medicine,* March 15, 1995, https://doi.org/10.7326 /0003-4819-122-6-199503150-00009.

26   Peter Barton Hutt, "Philosophy of Regulation Under the Federal Food, Drug and Cosmetic Act," *Food, Drug and Cosmetic Law Journal* 28 (1973): 177–87.

27   Alexander Fleming, "Penicillin," *British Medical Journal*, 2, no. 4210 (1941): 386–7, https://www.ncbi.nlm.nih.gov/pmc/articles/PMC2162878/.

28   "Thalidomide's Secret Past: The Link with Nazi Germany," Oncozine, accessed June 17, 2020, https://www.oncozine.com/thalidomides-secret-past-the-link-with-nazi-germany/.

29   Roger Williams, "The Nazis and Thalidomide: The Worst Drug Scandal of All Time," *Newsweek*, September 10, 2012, https://www.newsweek.com/nazis-and-thalidomide-worst -drug-scandal-all-time-64655.

30   Harold Evans, "Thalidomide: How Men Who Blighted Lives of Thousands Evaded Justice," *The Guardian*, November, 14, 2014, https://www.theguardian.com/society/2014/nov/14/-sp -thalidomide-pill-how-evaded-justice.

31   Brigid Lusk, "Dark Remedy, The Impact of Thalidomide and Its Revival as a Vital Medicine," *Nursing History Review* 14 (2006): 271–2.

32   Williams, "The Nazis and Thalidomide: The Worst Drug Scandal of all time."

33   Evans, "Thalidomide: How Men Who Blighted Lives of Thousands Evaded Justice."

34   Lusk, "Dark Remedy, The Impact of Thalidomide and Its Revival as a Vital Medicine."

35   Kinch, *A Prescription for Change*.

36   Charles L. Fontenay, *Estes Kefauver* (Knoxville, TN: University of Tennessee Press, 1980).

37   William W. Goodrich, "FDA's Regulation under the Kefauver-Harris Drug Amendments of 1962," *Food, Drug and Cosmetic Law Journal* 18, no. 10 (1963): 561–9.

38   "Drug Efficacy Study Implementation," FDA.gov, accessed June 17, 2020, https://www.fda .gov/drugs/enforcement-activities-fda/drug-efficacy-study-implementation-desi.

39   "Organized Collections," National Academy of Sciences, accessed June 17, 2020, http://www .nasonline.org/about-nas/history/archives/collections/des-1966-1969-1.html.

CHAPTER FOUR: I FOUGHT THE LAW (AND THE LAW WON)

1   "Fleming Discovers Penicillin," Public Broadcasting System (PBS), accessed June 17, 2020, http://www.pbs.org/wgbh/aso/databank/entries/dm28pe.html.

2   Kinch, *A Prescription for Change*.

3   This mechanism, known as Q-T prolongation, involves the perturbation of a type of calcium channel. The toxicity caused by Vioxx is shared by hydroxychloroquine, a drug that gained unwarranted notoriety as a potential therapeutic agent for COVID-19.

4   Although not the focus of this particular book, one might note the somewhat surprising fact that these earliest trials are not designed to convey evidence that the drug is working (known in the parlance as its efficacy). Although sometimes a sponsor might try to glean this information, such data should always be taken with the proverbial grain of salt.

5   An exception arises in diseases where withholding or delaying a drug for a particular patient population might be seen as unethical, such as cancer patients with no other recourse or patients with rare diseases.

6   Amit Pratap Singh Rathore, "Getting a Handle on Clinical Trial Costs," Clinical Leader, accessed June 17, 2020, https://www.clinicalleader.com/doc/gettingg-a-handle-on-clinical -trial-costs-0001.

7   "Insurance Coverage and Clinical Trials," National Cancer Institute, accessed July 16, 2020, https://www.cancer.gov/about-cancer/treatment/clinical-trials/paying/insurance.

8   "Steven Paul," *Nature Reviews Drug Discovery* 8 no. 14 (2009): https://doi.org/10.1038 /nrd2800.

9   Bernard Munos, "Lessons from 60 Years of Innovation," *Nature Reviews Drug Discovery*, 8 (2009): 959–68, https://www.nature.com/articles/nrd2961.

10 Jack W. Scannell, et al., "Diagnosing the Decline in Pharmaceutical R&D Efficiency," *Nature Reviews Drug Discovery* 11 (2012): 191–200, https://www.nature.com/articles /nrd3681?draft=marketing.

11 Naomi Freundlich, "The Microbes Are Back with a Vengeance," *Bloomberg News,* January 20, 1991, https://www.bloomberg.com/news/articles/1991-01-20/the-microbes-are-back-with -a-vengeance.

12 Harlan M. Krumholz, et al., "What Have We Learnt from Vioxx?" *British Medical Journal* 334, no. 7585 (2007): 120–3, https://www.ncbi.nlm.nih.gov/pmc/articles/PMC1779871/.

13 Ben Adams, "FDA's New Drugs Director Jenkins Retires, Months After Criticizing Regulator," Fierce Biotech, December 5, 2016, https://www.fiercebiotech.com/biotech/fda -new-drugs-director-jenkins-retires-months-after-criticising-regulator-raps.

14 Alfred H.J. Kim, "FDA Authorizes Emergency Use of Antimalarial Drugs for COVID-19," Healio, March 30, 2020, https://www.healio.com/infectious-disease/emerging-diseases/news /online/%7Bf58e6106-ed19-4ec7-9b2e-7f1769f01cc7%7D/fda-authorizes-emergency-use-of -antimalarial-drugs-for-covid-19.

15 Joshua Geleris, et al., "Observational Study of Hydroxychloroquine in Hospitalized Patients with COVID-19," *New England Journal of Medicine,* June 18, 2020, https://www.nejm.org /doi/full/10.1056/NEJMoa2012410.

16 "Prescription Drug Monitoring Programs," *Pew Charitable Trusts,* accessed June 16, 2020, https ://www.pewtrusts.org/~/media/assets/2016/12/prescription_drug_monitoring_programs.pdf.

17 The same fate also awaited MedImmune, which, despite ample revenues, would ultimately be integrated into a rival company, albeit at a higher cost and foreshadowing a subject we will detail in great detail later in our story.

CHAPTER FIVE: THE MAN BEHIND THE CURTAIN: WIZARD OF ODDS

1 Thomas Sullivan, "A Tough Road: Cost to Develop One New Drug is $2.6 Billion," *Policy & Medicine,* updated March 21, 2019, https://www.policymed.com/2014/12/a-tough-road -cost-to-develop-one-new-drug-is-26-billion-approval-rate-for-drugs-entering-clinical-de .html.

2 B. Booth, "New Blood Needed: Pharma R&D Leadership Tenure," *Forbes,* September 5, 2017, https://www.forbes.com/sites/brucebooth/2017/09/05/new-blood-needed-pharma-rd -leadership-tenure/#3dc6ab9c409a.

3 N. Krug, "L. Lasagna, Doctor, 80, and Expert on Placebos," *New York Times,* August 11, 2003, https://www.nytimes.com/2003/08/11/us/l-lasagna-doctor-80-and-expert-on-placebos.html.

4 Pearce Wright, "Louis Lasagna," *The Lancet,* accessed June 17, 2020, https://www.thelancet .com/pdfs/journals/lancet/PIIS0140673603146405.pdf.

5 Louis Lasagna, et al, "A Study of the Placebo Response," *American Journal of Medicine* 16, no. 6 (1954): 770–9, https://www.amjmed.com/article/0002-9343(54)90441-6/abstract.

6 Louis Lasagna, "The Placebo Effect," accessed June 17, 2020, https://www.jacionline.org /article/0091-6749(86)90008-4/pdf.

7 Janice Hopkins Tanne, "Louis Lasagna," *British Medical Journal* 327 no. 7414 (2003): 565.

8 David Healy, "The Tragedy of Louis Lasagna," accessed June 17, 2020, https://davidhealy .org/the-tragedy-of-lou-lasagna/.

9 Aaron E. Carroll, "$2.6 Billion to Develop a Drug?" *New York Times,* November 19, 2014, https://www.nytimes.com/2014/11/19/upshot/calculating-the-real-costs-of-developing-a -new-drug.html.

10 "Measuring the Return from Pharmaceutical Innovation 2014," Deloitte, accessed June 17, 2020, https://www2.deloitte.com/uk/en/pages/life-sciences-and-healthcare/articles/measuring -the-return-from-pharmaceutical-innovation-2014.html.

11   Alexander Schumacher, Oliver Gassmann, and Markus Hinder, "Changing R&D Models in Research-Based Pharmaceutical Companies," *Journal of Translational Medicine* 14 (2016): 105–10, https://www.ncbi.nlm.nih.gov/pmc/articles/PMC4847363/.

12   Don Seiffert, "Report suggests drug-approval rate now just 1 in 10," *Boston Business Journal*, May 2016, https://www.bizjournals.com/boston/blog/bioflash/2016/05/report-suggests -drug-approval-rate-now-just-1-in.html.

13   Bernard Munos, in discussion with Lori Weiman and Michael Kinch, August 19, 2020; topic: Drug Pricing.

14   Ben Adams, "Harvard, Tufts Med Students Stage Protest at 'Biased' $2.9B Drug Development Figure," Fierce Biotech, accessed June 17, 2020, https://www.fiercebiotech .com/r-d/harvard-tufts-med-students-stage-protest-at-biased-2-9b-drug-development-figure.

15   Andrew Dahlem, in discussion with Michael Kinch, November 7, 2020; topic: Drug Development.

16   David T. Wong, et al, "Prozac, the First Selective Serotonin Uptake Inhibitor and an Antidepressant Drug," *Life Sciences* 57, no. 5 (1995): 411–41, https://www.sciencedirect .com/science/article/abs/pii/0024320595002090?via%3Dihub.

17   That our society has reached a point where such a high frequency of its people require therapeutic intervention for depression is an entirely separate subject not to be addressed here.

18   Bethany McLean, "A Bitter Pill Prozac Made Eli Lilly," *Fortune,* August 13, 2001, https://archive .fortune.com/magazines/fortune/fortune_archive/2001/08/13/308077/index.htm.

19   Ransdell Pierson, "Special Report: Lilly's Survival Plan Is Far From Generic," *Reuters*, November 9, 2010, https://www.reuters.com/article/us-lily/special-report-lillys-survival-plan -is-far-from-generic-idUSTRE6A83TE20101109.

20   Jo Shorthouse, "From Y/Z to Goodbye: Lechleiter's Lilly Legacy," *Scrip*, accessed June 17, 2020, https://scrip.pharmaintelligence.informa.com/SC097708/From-YZ-To-Goodbye -Lechleiters-Lilly-Legacy.

21   Scott Hensley, "Failure of Lilly Drug is Latest Alzheimer's Setback," NPR, August 24, 2012, https://www.npr.org/sections/health-shots/2012/08/24/159997459/failure-of-lilly-drug-is -latest-alzheimers-setback.

22   Peter Loftus, "Eli Lilly to Cut 8% of Jobs, Invest More on New Drugs," *Wall Street Journal*, September 7, 2017, https://www.wsj.com/articles/eli-lilly-to-cut-8-of-global-workforce-or -3-500-jobs-1504790131.

23   Munos, "Lessons from 60 Years of Innovation."

24   Will Kenton, "Spillover Effect," Investopedia, accessed June 17, 2020, https://www.investopedia .com/terms/s/spillover-effect.asp.

CHAPTER SIX: FINDING A NEW PURPOSE IN LIFE

1   Keith Souter, *An Aspirin a Day* (London, UK: Michael O'Mara, 2012).

2   "WHO Model Lists of Essential Medicines," World Health Organization, accessed June 17, 2020, https://www.who.int/medicines/publications/essentialmedicines/en/.

3   As detailed in *A Prescription for Change*, the attribution of the discovery to Felix Hoffman was a tale of revisionist history by the Nazis during their reign. Eichengrun survived the war and was later rightfully recognized as the inventor.

4   The name "Aspirin" was trademarked by Bayer Pharmaceuticals for acetylsalicylic acid but the trademark was stripped from the German company with American entry into the First World War and has since become a pseudo-generic name for the valuable product.

5   "Dr. William D. Paul, Surgeon, Dies; Was Inventor of Buffered Aspirin," *New York Times*, December 21, 1977, https://www.nytimes.com/1977/12/21/archives/dr-william-d-paul -surgeon-dies-was-inventor-of-buffered-aspirin.html.

6 David McCartney, "Old Gold: Good Medicine: Pain Relief's Iowa Roots," University of Iowa, accessed June 17, 2020, https://spectator.uiowa.edu/2011/january/oldgold.html.

7 Neither Routh nor Paul received royalties from their invention. Routh would later go on to develop Rolaids but, again, did not receive royalties.

8 Francesca Selman, et al, "Regulatory Aspects and Quality Controls of Polymer-Based Parenteral Long-Acting Drug Products," *Drug Discovery Today* 25, no. 2 (2020): 321–9, https://www.sciencedirect.com/science/article/pii/S1359644619304672.

9 Antonoi M. Gualandi-Signorini and G. Giorgi, "Insulin Formulation—A Review," *European Review of Medical Pharmacology Science* 5, no.3 (2001): 73–83, https://www.ncbi .nlm.nih.gov/pubmed/12004916.

10 Nate Raymond, "Jury Convicts Ex-Employees of Pharmacy in U.S. Meningitis Outbreak," *Reuters*, December 13, 2018, https://www.reuters.com/article/us-massachusetts-meningitis -idUSKBN1OC28N.

11 Jennifer Gudeman, et al., "Potential Risks of Pharmacy Compounding," *Drugs in R&D* 13, no. 1 (2013): 1–8, https://www.ncbi.nlm.nih.gov/pmc/articles/PMC3627035/.

12 Mel Seabright, "The Crackdown on Pharmacy Compounding," *Pharmacy Times*, accessed June 17, 2020. https://www.pharmacytimes.com/contributor/mel-seabright- pharmd-mba/2016/02/the-crackdown-on-pharmacy-compounding.

13 Judah Folkman, "Tumor Angiogenesis: Therapeutic Implications," *New England Journal of Medicine* 285(1971): 1182–6, https://www.nejm.org/doi/full/10.1056/NEJM197111182852108.

CHAPTER SEVEN: SELF-INFLICTED WOUNDS

1 Bernard Munos, in discussion with Lori Weiman and Michael Kinch, August 19, 2020; topic: Drug Development Trends.

2 Charles Muscoplat, in discussion with Lori Weiman and Michael Kinch, August 19, 2020; topic: Drug Development Trends.

3 Bernard Munos, in discussion with Lori Weiman and Michael Kinch, August 19, 2020; topic: Drug Development Trends.

4 Michael S. Kinch and Ryan Moore, "Innovator Organizations in New Drug Development," *Cell Chemical Biology* 23, no. 6 (2016): 644–53, https://www.ncbi.nlm.nih.gov/pubmed/27341432.

5 William Stevenson, "Charles Pfizer (1824–1906)," Immigrant Entrepreneurship, accessed June 17, 2020, https://www.immigrantentrepreneurship.org/entry.php?rec=31.

6 Ludmila Birladeanu, "The Stories of Santonin and Santonic Acid," *Angewandte Chemie*, March 13, 2003, https://onlinelibrary.wiley.com/doi/full/10.1002/anie.200390318.

7 David Goetzl, "Pfizer Aces Its Advertising Test," Ad Age, accessed June 17, 2020, https://adage.com/article/special-report-tv-upfront/pfizer-aces-advertising-test/53181.

8 Melody Petersen, "Pfizer Gets Its Deal to Buy Warner-Lambert for $90.2 Billion," *New York Times*, August 2, 2000, https://www.nytimes.com/2000/02/08/business/pfizer-gets-its-deal -to-buy-warner-lambert-for-90.2-billion.html.

9 John Carroll, "Dealmaking Spiked To Record Levels in April as COVID-19 Triggered a Fever in Partnering. But What Happens to Collaborations in a New World Seen Through Zoom," Endpoints, accessed June 17, 2020, https://endpts.com/dealmaking-spiked-to -record-levels-in-april-as-covid-19-triggered-a-fever-of-partnering-but-what-happens -to-collaborations-in-a-new-world-seen-through-zoom/.

10 Jay Hancock, "Drugmakers Tout COVID-19 Vaccines to Refurbish Their Public Image," Kaiser Health News, accessed June 17, 2020, https://khn.org/news/drugmakers -tout-covid-19-vaccines-to-refurbish-their-public-image/.

11 Kinch, *A Prescription for Change*.

12 Bernard Munos, in discussion with Michael Kinch, October 9, 2019; topic: Drug Development Trends.

13   "The Top 21 . . .Wealthiest Pharma Companies," *European Pharmaceutical Review,* accessed June 17, 2020, https://www.europeanpharmaceuticalreview.com/article/47001/top-21 -wealthiest-pharma-companies/.

14   Angela Shah, "Five Questions for Melinda Richther, Global Head at JLabs," XConomy, accessed June 17, 2020, https://xconomy.com/national/2018/03/06/ five-questions-for-melinda-richter-global-head-at-jlabs/.

15   Ravi Veloor, "Good Company: JLabs' Melinda Richter Finds A New Life in Healing," *Straits Times,* accessed June 2017, https://www.straitstimes.com/world/jlabs-richter-finds -a-new-life-in-healing.

16   Melanie Richter, "Bitten by the Bug—Melinda Richter at TEDxAmericasFinestCity." *YouTube,* https://www.youtube.com/watch?v=pzjYbj6CkLM.

17   "Melinda Richter on breaking down the barriers to healthcare innovation," MaRS, accessed June 17, 2020, https://www.marsdd.com/news/melinda-richter-healthkick-breaking -barriers-healthcare-innovation/.

18   "Pfizer simplifies contract research with Parexel and Icon," Pharmafile, accessed June 17, 2020, http://www.pharmafile.com/news/157913/pfizer-simplifies-contract-research-parexel -and-icon.

19   Rebekah H. Griesenauer, et al, "CDEK: Clinical Drug Experience Knowledgebase," Database (2019), https://doi.org/10.1093/database/baz087.

CHAPTER EIGHT: AS SEEN ON TV

1   Zachary Brennan, "Do Biopharma Companies Really Spend More on Marketing than R&D?" Regulatory Affairs Professionals Society, accessed June 17, 2020, https://www.raps .org/news-and-articles/news-articles/2019/7/do-biopharma-companies-really-spend-more -on-market.

2   Mabel Kabaini and Alec Burlakoff, "The rise and fall of a pharmaceutical opioid sales executive," *CBS News 60 Minutes,* June 21, 2020, https://www.cbsnews.com/news/alec -burlakoff-rise-and-fall-of-a-pharmaceutical-opioid-sales-executive-60-minutes-2020-06-21.

3   "Outrageous vintage cigarette ads," CBSNews.com, accessed June 17, 2020, https://www .cbsnews.com/pictures/outrageous-vintage-cigarette-ads/3/.

4   Mark Jackson, "Divine Stramonium," *Medical History* 54, no. 2 (2010): 171–94, https://www .ncbi.nlm.nih.gov/pmc/articles/PMC2844275/.

5   Marcel Proust, "Marcel Proust; Letters to his Mother," WorldCat, accessed June 17, 2020, https://www.worldcat.org/title/marcel-proust-letters-to-his-mother/oclc/1300196.

6   AC Hardman, "Abuse of Belladonna Alkaloids," *Canadian Medical Association Journal* 98, no. 9 (1968): 466–68, https://www.ncbi.nlm.nih.gov/pubmed/20329171.

7   The active ingredient in stramonium leaves is belladonna (atropine), which can cause hallucinations.

8   Gyvel Young-Witzel, *The Sparkling Story of Coca-Cola* (New York: Crestline, 2012).

9   The origins of the name Dr Pepper have been lost to time, but a legend that the moniker was meant to honor a lost love are, to be polite, utterly bogus.

10   "United States V. Johnson." Legal Information Institute, accessed June 17, 2020, https ://www.law.cornell.edu/supct/html/98-1696.ZS.html.

11   Nicola Davies, "FDA Focus: The Sherley Amendments," The Pharma Letter, accessed June 17, 2020, https://www.thepharmaletter.com/article/fda-focus-the-sherley-amendment.

12   Julie Donohue, "A History of Drug Advertising," *Milbank Quarterly* 84, no.4 (2006): 659–99, https://www.ncbi.nlm.nih.gov/pmc/articles/PMC2690298/#b34.

13   Shayne Cox Gad, *Drug Safety Evaluation* (Hoboken, NJ: Wiley, 2009).

14   "The Durham-Humphrey Amendment," *Journal of the American Medical Association* 149, no. 4 (1952): 371, https://jamanetwork.com/journals/jama/fullarticle/314797.

ENDNOTES

15   Richard Harris, *The Real Voice* (New York: MacMillan, 1964).

16   "AMA Calls for Ban on DTC Ads of Prescription Drugs and Medical Devices," American Medical Association, accessed June 17, 2020, https://www.ama-assn.org/press-center/press-releases/ama-calls-ban-dtc-ads-prescription-drugs-and-medical-devices.

17   Subcommittee on Antitrust and Monopoly, United States Senate, *Part 17: Administered Prices in the Drug Industry* (Washington, DC: United States Printing Office, 1960).

18   Edwin L. Rothfield, et al., "Severe Chlorpropamide Toxicity," *Journal of the American Medical Association* 172, no. 1 (1960): 54–6, https://jamanetwork.com/journals/jama/article-abstract/327342.

19   Louis A. Morris, "The Attitudes of Consumers toward Direct-to-Consumer Advertising of Prescription Drugs," *Public Health Reports* 101, no. 1 (1974): 82–9, https://www.jstor.org/stable/4627779?seq=1#metadata_info_tab_contents.

20   Julie Donohue, "A History of Drug Advertising," *Milbank Quarterly* 84, no. 4 (2006): 659–99, https://www.ncbi.nlm.nih.gov/pmc/articles/PMC2690298/#b34.

21   Subcommittee on Small Business, United States Senate, *Hearings Before the Subcommittee on Government Regulation* (Washington, DC: U.S. Government Printing Office, 1972).

22   This form of Strep infection is not to be confused with its more famous cousin, which causes "strep throat": an acute infection characterized by a spiking fever, swollen lymph nodes in the neck, and a very raw throat. Generally responsive to antibiotics, the painful infection is prominent among school-age children and highly contagious though rarely life-threatening.

23   John M. Barry, *The Great Influenza: The Story of the Deadliest Pandemic in History* (New York: Penguin, 2005).

24   Almea Matanock, "Use of 13-Valent Pneumococcal Conjugate Vaccine and 23-Valent Pneumococcal Polysaccharide Vaccine Among Adults Aged ≥65 Years: Updated Recommendations of the Advisory Committee on Immunization Practices," *Morbidity and Mortality Weekly Report* 68, no. 46 (2009): 1069–75, https://www.cdc.gov/mmwr/volumes/68/wr/mm6846a5.htm.

25   C. Lee Ventola, "Direct-to-Consumer Pharmaceutical Advertising," *Pharmacy and Therapeutics* 36, no. 10 (2011): 681–4, https://www.ncbi.nlm.nih.gov/pmc/articles/PMC3278148/.

26   Subcommittee on Oversight Investigations, Committee on Energy and Commerce, House of Representatives, *Prescription Drug Advertising to Consumers* (Washington, DC: U.S. Government Printing Office, 1984).

27   Lawrence K. Altman, "Prescription Drugs are Advertised to Patients," *New York Times,* February 23, 1982, https://www.nytimes.com/1982/02/23/science/prescription-drugs-are-advertised-to-patients-breaking-with-tradition.html.

28   Dylan Scott, "The Untold Story of TV's First Prescription Drug Ad," STAT, accessed June 17, 2020, https://www.statnews.com/2015/12/11/untold-story-tvs-first-prescription-drug-ad/.

29   "Prescription for Profit," Ad Age, accessed June 17, 2020, https://adage.com/node/1803331/printable/print.

30   "Top Spenders," Open Secrets, accessed June 24, 2020, https://www.opensecrets.org/federal-lobbying/top-spenders?cycle=2019.

31   Kerry Segrave, *Baldness: A Social History* (Jefferson, NC: McFarland, 2008).

32   John Crudele, "Hair Drug Seen as a Wonder for Upjohn," *New York Times,* May 28, 1985, https://www.nytimes.com/1985/05/28/business/hair-growth-drug-seen-as-a-wonder-for-upjohn.html.

33   Gersh Kuntzman, *Hair!: Mankind's Historic Quest to End Baldness* (New York: Random House, 2001).

34   Stuart Elliott, "F.D.A. Criticizes Viagra Ads, Prompting Pfizer to Halt Them," *New York Times,* November 16, 2004, https://www.nytimes.com/2004/11/16/business/media/fda-criticizes-viagra-ads-prompting-pfizer-to-halt-them.html.

35 Carl Jensen, *Censored 1996: The News that Didn't Make the News* (New York: Seven Stories Press, 1996).

36 Marian Burros, "F.D.A. Commissioner Is Resigning After 6 Stormy Years in Office." *New York Times,* November 26, 1996, https://www.nytimes.com/1996/11/26/us/fda-commissioner -is-resigning-after-6-stormy-years-in-office.html.

37 L.M. Schwartz, S. Woloshin, "Medical Marketing in the United States, 1997–2016," *Journal of the American Medical Association* 321, no. 1 (2019): 80–96, https://jamanetwork .com/journals/jama/fullarticle/2720029.

38 C. Lee Ventola, "Direct-to-Consumer Pharmaceutical Advertising,"*Pharmacy and Therapeutics* 36, no. 10 (2011): 681–4, https://www.ncbi.nlm.nih.gov/pmc/articles/PMC3278148/.

39 Schwartz and Woloshin, "Medical Marketing in the United States, 1997–2016."

40 Katherine Ellen Foley, "Big Pharma spent an additional $9.8 billion on marketing in the past 20 years," Quartz, January 9, 2019, https://qz.com/1517909/big-pharma-spent-an -additional-9-8-billion-on-marketing-in-the-past-20-years-it-worked/.

41 Richard Anderson, "Pharmaceutical Industry Gets High on Fat Profits," BBC, November 6, 2014, https://www.bbc.com/news/business-28212223.

42 For Eli Lilly, the expenditures were virtually identical, with S&M barely beating R&D (pun intended).

43 Ana Swanson, "Big Pharmaceutical Companies Are Spending Far More on Marketing than Research," *Washington Post,* February, 11, 2015, https://www.washingtonpost.com/news/wonk /wp/2015/02/11/big-pharmaceutical-companies-are-spending-far-more-on-marketing-than -research/.

44 German Lopez, "9 of 10 Top Drugmakers Spend More Money on Marketing than Research," Vox, February 11, 2015, https://www.vox.com/2015/2/11/8018691/big-pharma -research-advertising.

CHAPTER NINE: I'M FROM THE GOVERNMENT, AND AM HERE TO HELP . . .

1   Randy Shilts's "And the Band Played On" conveys a raw and outstanding overview of this critical time period.

2   Kinch, *A Prescription for Change.*

3   Robert Pear, "Faster Approval of AIDS Drugs is Urged," *New York Times*, August 16, 1990, https://www.nytimes.com/1990/08/16/us/faster-approval-of-aids-drugs-is-urged.html.

4   Dexatrim, 1938; Seldane, 1985; Hismanal, 1977; the components of Fen-Phen, 1973 and 1959; Both Vioxx and Bextra were approved in 2004.

5   Linda Peters in discussion with Lori Weiman and Michael Kinch, September 4, 2020.

6   Philip Routledge, "150 Years of Pharmacovigilance," *Department of Medical History* 351, no. 9110 (1998): 1200–1, https://doi.org/10.1016/S0140-6736(98)03148-1.

7   Paul Beninger, "Pharmacovigilance: An Overview," *Clinical Therapeutics* 40, no. 12 (2018): 1991–2004, https://www.clinicaltherapeutics.com/article/S0149-2918(18)30317-5/fulltext.

8   "Prescription Drug Labeling Resources," FDA.gov, accessed June 17, 2020, https://www.fda .gov/drugs/laws-acts-and-rules/prescription-drug-labeling-resources.

9   Syed Rizwanuddin Ahmad, "Adverse Drug Event Monitoring at the Food and Drug Administration," *Journal of General Internal Medicine* 18, no. 1 (2003): 57–60, https://www .ncbi.nlm.nih.gov/pmc/articles/PMC1494803/.

10 H.D. Scott, et al, "Rhode Island Physicians; Recognition and Reporting of Adverse Drug Reactions," *Rhode Island Medical Journal* 70, no. 7(1987): 311–6, https://www.ncbi.nlm.nih .gov/pubmed/3476980.

11 110th Congress, H.R.3580—Food and Drug Administration Amendment Act of 2007, accessed June 17, 2020, https://www.congress.gov/bill/110th-congress/house-bill/3580.

12 Not be confused with Title IX of the Education Amendments Act of 1972, which banned educational discrimination based on sex.

13   Viraj Suvarna, "Phase IV of Drug Development," *Perspectives on Clinical Research* 1, no. 2 (2010): 57–60, https://www.ncbi.nlm.nih.gov/pmc/articles/PMC3148611/.

14   Phil B. Fontanarosa, "Postmarketing Surveillance-Lack of Vigilance, Lack of Trust," *Journal of the American Medical Association* 292, no. 21 (2004): 2647–50. https://jamanetwork.com /journals/jama/fullarticle/199884.

15   Xinji Zhang, et al., "Overview of Phase IV Clinical Trials for Postmarket Drug Safety Surveillance," *British Medical Journal* 6, no. 11 (2016), https://bmjopen.bmj.com/content /6/11/e010643.

16   The three larger lobbyists represented aggregate causes such as the chamber of commerce, immigration, and real estate issues.

17   Michael D. Hogue, et al., "Pharmacist Involvement with Immunizations: A Decade of Professional Advancement," *Journal of the American Pharmacists Association* 46, no. 2 (2006): 168–82, https://www.sciencedirect.com/science/article/abs/pii/S1544319115315521.

CHAPTER TEN: ODD COUPLINGS

1   Roger Ebert, "Lorenzo's Oil," RogerEbert.com, accessed June 17, 2020, https://www .rogerebert.com/reviews/lorenzos-oil-1993.

2   Joshua Green, "Jack Klugman's Secret, Lifesaving Legacy," *Washington Post*, December 25, 2012, https://www.washingtonpost.com/news/wonk/wp/2012/12/25/jack-klugmans-secret -lifesaving-legacy/.

3   Karen de Witt, "House Told of Need for 'Orphan Drugs,'" *New York Times*, March 10, 1981, https://www.nytimes.com/1981/03/10/us/house-told-of-need-for-orphan-drugs.html.

4   Henry Waxman, *The Waxman Report: How Congress Really Works* (New York: Hachette, 2009).

5   Ezra Klein, "'The Rachel Maddow Show' for Wednesday, December 26th, 2012," NBCNews.com, accessed June 17. 2020, http://www.nbcnews.com/id/50306206/ns/msnbc -rachel_maddow_show/.

6   This particular approach proved so valuable that Henry Waxman and Orrin Hatch, the same antagonists confronting on the opposite sides of the Orphan Drug Act in 1983, would this time team up a year later to pass the Drug Prices Competition and Patent Term Restoration Act, better known colloquially as the Hatch-Waxman Act. We will return to this key piece of legislation in a future chapter, but for now, it suffices to say that the 1984 law granted a five-year period of exclusivity for any new medicine introduced to the public, even if the product utterly lacked patent coverage.

7   Rich Daly, "House Offers Incentives For Development of 'Orphan' Drugs," *Congressional Quarterly Daily Monitor*, September 5, 2002.

8   Michael S. Kinch and Rebekah H. Griesenauer, "2018 in Review: FDA Approvals of New Molecular Entities," *Drug Discovery Today* 24, no. 9 (2019): 1710–4, https://www.science direct.com/science/article/pii/S135964461930114X?via%3Dihub.

9   "High Blood Pressure," Centers for Disease Control and Prevention, accessed June 18, 2020, https://www.cdc.gov/bloodpressure/faqs.htm.

10   "Cholesterol," Centers for Disease Control and Prevention, accessed June 18, 2020, https ://www.cdc.gov/cholesterol/cholesterol_education_month.htm.

11   Ken Alltucker, "A New Drug Costs $2.1 Million for Children with a Muscle-Wasting Disease," *USA Today*, May 24, 2019, https://www.usatoday.com/story/news/health/2019 /05/24/zolgensma-2-1-million-drug-nations-most-expensive/1223666001/.

12   Prominent exceptions to this rule include measures to limit the overuse of certain addictive substances of abuse or exceptionally toxic medicines.

13   Deena Beasley, "The Cost of Cancer: New Drugs Show Success At a Steep Price," *Reuters*, April 3, 2017, https://www.reuters.com/article/us-usa-healthcare-cancer-costs/the-cost -of-cancer-new-drugs-show-success-at-a-steep-price-idUSKBN1750FU.

14   Jonathan Gardner, "In Rare Move, Gilead Gives Up 'Orphan Status' for Experimental Coronavirus Drug," BiopharmaDive, accessed June 18, 2020, https://www.biopharmadive.com/news/coronavirus-gilead-remdesivir-orphan-drug/574882/.

15   Alex Keown, "Following Outcry, Gilead Sciences Seeks to Rescind Orphan Drug Designation for COVID-19 Drug," Biospace, accessed June 18, 2020, https://www.biospace.com/article/following-outcry-gilead-sciences-seeks-to-rescind-orphan-drug-designation-for-covid-19-drug/

16   Sarah Jane Tribble and Sydney Lupkin, "Drugs for Rare Diseases Have Become Uncommonly Rich Monopolies," NPR, January 17, 2017, https://www.npr.org/sections/health-shots/2017/01/17/509506836/drugs-for-rare-diseases-have-become-uncommonly-rich-monopolies.

CHAPTER ELEVEN: GENERIC, BUT NOT UNINTERESTING

1   Bernard Munos, in discussion with Michael Kinch, October 9, 2020; topic: Drug Development.

2   "11th Annual Edition of AAM Access & Savings," Association for Accessible Medicines, accessed June 19, 2020, https://accessiblemeds.org/resources/reports/209828-generic-drug-access-and-savings-report.

3   Kinch, *A Prescription for Change.*

4   Robert A Buerki and Louis D. Vottero, *Ethical Practices in Pharmacy* (Madison, WI: American Institute of the History of Pharmacy, 1997).

5   The FDA settled on acetylsalicylic acid but later changed it to aspirin (without a capital) after the product was confiscated from German-owned Bayer, which had been labeled an enemy combatant.

6   "Drug Antisubstitution Laws," *Journal of the American Medical Association* 221, no. 7 (1972): 711, https://jamanetwork.com/journals/jama/fullarticle/343935.

7   "The Plea of a Jacksonville Druggist," *Journal of the American Medical Association* 220, no. 6 (1972): 853–4, https://jamanetwork.com/journals/jama/article-abstract/342334.

8   The PDA and NAPM would later merge in 2001 to become the Generic Pharmaceutical Association and, sensing the political wind at their backs, changed their name to the Association for Accessible Medicines in 2017.

9   John Jacobs, "Drug Anti-Substitution Laws Attacked," *Washington Post,* November 16, 1977, https://www.washingtonpost.com/archive/politics/1977/11/16/drug-anti-substitution-laws-attacked/e0cc6a94-cc77-45fd-808d-bd8e0858bed1/.

10   Michael McCaughan, "The REMS Pioneers: Amgen's Nplate Sets Another New Standard," In Vivo, accessed June 18, 2020, http://invivoblog.blogspot.com/2008/09/rems-pioneers-amgens-nplate-sets.html.

11   Bioequivalence is normally measured by assessing concentrations in the blood over time and comparing the experimental generic medicine with the branded drug.

12   Emmarie Huetteman, "Klobuchar Wants to Stop 'Pay for Delay' Deals that Keep Drug Prices High," Kaiser Health News, accessed June 18, 2020, https://khn.org/news/klobuchar-wants-to-stop-pay-for-delay-deals-that-keep-drug-prices-high/.

13   Bernie Sanders, "Sign the Petition: Stand with Bernie to Stop Skyrocketing Drug Prices," Bernie Sanders, U.S. Senator for Vermont, accessed June 18, 2020, https://www.sanders.senate.gov/petition/drug-prices.

14   Elizabeth Warren, "As Health Care Debate Shits, Senator Warren Joins Senator Franken and Senate Colleagues in Milestone Effort to Bring Down Prescription Drug Prices," Elizabeth Warren Senate, accessed June 18, 2020, https://www.warren.senate.gov/newsroom/press-releases/as-health-care-debate-shifts-senator-warren-joins-senator-franken-and-senate-colleagues-in-milestone-effort-to-bring-down-prescription-drug-prices.

15   National Archives and Record Administration, "62 FR 43535—Prescription Drug Products; Levothyroxine Sodium." *Federal Register* 62, no. 157 (August 14, 1997).

16   Philip J. Hilts, "After 46 Years of Sales, Thyroid Drug Needs F.D.A. Approval," *New York Times,* July 24, 2001, https://www.nytimes.com/2001/07/24/science/after-46-years-of-sales -thyroid-drug-needs-fda-approval.html.

17   Sheldon Kaplan, et al., "Hypodermic Injection Device Having Means for Varying the Medicament Capacity Thereof," United States Patent and Trade Office, Patent number: US4031893A, accessed June 18, 2020, https://www.google.com/patents/US4031893.

18   "Chemical Warfare Experience in the Iran/Iraq War," United States Army, accessed June 18, 2020, https://gulflink.health.mil/declassdocs/dia/19970129/123096_8061115 _mic_0001.html.

19   Not to be confused with its American counterpart, Merck KGaA is the original parent company, headquartered in Germany and sometimes referred to as "German Merck."

20   Aaron E. Carroll, "The EpiPen, a Case Study in Health System Dysfunction," *New York Times,* August 24, 2016, https://www.nytimes.com/2016/08/24/upshot/the-epipen-a-case -study-in-health-care-system-dysfunction.html.

21   Matt Reimann, "The Story of the EpiPen," Timeline, accessed June 18, 2020, https://timeline .com/epipen-technology-drug-industry-b28d19036dee.

22   Adam Feuerstein, "Retrophin CEO Under Fire for Twitter Faux Pas," The Street, accessed June 17, 2020, https://www.thestreet.com/story/12839330/1/retrophin-ceo-under-fire-for -twitter-faux-pas.html.

23   Adam Feuerstein, "Shkreli's Inability to Focus, Immaturity Cost Him Retrophin CEO Job," The Street, accessed June 18, 2020, https://www.thestreet.com/story/12897910/1 /shkrelis-inability-to-focus-immaturity-cost-him-retrophin-ceo-job.html.

24   Yoram Unguru, "Drug Shortages Jeopardize the Lives of Children with Cancer," STAT, March 19, 2019, https://www.statnews.com/2019/03/19/drug-shortages-jeopardize -children-cancer/.

25   Keerthi Gogineni, et al., "Survey of Oncologists About Shortages of Cancer Drugs," *New England Journal of Medicine* 369 (2013): 2463–4, https://www.nejm.org/doi/full/10.1056 /NEJMc1307379.

26   Roni Caryn Rabin, "Faced with a Drug Shortfall, Doctors Scramble to Treat Children with Cancer," *New York Times*, October, 14, 2019, https://www.nytimes.com/2019/10/14/health /cancer-drug-shortage.html.

CHAPTER TWELVE: THE COSTS OF COMPLEXITY

1   The placebo effect is quite a real phenomenon providing benefits to many. This outcome reflects a fascinating and poorly understood consequence of how the brain and body work in utterly mysterious ways.

2   Irvin Molotsky, "U.S. Issues Rules on Diet Supplement Labels," *New York Times*, December 30, 1993, https://www.nytimes.com/1993/12/30/us/us-issues-rules-on-diet-supplement -labels.html.

3   "Success Story: Taxol," National Cancer Institute, accessed June 18, 2020, https://dtp .cancer.gov/timeline/flash/success_stories/S2_Taxol.htm.

4   Yi Li, et al., "Current and Emerging Options for Taxol Production," *Advances in Biochemical Engineering and Biotechnology* 148 (2015):405–25, https://pubmed.ncbi.nlm.nih.gov/25528175/.

5   David G.I. Kingston, "Taxol, a Molecular for All Seasons," *Chemical Communications* 10 (2001), https://doi.org/10.1039/B100070P.

6   Josh Bloom, "Semisynthetic: A 'Real' Word that Saves Lives," American Council on Science and Health, December 28, 2016, https://www.acsh.org/news/2016/12/28/semisynthetic -real-word-saves-lives-10605.

7   Nick Mulcahy, "Strong Case for Weekly Paclitaxel in Breast Cancer," Medscape, accessed June 18, 2020, https://www.medscape.com/viewarticle/805220.

ENDNOTES

8   Caroline F. Thorn, et al., "Doxorubicin Pathways: Pharmacodynamics and Adverse Effects," *Pharmacogenetics and Genomics* 7 (2011): 440–6, https://www.ncbi.nlm.nih.gov/pmc/articles/PMC3116111/.

9   Type-1 diabetes is often referred to as "juvenile diabetes."

10   Arthur Ainsberg, "Miracle on Bloom Street," *Toronto Star*, January 7, 2012, https://www.thestar.com/opinion/editorialopinion/2012/01/07/miracle_on_bloor_street.html.

11   "Patient Records for Leonard Thompson," University of Toronto, accessed June 18, 2020, https://insulin.library.utoronto.ca/islandora/object/insulin%3AM10015.

12   Charles H. Best, "The First Clinical Use of Insulin," *Diabetes* 5, no. 1 (1956): 65–7.

13   Michael Bliss, *Banting: A Biography* (Toronto: University of Toronto Press, 1993).

14   Kinch, *A Prescription for Change.*

15   Austin Bunn, "The Bittersweet Science," *New York Times Magazine,* March 16, 2003, https://www.nytimes.com/2003/03/16/magazine/the-way-we-live-now-3-16-03-body-check-the-bittersweet-science.html.

16   "New Medical Institute," *New York Times,* April 27, 1921, https://timesmachine.nytimes.com/timesmachine/1921/04/27/98676601.pdf.

17   The average survival of patients diagnosed with type-1 diabetes was less than a year.

18   Henry B.M. Best, *Margaret and Charley: The Personal Story of Dr. Charles Best, to Co-Discoverer of Insulin* (Toronto: Dundurn, 2003).

19   Abigail Zuger, "Rediscovering the First Miracle Drug," *New York Times,* October 5, 2010, https://www.nytimes.com/2010/10/05/health/05insulin.html?.

20   Thea Cooper and Arthur Ainsberg, *Breakthrough: Elizabeth Hughes, the Discovery of Insulin and the Making of a Medical Miracle* (New York: St. Martin's Press, 2010).

21   Darby Herkert, et al., "Cost-Related Insulin Underuse Among Patients with Diabetes," *JAMA Internal Medicine* 179, no. 1 (2019): 112–4, https://jamanetwork.com/journals/jamainternalmedicine/fullarticle/2717499.

22   Elisabeth Rosenthal, "When High Prices Mean Needless Death," *JAMA Internal Medicine* 179, no. 1 (2019): 114–5.

23   M. E. Krahl, "George Henry Alexander Clowes: 1877–1958," *Cancer Research* 19 (1959): 334–6.

24   Louis Rosenfeld, "Insulin: Discovery and Controversy," *Clinical Chemistry* 48, no. 12 (2002): 2270–88, http://clinchem.aaccjnls.org/content/48/12/2270#sec-19.

25   A trade secret is information kept restricted to a particular company, as exemplified by Colonel Sanders's seven herbs and spices or the recipe for Coca-Cola. Trade secrets can remain protected for generations but are subject to the risk that the secret is discovered or revealed.

26   Andrew Dahlem, in discussion with Michael Kinch, November 7, 2019; topic: Drug Development.

27   The official journal of the most prestigious organization of American scientists, which would eventually include both men.

28   The term "recombinant DNA technology" reflects the fact that a human gene could be combined with bacterial DNA to enable the ability to produce a human molecule in a non-human cell.

29   Periodic disruptions in supply had occurred as a result of unplanned outbreaks of various infections in livestock populations.

30   We will selectively ignore exotic forms of hydrogen that weigh more due to the presence of pesky neutrons.

31   An individual "skilled in the art" is not a novice, who would be unskilled, but also not someone of extraordinary skill. This could include a trained PhD but not the one person who is the leader who spent a lifetime studying that particular field/art.

32   American law only recently changed so that an invention has to remain non-obvious until at least the day a particular patent is filed. Prior to the current rules, American law would

support non-obvious to include the time in which an idea was conceived but this led to many lawsuits among those claiming to be the true originator of an idea. As it now stands, the winner is the one with the fastest patent attorney and the ability to file a patent first.

CHAPTER THIRTEEN: SMART BOMBS AND DUMB MONEY

1   Daniel Dykhuizen, "Species Numbers in Bacteria," *Proceedings of the California Academy of Sciences* 56, no. 6 (2005): 62–71, https://www.ncbi.nlm.nih.gov/pmc/articles/PMC3160642/.

2   Jerry W. Shay and Woodring E. Wright, "Hayflick, His Limit, and Cellular Aging," *Nature Reviews Molecular Cell Biology* 1 (2000): 72–6, https://www.nature.com/articles/35036093?draft=journal.

3   "A Missed Opportunity," What is Biotechnology? accessed June 18, 2020, https://www.what isbiotechnology.org/index.php/exhibitions/milstein/patents/The-monoclonal-antibody -patent-saga.

4   "The Nobel Prize in Physiology or Medicine 1984," NobelPrize.org, accessed June 18, 2020, https://www.nobelprize.org/prizes/medicine/1984/summary/.

5   Lara C. Marks, *The Lock and Key of Medicine: Monoclonal Antibodies and the Transformation of Healthcare* (New Haven, CT: Yale University Press, 2015).

6   The name chimera refers back to ancient legends fantastic creatures from Greco-Roman mythologies.

7   While the employee may have been released from service, they were not necessarily released from control. While this results in less control over the individual, the contract and non-disclosure agreement would persist indefinitely, even after the termination. This gives a legal remedy if there is a breach of the confidentiality obligation (injunction being the most important, assuming the breach is discovered), but less control than for a current employee and, according to a wise attorney, "There's no honor in contracts," as they can be broken, especially if the fine might be compensated by a new employer.

8   MedImmune, 1999 Annual Report to Shareholders, page 7.

9   "Global Therapeutic Monoclonal Antibody Products Market to 2021—Sales to Reach Approximately $110 Billion by 2018 and Nearly $150 Billion by 2021," Research and Markets, accessed June 18, 2020, https://www.researchandmarkets.com/research/b3gj4m /the_development.

10   Charles Muscoplat, in discussion with Lori Weiman and Michael Kinch, August 19, 2020; topic: Drug Development Trends.

11   A biologic is a term generally meant to capture medical products developed using genetic engineering techniques and/or manufactured using living cells (the micro-factories mentioned in the text).

12   J. H. DeVries, et al., "Biosimilar insulins: a European perspective" *Diabetes, Obesity and Metabolism* 17, no. 5 (2015): 445–51, https://www.ncbi.nlm.nih.gov/pmc/articles/PMC4403967/.

13   Lutz Heinemann and Marcus Hompesch, "Biosimilar Insulins: Basic Considerations," *Journal of Diabetes Science and Technology* 8, no. 1 (2014): 6–13, https://www.ncbi.nlm.nih .gov/pmc/articles/PMC4454103/.

14   The name Hospira is an amalgamation of "hospital" with the Latin term *spero*, which translates in English to "hope."

15   As a postscript, years after the cocaine project was shut down, the company moved the location of its headquarters. Despite exhaustive searches, the remaining cocaine in the safe was never located (admittedly, this was a trivial amount but compelled much speculation).

16   "Trump Administration Makes CAR T-Cell Cancer Therapies Available to Medicare Beneficiaries Nationwide," CMS.gov, accessed June 18, 2020, https://www.cms.gov/newsroom /press-releases/trump-administration-makes-car-t-cell-cancer-therapy-available-medicare -beneficiaries-nationwide.

17   Olivia Wilkins, et al., "CAR T-Cell Therapy: Progress and Prospects," *Human Gene Therapy Methods* 28, no. 2 (2017): 61-6, https://www.ncbi.nlm.nih.gov/pmc/articles /PMC5429042/

18   Raymond J. March, "Why This New Gene Therapy Costs $2.1 Million," Foundation for Economic Education, accessed June 18, 2020. http,://fee.org/articles/why-this-new-gene -therapy-drug-costs-21-million/.

19   Justin McCarthy, "Big Pharma Sinks to the Bottom of US Industry Ratings," Gallup, September 3, 2019, https://news.gallup.com/poll/266060/big-pharma-sinks-bottom -industry-rankings.aspx.

CHAPTER FOURTEEN: REPUTATION DECIMATION

1   Andrew Dahlem, in discussion with Michael Kinch, November 7, 2019; topic: Drug Development.

2   Lydia Ramsey Pflanzer, "Pharma CEOs Got Into a Heated Debate Over Why People Hate the Industry," *Business Insider,* accessed December 1, 2016, https://www.businessinsider .com/pfizer-and-regeneron-ceos-on-drug-pricing-and-reputation-2016-12.

3   Julia Sheppard, "Burroughs, (Silas) Mainville," Oxford Dictionary of National Biography, accessed June 18, 2020, https://www.oxforddnb.com/view/10.193/ref:odnb/9780198614128.001 .0001/odnb-9780198614128-e-50641;jsessionid=1CEBDA0214B08D4A7E047F83C401E530.

4   Roy Church and E. M. Tansey, *Burroughs Wellcome & Co.: Knowledge, Trust, Profit, and the Transformation of the British Pharmaceutical Industry, 1880–1940* (Swindon, England: Crucible Books, 2007).

5   E. M. Tansey, "Medicines and Men: Burroughs, Wellcome & Co, and the British Drug Industry Before the Second World War," *Journal of the Royal Society of Medicine* 95, no. 8 (2002): 411-6, https://www.ncbi.nlm.nih.gov/pmc/articles/PMC1279970/.

6   "AZT's Inhuman Cost," *New York Times*, August 28, 1989, https://www.nytimes.com /1989/08/28/opinion/azt-s-inhuman-cost.html.

7   Irvin Molotsky, "U.S. Approves Drug to Prolong Lives of AIDS Patients," *New York Times*, March 21, 1987, https://www.nytimes.com/1987/03/21/us/us-approves-drug-to-prolong -lives-of-aids-patients.html.

8   "AIDS Drug Costs to Be Cut for Poor Women," *New York Times,* March 6, 1998, https://www .nytimes.com/1998/03/06/world/aids-drug-cost-to-be-cut-for-poor-women.html.

9   Joseph Walker, "COVID-19 Drug Remdesivir to Cost $3,120 for Typical Patient," *Wall Street Journal,* June 29, 2020, https://www.wsj.com/articles/covid-19-drug-remdesivir-to -cost-3-120-for-typical-patient-11593428402.

10   Bill Whitaker, "Money, Dinners and Strip Clubs," *CBS News*, June 21, 2020, https://www .cbsnews.com/news/opioid-epidemic-pharmaceutical-executives-60-minutes-2020-06-21/.

11   Recall that Eroom's Law was derived from data generated by companies and submitted in confidence to Tufts University. As such, these findings are not available for independent scrutiny.

12   Aaron S. Kesselheim, et al., "The High Cost of Prescription Drugs in the United States: Origins and Prospects for Reform," *Journal of the American Medical Association* 316, no. 8 (2016): 858–71, https://www.ncbi.nlm.nih.gov/pubmed/27552619.

13   Sheryl Gay Stolberg and Margot Sanger-Katz, "Trump Keeps Promoting a Drug Order that No One Has Seen," *New York Times*, August 24, 2020, https://www.nytimes.com/2020/08 /24/us/politics/trump-drug-prices.html.

14   Lori Robertson, "Trump's Executive Order on Prescription Drugs," FactCheck.org, accessed September 15, 2020, https://www.factcheck.org/2020/07/trumps-executive-orders-on -prescription-drugs/.

15   Sarah Overmohle, "Drugmakers Refuse to Attend White House Meeting After Trump Issues Executive Orders on Costs," Politico, July 27, 2020, https://www.politico.com /news/2020/07/27/drugmakers-trump-meeting-canceled-382847.

16   "PhRMA Statement on Drug Pricing Executive Orders," Phrma.org, accessed September 15, 2020, https://phrma.org/Press-Release/PhRMA-Statement-on-Drug-Pricing-Executive-Orders.

17   Robertson, "Trump's Executive Orders on Prescription Drugs."

18   Ed Silverman, "Most Americans believe prescription drug prices are unreasonable, " Stat News, September 29, 2016, https://www.statnews.com/pharmalot/2016/09/29/americans-believe-drug-prices-unreasonable/.

19   Carey Sagon, "Survey Shows Growing Worry Among 50+ Over Drug Prices," AARP, April 19, 2016, https://www.aarp.org/health/drugs-supplements/info-2016/prescription-cost-worry-older-adults.html.

20   Linda Peters, in discussion with Michael Kinch and Lori Weiman, September 4, 2020.

CHAPTER FIFTEEN: HOW ARE DRUG PRICES DETERMINED?

1   John Carroll, "Blueprint Scores First FDA OK for a Precision GIST Cancer Drug, Just Ahead of a Rival Treatment. And the Price Is a Big Surprise," Endpoints, accessed June 18, 2020, https://endpts.com/blueprint-scores-first-fda-ok-for-a-precision-gist-cancer-drug-just-ahead-of-a-rival-treatment/.

2   Herbert E. Klarman, et al., "Cost-Effectiveness Analysis Applied to the Treatment of Chronic Renal Disease," *Medical Care* 6, no. 1 (1968): 48–54, https://journals.lww.com/lww-medicalcare/Citation/1968/01000/Cost_Effectiveness_Analysis_Applied_to_the.5.aspx.

3   William S. Smith, "The U.S. Shouldn't Use the 'QALY' in Cost-Effectiveness Reviews," Stat News, February 22, 2019, https://www.statnews.com/2019/02/22/qaly-drug-effectiveness-reviews/.

CHAPTER SIXTEEN: AND YOU THOUGHT PHARMA WAS OPAQUE

1   The first vaccine, derived from blood donated by gay men and intravenous drug users, was replaced by a safer, recombinant DNA form of vaccine a few years later.

2   For those counting viruses, hepatitis A is an acute disease, often associated with food, caused by a third virus, known as hepatitis a. Although this disease can be debilitating, it is less deadly than that caused by hepatitis B and C viruses.

3   Caroline Humer, "Express Scripts Drops Gilead Hep C Drugs for Cheaper AbbVie Rival," *Reuters*, December 22, 2014, https://www.reuters.com/article/us-express-scripts-abbvie-hepatitisc/express-scripts-drops-gilead-hep-c-drugs-for-cheaper-abbvie-rival-idUSKBN0K007620141222.

4   Permanent Select Committee on Small Business, "Problems on Third Party Prepaid Prescription Programs," United States House of Representatives, accessed June 18, 2020, https://books.google.com/books?id=vrUVAAAAIAAJ&pg.

5   Permanent Select Committee on Small Business, United States Senate, "Competitive Problems in the Drug Industry," 92nd Congress (Washington, DC: U.S. Government Printing Office, 1971), https://play.google.com/store/books/details?id=yQ02AAAAIAAJ&rdid=book-yQ02AAAAIAAJ&rdot=1.

6   Select Committee on Small Business, United States House of Representatives "Competitive Problems in the Drug Industry," 92nd Congress (Washington, DC: U.S. Government Printing Office, 1971), https://books.google.com/books?id=YRn9lLsXg5AC&pg=PT78&lpg=PT78&dq=%22Pharmaceutical+Card+System%22++phoenix+1969&source=bl&ots=Sq4Z2RIKiU&sig=ACfU3U2RShrN37nVlnXmjtPTZBJtBQZ54Q&hl=en&sa=X&ved=2ahUKEwiDnMHPwebpAhXZLc0KHQeBCHYQ6AEwAnoECAgQAg#v=onepage&q&f=false.

7   Ibid.

8   Barnaby J. Feder, "McKesson: No.1 But a Doze on Wall Street," *New York Times*, March 17, 1991, https://www.nytimes.com/1991/03/17/business/mckesson-no-1-but-a-doze-on-wall-street.html.

9   "Lilly Buys McKesson's PCS Unit for $4 Billion," The Pharma Letter, accessed June 18, 2020. https://www.thepharmaletter.com/article/lilly-buys-mckesson-s-pcs-unit-for-4-billion.

10 "Rite Aid to Buy PCS," *RiteAid.com*, accessed June 18, 2020, https://www.riteaid.com /corporate/news/-/pressreleases/news-room/1998/rite-aid-to-buy-pcs.

11 "Caremark Rx and AdvancePCS Announce Strategic Combination Creating $23 Billion Revenue Company," BusinessWire, accessed June 18, 2020, https://www.businesswire.com /news/home/20030902005918/en/Caremark-Rx-AdvancePCS-Announce-Strategic -Combination-Creating.

12 "Caremark in $6 Billion Deal to Buy AdvancePCS," The Street, accessed June 18, 2020, https://www.thestreet.com/opinion/caremark-in-6-billion-deal-to-buy-advancepcs -10111306.

13 Andrew Ross Sorkin, "CVS to Buy Caremark in All-Stock Deal," *New York Times*, November 1, 2006, https://www.nytimes.com/2006/11/01/business/01cnd-drug.html.

14 Lydia Ramsey Pflanzer, "Big Pharma's Lobby Is Blaming America's Soaring Drug Costs of Middlemen," *Business Insider*, March 29, 2017, https://www.businessinsider.com/phrma -report-on-percent-of-americans-paying-full-list-price-2017-3.

15 Serena Gordon, "Why are Insulin Prices So High for US Patients?" US News and World Report, November 7, 2019, https://www.usnews.com/news/health-news/articles/2019-11-07 /why-are-insulin-prices-still-so-high-for-us-patients.

16 Eric Pachman, Response to Steve Miller comments to authors, September 6, 2020, e-mail message.

CHAPTER SEVENTEEN: AMERICAN EXCEPTIONALISM

1   Sarnak, Squires, and Bishop, "Paying For Prescription Drugs Around The World."

2   "The World Factbook," United States Central Intelligence Agency (CIA), accessed June 18, 2020, https://www.cia.gov/library/publications/resources/the-world-factbook/fields /343rank.html.

3   P. O'Neill and J. Sussex, "International Comparison of Medicines Usage: Quantitative Analysis Association of the British Pharmaceutical Industry," Office of Health Economics, accessed June 18, 2020, http://www.lif.se/contentassets/a0030c971ca6400e9fbf09a61235263f /international-comparison-of-medicines-usage-quantitative-analysis.pdf.

4   "International Pharmaceutical Price Differences," Productivity Commission (Australia), accessed September 3, 2020, https://www.pc.gov.au/inquiries/completed/pharmaceutical -prices/report/pbsprices.pdf.

5   Sarnak, Squires, and Bishop, "Paying For Prescription Drugs Around The World."

6   Dana Goldman and Darius Kakdaalla, "The Global Burden of Medical Innovation," Brookings Institution, accessed June 18, 2020, https://www.brookings.edu/research /the-global-burden-of-medical-innovation.

7   N. Sood, et al., "The effect of regulation on pharmaceutical revenues: experience in nineteen countries," *Health Affairs* 28, no. 1 (2009): w125-w137.

8   C. Henschke, et al., "Structural changes in the German pharmaceutical market: price setting mechanisms based on the early benefit evaluation," *Health Policy* 109 (2003): 263–9.

9   Henschke, "Structural Changes in the German Pharmaceutical Market."

10 Martin Wenzl and Valerie Paris, "Pharmaceutical Reimbursement and Pricing in Germany," Organization for Economic Cooperation and Development (OECD), accessed June 18, 2020, https://www.oecd.org/health/health-systems/Pharmaceutical-Reimbursement-and-Pricing-in-Germany.pdf.

11 FDA, "FDA Approves Ravicti," Drugs.com, accessed July 6, 2020, https://www.drugs.com /newdrugs/fda-approves-ravicti-chronic-management-some-urea-cycle-disorders-3676.html.

12 Lota Zoth, phone conversation with Lori Weiman, September 9, 2020.

13   K. Douglas and C. Jutras, "Patent protection for pharmaceutical products in Canada—chronology of significant events," Ottawa (ON): Parliament of Canada, accessed June 18, 2020, www.parl.gc.ca /content/LOP/ResearchPublications/prb9946-e.htm.

14   Paul Grootendorst, "Canada's Laws on Pharmaceutical Intellectual Property," *Canadian Medical Association Journal* 184, no. 5 (2012): 543–9, https://www.ncbi.nlm.nih.gov/pmc /articles/PMC3307559/pdf/1840543.pdf.

15   Allison Martell, "Canada Enacts, Drug Price Crackdown, In Blow to Pharmaceutical Industry," *Reuters*, August 9, 2019, https://www.reuters.com/article/us-canada-pharmaceuticals/canada -enacts-drug-price-crackdown-in-blow-to-pharmaceutical-industry-idUSKCN1UZ0XH.

16   "Government of Canada Announces Changes to Lower Drug Prices and Lay the Foundation For National Pharmacare," Health Canada, accessed June 18, 2020, https://www .canada.ca/en/health-canada/news/2019/08/government-of-canada-announces-changes-to -lower-drug-prices-and-lay-the-foundation-for-national-pharmacare.html.

17   Reuters, "Canada Announces Regulation to Cut Prices of Prescription Drugs," The Guardian, August 9, 2020, https://www.theguardian.com/world/2019/aug/09/canada-prescription -drugs-cut-cost.

CHAPTER EIGHTEEN: A STOMACH-CHURNING STORY

1   Carol Reed, et al., *The Third Man.* (UK: London Film Productions, 1949.)

2   Theodoros Kelesidis and Matthew E. Falagas, "Substandard/Counterfeit Antimicrobial Drugs," *Clinical Microbiology Reviews* 28, no. 2 (2015): 443–64, https://pubmed.ncbi.nlm .nih.gov/25788516/.

3   "Purple Haze: How a Little Purple Pill Called Nexium Exposes Big Problems in the US Drug Supply Chain," 3 Axis Advisors, accessed June 18, 2020, https://www.3axisadvisors.com/projects /2019/12/10/purple-haze-how-a-little-purple-pill-called-nexium-exposes-big-problems-in-the-us -drug-supply-chain.

4   Some claim Napoleon died from gastric cancer (which can be triggered by ulcers) or as a victim of poisoning, intentionally or otherwise.

5   The company was able to get the name "Losec" approved in many European countries.

6   Tim Spector, *Identically Different* (New York: Harry N. Abrams, 2013).

7   "Purple Haze: How a Little Purple Pill Called Nexium Exposes Big Problems in the US Drug Supply Chain."

8   Ibid.

9   These different forms are known to chemists as enantiomers. A right-handed molecule is known as an R- or dextro-form of a molecule whereas a left-handed molecule is designated as an S- or levo-form.

10   Gardiner Harris, "Prilosec's Maker Switches Users to Nexium, Thwarting Generics," *Wall Street Journal,* June 6, 2002, https://www.wsj.com/articles/SB1023326369679910840.

11   Stuart Elliott and Nat Ives, "Questions on the $3.8 Billion Drug Ad Business," *New York Times,* October 12, 2004, https://www.nytimes.com/2004/10/12/business/media/questions -on-the-38-billion-drug-ad-business.html.

12   Alex Berenson. "Where Has All the Prilosec Gone?" *New York Times,* March 2, 2005, https://www.nytimes.com/2005/03/02/business/where-has-all-the-prilosec-gone.html.

13   Elliott and Ives, "Questions on the $3.8 Billion Drug Ad Business."

14   Brendan Pierson, "U.S. Court Upholds AstraZeneca, Ranbaxy Win in Nexium Antitrust Law," *Reuters,* November 21, 2016, https://www.reuters.com/article/astrazeneca -nexium-appeal/u-s-court-upholds-astrazeneca-ranbaxy-win-in-nexium-antitrust-trial -idUSL1N1DM1W2.

15   "Purple Haze: How a Little Purple Pill Called Nexium Exposes Big Problems in the US Drug Supply Chain."

16   LeAnn W. O'Neill, et al., "Long-Term Consequences of Chronic Proton Pump Inhibitor Use," *US Pharmacist* 38, no. 12 (2013): 38–422, https://www.uspharmacist.com/article/longterm-consequences-of-chronic-proton-pump-inhibitor-use.

17   "By the Way, Doctor: Does the Long Term Use of Prilosec Cause Stomach Cancer?" Harvard Health Publishing, accessed June 18, 2020, https://www.health.harvard.edu/diseases-and-conditions/by_the_way_doctor_does_long_term_use_of_prilosec_cause_stomach_cancer.

18   "Purple Haze: How a Little Purple Pill Called Nexium Exposes Big Problems in the US Drug Supply Chain."

CHAPTER NINETEEN: VIEWS OF AN ARCHAEOLOGIST

1   Liz Tracey, "We're Living in a Post-Antibiotic World," *JSTOR Daily*, December 6, 2019, https://daily.jstor.org/were-living-in-a-post-antibiotic-world/.

2   Tatiana I Lobova, et al., "Multiple Antibiotic Resistance of Heterotrophic Bacteria Isolated from Siberian Lakes Subjected to Different Degrees of Anthropogenic Impact," *Microbial Drug Resistance* 17, no. 4 (2011): 583–91, https://www.researchgate.net/publication/51728648_Multiple_Antibiotic_Resistance_of_Heterotrophic_Bacteria_Isolated_from_Siberian_Lakes_Subjected_to_Differing_Degrees_of_Anthropogenic_Impact.

3   Kinch, *Between Hope and Fear.*

4   Umeh D. Parashar, et al., "Global Illness and Deaths Caused By Rotavirus Disease in Children," *Emerging Infectious Diseases* 9, no. 5 (2003): 565–72, https://wwwnc.cdc.gov/eid/article/9/5/02-0562_article.

5   "The Dutch Disease," *The Economist*, November 26, 1977, 82–3.

CHAPTER TWENTY: ALL ROADS LEAD TO WASHINGTON

1   "Kansas," Walmart.com, accessed June 18, 2020, https://corporate.walmart.com/our-story/locations/united-states/kansas.

2   Herbert E. Klarman, et al., "Cost-Effectiveness Analysis Applied to the Treatment of Chronic Renal Disease," *Medical Care* 6, no. 1 (1968): 48–54, https://journals.lww.com/lww-medicalcare/Citation/1968/01000/Cost_Effectiveness_Analysis_Applied_to_the.5.aspx.

3   S. Fanshel and J.W. Bush, "A Health-Status Index and Its Application To Health-Services Outcome," 1970, 1021–66, http://www.eurohex.eu/bibliography/pdf/0990244687/Fanshel_1970_OR.pdf.

4   "Welcome to the Global Health Cost-Effectiveness Analysis Registry," CEA Registry, accessed June 18, 2020. http://ghcearegistry.org/ghcearegistry/.

5   "How We Work: Grant, University of Washington," Gates Foundation, accessed June 18, 2020, https://www.gatesfoundation.org/How-We-Work/Quick-Links/Grants-Database/Grants/2017/11/OPP1186830.

6   Weekend Edition Sunday, "Putting a Price on COVID-19 Treatment—Remdesivir," NPR, May 8, 2020, https://www.npr.org/sections/health-shots/2020/05/08/851632704/putting-a-price-on-covid-19-treatment-remdesivir.

7   Angus Liu, "Fair Price for Gilead's COVID-19 Med Remdesivir? $4,460, Cost Watchdog Says," Fierce Pharma, accessed June 18, 2020, https://www.fiercepharma.com/marketing/gilead-s-covid-19-therapy-remdesivir-worth-4-460-per-course-says-pricing-watchdog.

8   "AHF Demands Gilead Price Remdesivir at $1.00 Per Dose," BusinessWire, May 12, 2020, https://www.businesswire.com/news/home/20200512005240/en/AHF-Demands-Gilead-Price-Remdesivir-1.00-Dose.

9   Damian Garde, "Less Than a Movie Ticket of 'Impossible to Overpay'? Experts Name Their Price For Remdesivir," Stat News, May 15, 2020, https://www.statnews.com/2020 /05/15/gilead-remdesivir-pricing-coronavirus/.

10   Peter Walker, "Investors to Pay for Prisoner Rehabilitation," The Guardian, March 19, 2010, https://www.theguardian.com/society/2010/mar/19/investors-pay-for-prisoner-rehabilitation.

11   Rebekah H. Griesenauer, et al., "NIH Support for FDA-Approved Medicines," *Cell Chemical Biology* 24, no. 11 (2017): 1315–6, https://pubmed.ncbi.nlm.nih.gov/29149588/.

12   Jocelyn Kaiser, "NIH Grapples with Rush to Claim Billions in Pandemic Research Funds," Science, June 3, 2020, https://www.sciencemag.org/news/2020/06/nih-grapples-researchers -rush-claim-billions-pandemic-research-funds.

13   "S.881—Small Business Innovation Development Act of 1982," Congress.gov, accessed June 18, 2020, https://www.congress.gov/bill/97th-congress/senate-bill/881.

14   Kinch and Moore, "Innovator Organizations in New Drug Development: Assessing the Sustainability of the Biopharmaceutical Industry."

15   Nora Kelly Lee, "Trump's Budget Proposal," *The Atlantic*, March 16, 2017, https://www .theatlantic.com/politics/archive/2017/03/trumps-budget-cuts-nih-funding-by-20-percent /519771/.

16   Kinch and Moore, "Innovator Organizations in New Drug Development: Assessing the Sustainability of the Biopharmaceutical Industry."

17   Marianna Mazzucato, *The Entrepreneurial State* (London: Anthem Press, 2013).

18   National Institutes of Health mission statement, NIH.gov, accessed June 18, 2020, https ://www.nih.gov/about-nih/what-we-do/nih-turning-discovery-into-health.

19   Andrew A. Toole, "Does Public Scientific Research Complement Private Investment in Research and Development in the Pharmaceutical Industry?" *Journal of Law and Economics* 50, no. 1 (2007): 81–104.

20   Pierre Azoulay, et al., "Public R&D Investments and Private-Sector Patenting: Evidence from NIH Funding Rules," The National Bureau of Economic Research, accessed June 18, 2020, www.nber.org/papers/w20889.

21   Juliette Cubanski, "What's the Latest on Medicare Drug Price Negotiations?" Kaiser Family Foundation, accessed June 18, 2020, https://www.kff.org/medicare/issue-brief/whats-the -latest-on-medicare-drug-price-negotiations/.

22   John F. Wasik, "Why Medicare Can't Get the Lowest Drug Prices," Forbes, August 10, 2018, https://www.forbes.com/sites/johnwasik/2018/08/10/why-medicare-cant-get-the-lowest -drug-prices/#73fe216b302b.

23   Alicia H. Munnell, "Opinion: Should the Government Be Allowed to Negotiate Drug Prices?" MarketWatch.com, January, 8, 2019, https://www.marketwatch.com/story /should-the-government-be-allowed-to-negotiate-drug-prices-2019-01-08.

24   Stacie B. Dusetzina, et al., "Sending the Wrong Price Signal: Why Do Some Brand-Name Drugs Cost Medicare Beneficiaries Less Than Generics?" Health Affairs, July 2019, https ://doi.org/10.1377/hlthaff.2018.05476.

25   Mike McCaughan, "Veterans Health Administration," Health Affairs, 2017, https://www .healthaffairs.org/do/10.1377/hpb20171008.000174/full/.

26   "International reference pricing: Discounts Down Under far surpass U.S. drug price concessions," 46brooklyn, accessed September 1, 2020, https://www.46brooklyn.com /research/2020/8/26/international-reference-pricing-discounts-down-under-far-surpass-us -drug-price-concessions.

27   Sarnak, Squires, and Bishop, "Paying For Prescription Drugs Around The World."

28   Sebastian Sieler, et al., "AMNOG Revisited," McKinsey.com, accessed June 18, 2020, https ://www.mckinsey.com/industries/pharmaceuticals-and-medical-products/our-insights /amnog-revisited.

29   Paige Winfield Cunningham, "The Health 202," *Washington Post*, August 12, 2017, https
      ://www.washingtonpost.com/news/powerpost/paloma/the-health-202/2017/12/08/the
      -health-202-the-orphan-disease-tax-credit-may-soon-be-out-in-the-cold/5a29644330fb046
      9e883fa84/.

30   Kao-Ping Chua and Rena M. Conti, "Orphan Drugs for Opioid Use Disorder: An Abuse of
      the Orphan Drug Act," Health Affairs Blog, July 26, 2019, https://www.healthaffairs.org
      /do/10.1377/hblog20190724.795814/full/.

CHAPTER TWENTY-ONE: FUTURE SHOCK ALREADY HAPPENED

1   Peter Frost, "More than Splitting Pills: Healthcare Giant Abbott Laboratories Ready to Spin
      off AbbVie," *Chicago Tribune,* December 30, 2012, https://www.chicagotribune.com
      /business/ct-xpm-2012-12-30-ct-biz-1230-bf-abbott-spin-20121230-story.html.

2   "Pfizer to Acquire Allergan for $160B," Genengnews.com, accessed June 17, 2020, https
      ://www.genengnews.com/news/pfizer-to-acquire-allergan-for-160b/.

3   Caroline Humer and Ankur Banerjee, "Pfizer, Allergan Scrap $160 Billion Deal After U.S.
      Tax Rule Change," *Reuters,* April 6, 2016, https://www.reuters.com/article/us-allergan-m-a
      -pfizer-idUSKCN0X3188.

4   Trefis Team, "Can Biosimilars Be the Next Growth Driver for Pfizer?" Forbes, August 30,
      2019, https://www.forbes.com/sites/greatspeculations/2019/08/30/can-biosimilars-be-the
      -next-growth-driver-for-pfizer/#1997051d6a5a.

5   David Setal and Isabel Kirshner, "Nobody Thought It Would Come to This: Drug Maker
      Teva Faces a Crisis," *New York Times*, December 27, 2017, https://www.nytimes.com/2017
      /12/27/business/teva-israel-layoffs.html.

6   Joseph Walker and Jonathan D. Rockoff, "Cystic Fibrosis Foundation Sells Drug's Rights
      for $3.3 Billion," *Wall Street Journal*, November 19, 2014, https://www.wsj.com/articles
      /cystic-fibrosis-foundation-sells-drugs-rights-for-3-3-billion-1416414300.

7   "ICER Slams Cost-Effectiveness of Three Vertex Cystic Fibrosis Drugs," FDA News,
      accessed June 17, 2020, https://www.fdanews.com/articles/186711-icer-slams-cost
      -effectiveness-of-three-vertex-cystic-fibrosis-drugs.

8   "Bill and Melinda Gates Foundation Global Access Statement," Gates Foundation, accessed
      June 17, 2020, https://www.gatesfoundation.org/How-We-Work/General-Information
      /Global-Access-Statement.

9   "History of Wellcome," Wellcome Foundation, accessed June 17, 2020, https://wellcome
      .ac.uk/about-us/history-wellcome.

10   "Drug Prices Based On Success Could Speed Up Cancer Patients' Treatment," Cancer
      Research UK, accessed June 17, 2020, https://www.cancerresearchuk.org/about-us/cancer
      -news/press-release/2019-02-21-drug-prices-based-on-success-could-speed-up-cancer
      -patients-treatment.

11   Reed Abelson and Katie Thomas, "Fed Up with Drug Companies, Hospitals Decide to
      Start Their Own," *New York Times,* January 18, 2018, https://www.nytimes.com/2018
      /01/18/health/drug-prices-hospitals.html.

12   Devon Pendleton, "The Meteoric Rise of Billionaire Len Blavatnik," *Bloomberg News*,
      April 26, 2019, https://www.bloomberg.com/news/features/2019-04-26/the-meteoric-rise
      -of-billionaire-len-blavatnik.

13   Alvin Powell, "A Gift to Turn Medical Discoveries into Treatments," *Harvard Gazette*,
      accessed June 17, 2020, https://news.harvard.edu/gazette/story/2018/11/a-gift-to
      -harvard-to-turn-medical-discoveries-into-treatments/.

14   "Gov. Pritzker Signs Legislation to Rein in Prescription Drug Costs," WSILTIV.com,
      accessed June 17, 2020, https://wsiltv.com/2019/08/31/gov-pritzker-signs-legislation-to-rein
      -in-prescription-drug-costs/.

15   Greg Orman, "Is Trump Bluffing on Rx Drugs? Dems Must Act Fast to Find Out," RealClear Politics, accessed July 29, 2020, https://www.realclearpolitics.com/articles /2020/07/28/is_trump_bluffing_on_rx_drugs_dems_must_act_fast_to_find_out.html.

16   "Cuyahoga River Fire," Ohio History Central, accessed July 29, 2020, https://ohio historycentral.org/w/Cuyahoga_River_Fire.

17   "The Story of Chesapeake Bay," Maryland Department of the Environment, accessed July 29, 2020, https://mde.maryland.gov/programs/Water/TMDL/TMDLImplementation /Pages/overview.aspx.

18   "History of Bald Eagle Decline, Protection and Recovery," US Fish and Wildlife Service, access July 29, 2020, https://www.fws.gov/midwest/eagle/history/index.html.

19   Daniel E. Estrin, "Clean Water Act 101—A bit of legislative history," Green Law, accessed July 29, 2020, https://greenlaw.blogs.pace.edu/2011/04/01/cwa101/.

20   Dustin Renwick, "Five years on, the Flint water crisis in nowhere near over," *National Geographic,* accessed July 29, 2020, https://www.nationalgeographic.com /environment/2019/04/flint-water-crisis-fifth-anniversary-flint-river-pollution/.

21   "Fair Disclosure, Regulation FD," US Securities and Exchange Commission, accessed July 29, 2020, https://www.sec.gov/fast-answers/answers-regfdhtm.html.

22   "Proposed Rule: Selective Disclosure and Insider Trading," US Securities and Exchange Commission, accessed July 29, 2020, https://www.sec.gov/rules/proposed/34-42259.htm.

23   Ibid.

24   Priya Cherian Huskins, Esq., "Regulation FD and Social Media: A Refresher on Social Updates and Risk," Woodruff Sawyer, December 16, 2014, https://woodruffsawyer.com /do-notebook/regulation-fd-social/.

25   James Naughton, "The Chilling Effect of Regulation FD: Evidence From Twitter," Harvard Law School Forum on Corporate Governance, June 20, 2019, https://corpgov.law.harvard .edu/2019/06/20/the-chilling-effect-of-regulation-fd-evidence-from-twitter/.

26   Dan Witters, "Nine in 10 Concerned About Rising Drug Costs Due to COVID-19," Gallup, accessed July 29, 2020, https://news.gallup.com/poll/312641/nine-concerned-rising -drug-costs-due-covid.aspx.

INDEX

INDEX

INDEX

INDEX